INSULIN RESISTANCE

Edited by **Sarika Arora**

Insulin Resistance
http://dx.doi.org/10.5772/3210
Edited by Sarika Arora

Contributors

Gabriella Pinto, Simonetta Caira, Marina Cuollo, Sergio Lilla, Lina Chianese, Francesco Addeo, Haiyan Sun, Håvard Jenssen, Teresa Treweek, Marcel Jøhnke, Torben E. Petersen, Tomoko Shimamura, Hiroyuki Ukeda, Bärbel Lieske, Simonetta Caira, Rosa Pizzano, Paolo Polidori, Silvia Vincenzetti, Joanna Barłowska, Anna Wolanciuk, Zygmunt Litwińczuk, Jolanta Król, Gema Lucia Zambrano-Burbano,Yohanna Melissa Eraso-Cabrera, Carlos Eugenio Solarte-Portilla, Carol Yovanna Rosero-Galindo, Massimo Bionaz, Walter Hurley, Juan Loor, Edyta Molik, Genowefa Bonczar, Tomasz Misztal, Aneta Żebrowska and Dorota Zięba

Published by InTech

Janeza Trdine 9, 51000 Rijeka, Croatia

Publishing Process Manager Romina Skomersic
Technical Editor InTech Prepress, Novi Sad
Cover InTech Design team

Additional hard copies can be obtained from orders@intechopen.com

Insulin Resistance, Edited by Sarika Arora
p. cm.
ISBN 978-953-51-0890-0

For EU product safety concerns:
IN TECH d.o.o., Prolaz Marije Krucifikse Kozulić 3, 51000 Rijeka, Croatia,
info@intechopen.com or visit our website at intechopen.com.

Meet the editor

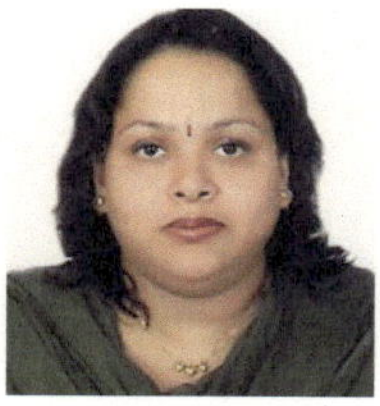

Dr Sarika Arora is currently working as an Associate Professor in the Department of Biochemistry, ESI Postgraduate Institute of Medical Sciences & Research, New Delhi, India. She received graduation and M.D. in Biochemistry from Lady Hardinge Medical College, New Delhi. She also worked in Gobind Ballabh Pant Hospital and Lady Hardinge Medical College as Assistant Professor. She has more than ten years of teaching and research experience. Dr Sarika Arora has more than forty publications in national and international journals. Her areas of expertise are mainly Insulin resistance, neuropeptides and their role in obesity, iron metabolism, oxidative stress and studies on cardiovascular risk factors.

Contents

Preface

Insulin resistance refers to reduced insulin action in metabolic and vascular target tissues, hence higher than normal concentration of insulin is required to maintain normoglycemia and other actions of insulin, hence it may be considered as a euglycemic pre-diabetic state. The growing incidence of insulin resistance and type 2 diabetes is seriously threatening human health globally. The development of insulin resistance leads to many of the metabolic abnormalities associated with this syndrome. The syndrome includes a cluster of clinical problems such as hypertension, dyslipidemia and obesity along with insulin resistance leading to a substantial increase in cardiovascular risk. These patients tend to have impaired fasting plasma glucose levels, which increase the prevalence of more atherogenic, small dense low-density lipoprotein (LDL) particles.

During last decade several studies have been conducted to understand the mechanisms contributing to the state of insulin resistance. Insulin signalling pathways have been dissected in different insulin responsive tissues such as skeletal muscles, adipose tissues, fibroblasts as well as ovaries to elucidate the mechanism. These studies suggest a post receptor signalling defect where metabolic action of insulin is affected. The first chapter on Molecular mechanisms in Insulin resistance describes the insulin signaling pathways and broadly describes various mechanisms capable of producing an Insulin resistant state.

Metabolic regulation in cells is largely dependent on mitochondria, which play an important role in energy homeostasis by metabolizing nutrients and producing ATP. Imbalance between energy intake and expenditure leads to mitochondrial dysfunction, characterized by a reduced ratio of energy production (ATP production) to respiration. Genetic and environmental factors including diet, exercise, aging, and stress affect both mitochondrial function and insulin sensitivity. Recently, it has been shown that mitochondrial dysfunction is associated with insulin resistance in skeletal muscle, as well as in other tissues, including liver, fat, heart, vessels, and pancreas. Thus, insulin resistance caused in part by mitochondrial dysfunction may contribute to a common pathophysiologic etiology for many chronic diseases. Notably, SIRT3, a member of sirtuins located in mitochondria, can regulate the function of mitochondrial proteins via reversible posttranslational modification in response to metabolic stress. Imbalanced acetylation status of mitochondrial proteins by decreased expression and activity of SIRT3 has been demonstrated as one of the factors in the pathogenesis of insulin resistance in mice and human. The chapter by author Wang CH et al., describes the effect of mitochondrial dysfunction on Insulin sensitivity.

Genetic and epidemiological studies strongly suggest that insulin resistance is, at least in part, genetically determined. However, the involved genes and their effective variants are mostly unknown. The numerous genes have been suggested as a potential candidate gene for insulin resistance. The chapter titled 'Impact of genetic polymorphisms on Insulin resistance' by author Evrim Komurcu-Bayrak provides an update on the genetics of Insulin resistance.

The mechanisms that underlie metabolic syndrome and its cardiometabolic consequences may very well vary between ethnicities. It has been a recurring theme that the interactions between poor nutritional status, physical inactivity, and genetic predisposition might contribute to the disparities in the prevalence and characteristics of MetS and its components between ethnicities and the subgroups within. The incidence, component characteristics and complications of the metabolic syndrome in Puerto Ricans has been described in the chapter titled 'The Metabolic Syndrome in Hispanics - The Role of Insulin Resistance and Inflammation' by author Dr Altieri et al. wherein, they have highlighted the fact that the metabolic syndrome may be milder in Puerto Rico than in the mainland United States because it is characterized by less aggressive coronary artery disease and a relatively normal lipid profile.

The role of white adipose tissue (WAT) as an ordinary tissue responsible for lipid energy storage has been replaced due to studies that demonstrate the central activity of WAT in lipid and glucose metabolism and its ability to secrete factors with endocrine, paracrine and autocrine effects. For example, recent studies suggest that pro-inflammatory and anti-inflammatory substances produced by WAT contribute to the development of insulin resistance. The pro-inflammatory role of adipose tissue and association of appetite regulatory peptides with Insulin resistance have been covered in detail in the two chapters by authors Torres-Leal et al. and Maria Orbetzova.

The next section focuses on the systemic effects of Insulin Resistance. The chapter titled 'Cardiovascular and renal complications in obesity and obesity-related medical conditions' by Prof. Masuo and Lambert GV focuses on the sympathetic nervous system activity and insulin resistance in metabolic and their role in the etiopathogenesis of cardiovascular and renal complications in these patients. Another chapter in the same section focuses on the Myocardial Insulin Resistance, wherein the authors Eugene F du Toit and Daniel G Donner have beautifully described how myocardial insulin resistance translates to compromised intracellular insulin signalling and reduced glucose oxidation rates and adversely affects myocardial mechanical function and tolerance to ischemia and reperfusion.

The chapter on Ultrasonographic measurement of visceral fat by author Alempijevic T et al. describes how Ultrasonography can be used as a simple and reliable method for measuring both subcutaneous and visceral fat in clinical settings.

Furthermore, the development of insulin resistance, is associated with increased tissue renin–angiotensin system activity and increasingly appears to be a nexus between components of the syndrome. The chapter titled 'Anti-hypertensive agents and their benefits beyond blood pressure control' by authors Nadya Merchant and Bobby V Khan describe the effect of various antihypertensive agents especially angiotensin receptor blockers on various biomarkers of insulin resistance.

The purpose of this book is to provide contemporary factual information on Insulin resistance. The articles in this issue provide a valuable overview of insulin resistance, by integrating the recent advances which have occurred in various seemingly disparate fields. Thus, I have relied on the expertise of several outstanding contributors who are recognized authorities in their respective areas. I hope that this book will serve as a valuable resource for all clinicians in the related fields and also for the students.

Dr. Sarika Arora
Lady Hardinge Medical College,
India

Section 1

Molecular and Genetic Basis of Insulin Resistance

Chapter 1

Molecular Basis of Insulin Resistance and Its Relation to Metabolic Syndrome

Sarika Arora

Additional information is available at the end of the chapter

http://dx.doi.org/10.5772/54620

1. Introduction

The metabolic syndrome is an agglomeration of interrelated risk factors that is associated with nearly 5-fold increased risk for type 2 diabetes mellitus (DM) and a 2-fold increased risk of coronary artery disease (CAD) [1]. Reaven first suggested this cluster of metabolic abnormalities in 1988. It is characterized by insulin resistance, visceral adiposity, dyslipidemia and a systemic pro-inflammatory and pro-coagulant state [2]. Insulin resistance is defined as reduced insulin action in metabolic and vascular target tissues, hence higher than normal concentration of insulin is required to maintain normoglycemia. On a cellular level, it indicates an inadequate strength of insulin signaling from the insulin receptor downstream to the final substrates of insulin action involved in multiple metabolic and mitogenic aspects of cellular function [3].

The development of insulin resistance leads to many of the metabolic abnormalities associated with this syndrome. Patients with insulin resistance tend to have impaired fasting plasma glucose levels, which increase the prevalence of more atherogenic, small dense low-density lipoprotein (LDL) particles. The growing incidence of insulin resistance and metabolic syndrome (MS) is seriously threatening human health globally. Individuals with MS have a 30%–40% probability of developing diabetes and/or CVD within 20 years, depending on the number of components present [4].

In the United States (US), the prevalence of the MS in the adult population was estimated to be more than 25%. Similarly, the prevalence of MS in seven European countries was approximately 23%. It was estimated that 20%–25% of South Asians have developed MS and many more may be prone to it [5,6]. The main reason why MS is attracting scientific and commercial interest is that the factors defining the syndrome are all factors associated with increased morbidity and mortality in general and from CVD in particular [7].

Though, Insulin resistance has been recognized as a basis of CVD and diabetes type II, its etiology still remains elusive. Recent studies have contributed to a deeper understanding of the underlying molecular mechanisms of Insulin resistance. This review provides a detailed understanding of these basic pathophysiological mechanisms which may be critical for the development of novel therapeutic strategies to treat/ prevent metabolic syndrome.

2. Signalling through Insulin receptor and its downstream Pathways

Insulin action is initiated by an interaction of insulin with its cell surface receptor [8]. The insulin receptor (IR) is a heterotetramer consisting of two α subunits and two β subunits that are linked by disulphide bonds. Insulin binds to the extracellular α subunit of the insulin receptor and activates the tyrosine kinase in the β subunit {figure 1). Binding of insulin to IR effects a series of intramolecular transphosphorylation reactions, where one β subunit phosphorylates its adjacent partner on a specific tyrosine residue. Once the tyrosine kinase of insulin receptor is activated, it promotes autophosphorylation of the β subunit itself, where phosphorylation of three tyrosine residues (Tyr-1158, Tyr-1162, and Tyr-1163) is required for amplification of the kinase activity [9]. It then recruits different substrate adaptors such as the Insulin Receptor Substrate (IRS) family of proteins. Although IRs are present on the surface of virtually all cells, their expression in classical insulin target tissues, i.e. muscle, liver and fat, is extremely high [10]. Tyrosine phosphorylated IRS then displays binding sites for numerous signaling partners. Phosphorylated IRS proteins serve as multisite docking proteins for various effector molecules possessing *src* homology 2 (SH2) domains, including phosphatidylinositol 3-kinase (PI 3-kinase) regulatory subunits (p85, p55 p50, p85, and $p55^{PIK}$), the tyrosine kinases Fyn and Csk, the tyrosine protein phosphatase SHP-2/Syp, as well as several smaller adapter molecules such as the growth factor receptor binding proteins Grb-2, Crk, and Nck [11]. Activation of these SH2 domain proteins initiates signaling cascades, leading to the activation of multiple downstream effectors that ultimately transmit the insulin signal to a branching series of intracellular pathways that regulate cell differentiation, growth, survival, and metabolism. Four members of the IRS family have been identified that are considerably similar in their general architecture [12-15]. IRS proteins share a similar structure characterized by the presence of an NH_2-terminal pleckstrin homology (PH) domain adjacent to a phosphotyrosine-binding (PTB) domain followed by a variable-length COOH-terminal tail that contains a number of Tyr and Ser phosphorylation sites. The PH domain is critical for IR-IRS interactions. Plasma membrane phospholipids, cytoskeletal elements, and protein ligands mediate these interactions [16, 17]. In contrast, the PTB domain interacts directly with the juxtamembrane (JM) domain of the insulin and IGF-I receptors [18, 19], and hindrance of these interactions (by Ser/Thr phosphorylation) negatively affects insulin signaling [19]. A third domain, the kinase regulatory loop binding (KRLB) is found only in IRS-2 [20, 21]. This domain interacts with the phosphorylated regulatory loop of the IR, whereas the phosphorylation of two Tyr residues within the KRLB are crucial for this interaction [22].

PI3 kinase is a target of the IRS proteins (IRS-1 and IRS-2) which phosphorylates specific phosphoinositides to form phosphatidylinositol 4,5 bisphosphate (PIP2) to phosphatidylinositol 3,4,5 triphosphate; in turn, this activates ser/thr kinase, i.e. phosphoinositide-dependent kinase-1 (PDK1) [23, 24]. Known substrates of the PDKs are the protein kinase B (PKB) and also atypical forms of protein kinase C (PKC) [25].

Downstream from PI 3-kinase, the serine/threonine kinase Akt (also called PKB) triggers insulin effects on the liver. Phosphatidylinositol-dependent kinase (PDK) and PKB/Akt have a pleckstrin homology domain that enables these molecules to migrate toward the plasma membrane [26]. Activated Akt induces glycogen synthesis, through inhibition of GSK-3; protein synthesis via mTOR and downstream elements; and cell survival, through inhibition of several pro-apoptotic agents (Bad, Forkhead family transcription factors, GSK-3). Insulin stimulates glucose uptake in muscle and adipocytes via translocation of GLUT4 vesicles to the plasma membrane [27- 29]. This suggests that the impairment of insulin activity leading to insulin resistance is linked to insulin signalling defects.

Recently, an alternative PI 3-kinase independent mechanism to enhance GLUT4 translocation and glucose uptake was described. According to this model, binding of insulin to its receptor finally activates the small G-protein TC10 via the scaffolding protein CAP (Cbl-associated protein) resulting in GLUT4 translocation and enhanced glucose uptake [30]. Insulin signaling also has growth and mitogenic effects, which are mostly mediated by the Akt cascade as well as by activation of the Ras/MAPK pathway. A negative feedback signal emanating from Akt/PKB, PKCZ, p70 S6K and the MAPK cascades results in serine phosphorylation and inactivation of IRS signaling [31, 32]. Insulin signalling molecules involved in metabolic and mitogenic action have been demonstrated to play a role in cellular insulin resistance. A few recent reports indicate that some PKC isoforms may have a regulatory effect on insulin signalling. The expression levels and activity of a few PKC isoforms are found to be associated with insulin resistance [33-35].

Recent data from PKB knockout animal models provide an insight into the role of PKB in normal glucose homeostasis. While disruption of PKB/Akt1 isoform in mice have not shown to cause any significant perturbations in metabolism, mice with a knock out of the PKB(Akt2) isoform show insulin resistance ending up with a phenotype closely resembling Type 2 diabetes in humans [36-37]. Subsequent studies [38- 40] in insulin-resistant animal models and humans have consistently demonstrated a reduced strength of insulin signaling via the IRS-1/PI 3-kinase pathway, resulting in diminished glucose uptake and utilization in insulin target tissues. Recent studies on inherited insulin post-receptor mutations in humans have detected a missense mutation in the kinase domain of PKB (Akt2) in a family of severely insulin resistant patients. The mutant PKB was unable to phosphorylate downstream targets and to mediate inhibition of phosphoenolpyruvate carboxykinase (PEPCK), a gluconeogenic key enzyme [41]. Another recent study, involving the stimulation of PI3K and Akt-1, -2, and -3 by insulin and epidermal growth factors (EGFs) in skeletal muscles from lean and obese insulin-resistant humans showed that Insulin activated all Akt isoforms in lean muscles, whereas only Akt-1 was activated in obese muscles. Insulin receptor substrate (IRS)-1 expression was reduced in obese muscles, and this was accompanied by decreased Akt-2 and -3 stimulation. In contrast, insulin- or EGF-stimulated phosphotyrosine-associated PI3K activity was not different between lean and obese muscles.

These results showed that a defect in the ability of insulin to activate Akt-2 and -3 may explain the impaired insulin-stimulated glucose transport in insulin resistance [42].

This suggests that the impairment of insulin activity leading to insulin resistance is linked to insulin signalling defects. These insulin signalling pathways are shown in figure1.

3. Mechanisms related to Insulin resistance

Two separate, but likely, complementary mechanisms have recently emerged as a potential explanations for Insulin resistance. First, changes in IRS-1 either due to mutations or serine phosphorylation of IRS proteins can reduce their ability to attract PI 3-kinase, thereby minimizing its activation. A number of serine kinases that phosphorylate serine residues of IRS-1 and weaken insulin signal transduction have been identified. Additionally, mitochondrial dysfunction has been suggested to trigger activation of several serine kinases, leading to a serine phosphorylation of IRS-1. Second, a distinct mechanism involving increased expression of p85α has also been found to play an important role in the pathogenesis of insulin resistance. Conceivably, a combination of both increased expression of p85α and increased serine phosphorylation of IRS-1 is needed to induce clinically apparent insulin resistance.

4. Mutations of IRS as a cause of Insulin resistance

IRS-1 protein is a gene product of IRS-1 gene. In humans, rare mutations of the IRS-1 protein are associated with insulin resistance [43] and disruption of the IRS-1 gene in mice results in insulin resistance mainly of muscle and fat [44]. The genetic analysis of the IRS-1 gene has revealed several base-pair changes that result in amino acid substitutions [45-47]. The most common amino acid change is a glycine to arginine substitution at codon 972 (G972R), which has an overall frequency of ≈6% in the general population [48], with a carrier prevalence of 9% among Caucasians [49]. This mutation has been reported to significantly impair IRS-1 function in experimental models [50], and clinical studies have shown that this genetic variant is associated with reduced insulin sensitivity [51]. Expression of this variant in 32-D cells is associated with a significant (20-30%) impairment of insulin-stimulated PI3-kinase activity, as well as reduced binding of IRS-1 to the p85 regulatory subunit of PI3-kinase. Genotype/phenotype studies stratified according to body mass index (BMI) indicate that obese subjects who are heterozygous for the mutant allele have a 50% decrease in insulin sensitivity, compared with wild-type obese subjects. This suggests that there may be an interaction between the mutant allele and obesity, such that, in the presence of obesity, the mutant variant may aggravate the obesity-associated insulin resistance [49]. Moreover, earlier observations have indicated that the presence of a mutated IRS-1 gene is associated with dyslipidemia, further suggesting that this gene variant may have a significant effect on several risk factors for CAD [48, 50-52].

Interestingly, IRS-2 knockout mice not only show insulin resistance of muscle, fat and liver, but also manifest diabetes as a result of cell failure [53]. This phenotype with severe hyperglycemia as a consequence of peripheral insulin resistance and insufficient insulin secretion due to a significantly reduced β-cell mass reveals many similarities to type 2 diabetes in man and outlines the role of IRS proteins for the development of cellular insulin resistance. Homozygous knockout mice lacking a single allele of IRS-1 gene lack any significant phenotype, whereas homozygous disruption of the *IRS-1* gene results in a mild form of insulin resistance [54]. IRS-1 homozygous null mice (IRS-1-/-) do not show a clear diabetic phenotypic expression, presumably because of pancreatic β cell compensation. IRS-$2^{-/-}$ mice, on the other hand, developed diabetes as a result of severe insulin resistance paired with β-cell failure [55, 56]. Even though β cell mass was reduced in IRS-$2^{-/-}$ mice, individual β cell showed normal or increased insulin secretion in response to glucose [55].

In regard to insulin signaling, experiments in immortalized neonatal hepatocytes show that the lack of IRS-2 is not compensated for by an elevation of IRS-1 protein content or an increase in tyrosine phosphorylation [57]. Previous experiments performed in peripheral tissues of IRS-$1^{-/-}$ mice by Yamauchi et al. [44] suggested that IRS-2 could be a major player in hepatic insulin action. However, to what extent reduced IRS-2 contributes to insulin resistance in the liver remains uncertain. In humans, a number of polymorphisms have been identified in the *IRS-2* gene. Among those, the amino acid substitution Gly1057Asp has been found in various populations with a prevalence sufficiently high to modulate a population's risk of type 2 diabetes. In Caucasians, Finns, and Chinese, however, this variant has not shown an associated with type 2 diabetes [58, 59]. Although the polymorphism was associated with decreased insulin sensitivity and impaired glucose tolerance in women with polycystic ovary syndrome [60], it showed no association with insulin sensitivity in other studies [59, 61, 62]. In contrast, another study in women with polycystic ovary syndrome found that homozygous carriers of the Gly1057 allele had higher 2-h plasma glucose concentrations during an oral glucose tolerance test (OGTT) [63]. Decreased serum insulin and C-peptide concentrations during an OGTT were reported in middle-aged glucose-tolerant Danish males carrying the Asp1057 allele [62]. However, using formal β-cell function tests, associations with insulin secretion were not reproduced in German, Finnish, and Swedish populations [59, 61, 62].

5. Serine phosphorylation of IRS as a cause of Insulin resistance

IRS-1 contains 21 putative tyrosine phosphorylation sites, several of which are located in amino acid sequence motifs that bind to SH-2 domain proteins, including the p85 regulatory subunit of PI 3-kinase, Grb-2, Nck, Crk, Fyn, Csk, phospholipase Cγ, and SHP-2 [64]. IRS-1 contains also > 30 potential serine/threonine phosphorylation sites in motifs recognized by various kinases such as casein kinase II, protein kinase C, protein kinase B/Akt, and mitogen-activated protein (MAP) kinases [12, 64].

Human IRS-2 contains 22 potential tyrosine phosphorylation sites, but only 13 are conserved in IRS-1. The amino acid sequence identity between IRS-1 and IRS-2 is 43%, with some domains such as the PH and PTB domains exhibiting higher degrees of identity (65 and 75%, respectively). The COOH-terminal domains of IRS-1 and IRS-2 are poorly conserved, displaying only 35% identity, which arises largely from similar tyrosine phosphorylation motifs surrounded by variable stretches of amino acid sequence. The middle of IRS-2 possesses a unique region comprising amino acids 591–786 that interacts specifically with the kinase regulatory loop binding (KRLB) domain of the insulin receptor β subunit [65]. Since this region is absent in IRS-1, this domain may contribute to the signaling specificity of IRS-2. In addition, IRS-1 and IRS-2 may regulate unique signaling pathways because of different tissue distribution, subcellular localization, kinetics of activation/deactivation, or specificity of interaction with downstream effectors [66-68]. For example, it has been shown that IRS-1 and IRS-2 differ in their subcellular localization since IRS-1 is twofold more concentrated in the intracellular membrane compartment than in cytosol, whereas IRS-2 is twofold more concentrated in cytosol than in the intracellular membrane compartment [69]. Further studies have shown that IRS-2 is dephosphorylated more rapidly and activates PI 3-kinase more transiently than IRS-1, thus indicating that differences in kinetics of activation may contribute to the diversity of the insulin signaling transduced by IRS-1 and IRS-2 [69,70].

Since, IRS-1 and IRS-2 have the longest tails, which contain ~20 potential Tyr phosphorylation sites. Many of the Tyr residues gather into common Tyr-phosphorylated consensus motifs (YMXM or YXXM) that bind SH2 domains of their effector proteins. Spatial matching is required for successful protein-protein interaction. Ser/Thr phosphorylation of IRS proteins in close proximity to their PTB (receptor-binding) region impedes the binding of the SH2 domains of these effectors, thus inhibiting insulin signaling [71].

Serine phosphorylation of IRS proteins can occur in response to a number of intracellular serine kinases [72].The causes of IRS-1 serine phosphorylation are-

1. mTOR- p70S6 kinase, Amino acids, Hyperinsulinemia
2. JNK- Stress, Hyperlipidemia, Inflammation
3. IKK- Inflammation
4. TNFα- Obesity, Inflammation
5. Mitochondrial dysfunction
6. PKC θ- Hyperglycemia, Diacylglycerol, Inflammation

Recent studies have demonstrated hyper-serine phosphorylation of IRS-1 on Ser^{302}, Ser^{307}, Ser^{612}, and Ser^{632} in several insulin-resistant rodent models [73- 76] as well as in lean insulin-resistant offspring of type 2 diabetic parents [77]. Further evidence for this hypothesis stems from recent studies in a muscle-specific triple serine to alanine mutant mouse (IRS-1 Ser $\rightarrow$ Ala^{302}, Ser $\rightarrow$ Ala^{307}, and Ser $\rightarrow$ Ala^{612}), which has been shown to be protected from high-fat diet–induced insulin resistance in vivo [78]. Based on in vitro studies, serine phosphorylation may lead to dissociation between insulin receptor/IRS-1 and/or IRS-1/PI 3-kinase, preventing PI 3-kinase activation [79, 80] or increasing degradation of IRS-1 [81].

Ser^{318} of IRS-1 is a potential target for PKCζ [82], JNK, and kinases along the PI3K-mTOR pathway [83]. It is located in close proximity to the PTB domain. Therefore, its phosphorylation presumably disrupts the interaction between IR and IRS-1.

Phosphorylation of Ser^{318} is not restricted to insulin stimulation. Elevated plasma levels of leptin, an adipokine produced by adipocytes [84], also stimulates the phosphorylation of Ser^{318}. This down regulates insulin-stimulated Tyr phosphorylation of IRS-1 and glucose uptake.

In a recent study using skeletal muscle biopsies from 11 humans, the mTOR-S6K pathway was shown to negatively modulate glucose metabolism under nutrient abundance [151]. In agreement with previous studies, phosphorylation of Ser^{312} and Ser^{636} of IRS-1 was implicated as part of this negative regulation [85, 86]. Increased phosphorylation of Ser^{636} of IRS-1 was observed in myotubes of patients with type 2 diabetes. Inhibition of ERK1/2 with PD-98059 reduced this phosphorylation, thereby implicating ERK1/2 in the phosphorylation of Ser^{636} in human muscle [87].

To unveil the importance of phosphorylated Ser/Thr residues of human IRS-1, Yi et al. [88] adopted a mass spectrometry approach. More than 20 Ser residues of IRS-1 were found to undergo insulin-stimulated phosphorylation in human muscle biopsies, three of which were newly identified sites: Thr^{495}, Ser^{527}, and Ser^{1005}. This report validates previous in vitro and in vivo studies in animal models and suggests that the same strategy could be employed to identify phosphorylated Ser/Thr sites under conditions of insulin resistance, obesity, or type 2 diabetes.

Impaired hepatic glycogen storage and glycogen synthase activity is a common finding in insulin resistance [89] and polymorphisms in the glycogen synthase gene have been described in insulin resistant patients. The most frequent mutations are the so-called *Xba*I mutations and Met416Val within intron 14 and exon 10, respectively. Currently, there are conflicting data on the correlation of these polymorphisms with insulin resistance and Type 2diabetes mellitus [90-92].

Recently, a hypothesis that mitochondrial dysfunction or reduced mitochondrial content accompanied by a decreased mitochondrial fatty acid oxidation and accumulation of fatty acid acyl CoA and diacylglycerol can cause insulin resistance has gained substantial experimental support [93- 95]. The mechanism of insulin resistance in these cases has been suggested to involve activation of a novel PKC that either by itself or via IKKβ or JNK-1 could lead to increased serine phosphorylation of IRS-1. Severe mitochondrial dysfunction can result in diabetes that is typically associated with severe β-cell dysfunction and neurological abnormalities [96]. In a study ,using $^{13}C/^{31}P$ MRS, it was found that in the healthy lean elderly volunteers with severe muscle insulin resistance, there is~40% reduction in rates of oxidative phosphorylation activity associated with increased intramyocellular and intrahepatic lipid content [94]. This study suggests that an acquired loss of mitochondrial function associated with aging predisposes elderly subjects to intramyocellular lipid accumulation, which results in insulin resistance [78]. Further, it was found that mitochondrial density was reduced by 38% in the insulin-resistant offspring [77].

[This topic has been dealt in details in subsequent chapter by Wang etal.]

The proinflammatory novel PKCθ has been found to cause serine phosphorylation of IRS-1 [97, 98], while PKCθ knockout mice have been shown to be protected from fat-induced insulin resistance [75]. Increased activity of PKCθ, along with increased activity of JNK, has also been found in skeletal muscle of obese and type 2 diabetic subjects [99, 100], supporting a potential role of these serine kinases in the pathogenesis of insulin resistance.

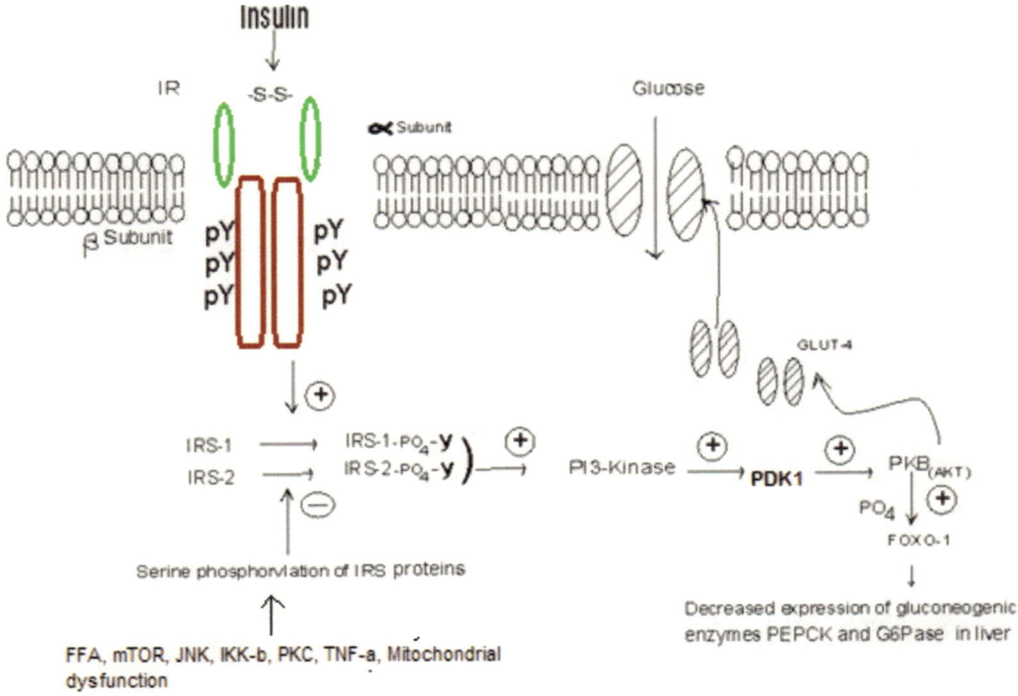

Figure 1. Insulin signaling pathway showing that the binding of insulin with Insulin receptor (IR) leads to phosphorylation of tyrosine residues followed by activation of downstream signalling pathways which result in recruitment in recruitment of GLUT-4 transporter to the plasma membrane and entry of glucose molecules within the cell. Serine phosphorylation of IRS protein has an inhibitory effect on downstream pathways resulting in insulin Resistance.

6. Increased expression of p85

A molecular mechanism that can potentially lead to insulin resistance is a disruption in the balance between the amounts of the PI 3-kinase subunits [101]. PI 3-kinase belongs to the class 1a 3-kinases [102], which exist as heterodimers, consisting of a regulatory subunit p85, which is tightly associated with a catalytic subunit, p110. Most tissues express two forms of regulatory subunit, p85α and p85β, and two forms of catalytic subunit, p110α and p110β [102]. p85α and p85β share the highest degree of homology in the C-terminal half of the molecules, which contains two SH2 domains that bind to tyrosine-phosphorylated proteins and an inter-SH2 domain that interacts with the catalytic subunit. The N-terminal halves of p85α and p85β contain an SH3 domain, a BCR homology region, and two proline-rich domains, but these domains are less well conserved between the two molecules. Two isoforms of p85α truncated in the N-terminal region, identified as AS53 (or p55α) [103, 104] and p50α [105, 106], as well as p85α itself, are derived from a single gene (*Pik3r1*). p85β and another short isoform with limited tissue distribution termed p55γ/p55^{PIK} are encoded by separate genes [107]. Normally, the regulatory subunit exists in stoichiometric excess to the catalytic one, resulting in a pool of freep85 monomers not associated with the p110 catalytic subunit. However, there exists a balance between the free p85 monomer and the p85-p110 heterodimer, with the latter being responsible for the PI 3-kinase activity [108-110]. Because the p85 monomer and the p85-p110 heterodimer compete for the same binding sites on the tyrosine-phosphorylated IRS proteins, an imbalance could cause either increased or decreased PI 3-kinase activity [111]. Increase or decrease in expression of p 85 would result in a shift in the balance either in the favour of free p85 or p85-p110 complexes [108-110].

One of the first indications that an imbalance between the abundance of p85 and p110 can alter PI 3-kinase activity came from experiments with 1-6 cultured skeletal muscle cells treated with dexamethazone [111]. This treatment significantly reduced PI 3-kinase activity, despite an almost fourfold increase in expression of p85α (no change in p85β) and only a minimal increase in p110. The authors concluded that p85α competes with the p85-p110 heterodimer, thus, reducing PI 3-kinase activity.

Subsequently, animals with a targeted disruption of *p85α* (p85$^{+/-}$ heterozygous mice) have been found to have a higher ratio of p85-p110 dimer to free p85 and to be more sensitive to insulin [101, 111-114].

The possibility of mismatch between free p85 and p85-p110 complexes has been recently supported by studies in insulin-resistant states induced by human placental growth hormone [115], obesity, and type 2 diabetes [100] and by short-term overfeeding of lean non-diabetic women [116]. Barbour etal [117] have demonstrated that insulin resistance of pregnancy is likely due to increased expression of skeletal muscle p85 in response to increasing concentrations of human placental growth hormone. Furthermore, women remaining insulin resistant postpartum have been found to display higher levels of p85 in the muscle [118].

Another small study of eight healthy lean women without a family history of diabetes, by Cornier et al showed that 3 days of overfeeding (50% above usual caloric intake) led to a significant increase in expression of p85α, ratio of p85α to p110, and a decline in insulin sensitivity. Within this experimental time frame, overfeeding did not cause any change in serine phosphorylation of either IRS-1 or S6K1, suggesting that increased expression of p85α may be an early molecular step in the pathogenesis of the nutritionally induced insulin resistance [116].

7. Role of the adipose tissue in insulin resistance

Insulin has 3 major target tissues—skeletal muscle, liver and adipose tissue. It has been postulated that the insulin receptor (IR) is overexpressed in the cells of these tissues. Also only these three organs in the body are capable of glucose deposition and storage; no other cells can store glucose. Removal of excess postprandial glucose by insulin occurs due to glucose uptake and storage in insulin sensitive target cells. About 75% of insulin-dependent postprandial glucose disposal occurs into the skeletal muscle [119]; therefore, it is the major target cell. While insulin-stimulated glucose disposal in adipose tissue is of little quantitative importance compared with that in muscle, regulation of lipolysis with subsequent release of glycerol and FFA into the circulation by insulin has major implications for glucose homeostasis.

It is widely accepted that increased availability and utilization of FFA contribute to the development of skeletal muscle insulin resistance [120-122]. Moreover, FFA have been shown to increase endogenous glucose production both by stimulating key enzymes and by providing energy for gluconeogenesis [123]. Finally, the glycerol released during triglyceride hydrolysis serves as a gluconeogenic substrate [124]. Consequently, resistance to the antilipolytic action of insulin in adipose tissue resulting in excessive release of FFA and glycerol would have deleterious effects on glucose homeostasis.

Patients suffering from insulin resistance and type 2 diabetes frequently display signs of abnormal lipid metabolism, increased circulatory concentration and elevated deposition of lipids in the skeletal muscle [125]. Increase in plasma FFA reduces insulin-stimulated glucose uptake, whereas a decrease in lipid content improves insulin activity in the skeletal muscle cells, adipocytes and liver [126]. Lipid-associated insulin resistance has also been shown to be linked to Glut4 translocation defects [27]. Studies have shown that raising plasma fatty acids in both rodents [75] and humans [127] abolishes insulin activation of IRS-1–associated PI 3-kinase activity in skeletal muscle where IRS-1 is most prevalent.

Adipose tissue can modulate whole body glucose metabolism by regulating levels of circulating free fatty acids (FFA) and also by secreting adipokines, thereby acting as an endocrine organ. However, the underlying mechanism of FFA-induced impairment of insulin signals is still unclear. The molecular mechanism underlying defective insulin-stimulated glucose transport activity can be attributed to increases in intramyocellular lipid metabolites such as fatty acyl CoAs and diacylglycerol, which in turn activate a serine/threonine kinase cascade, thus leading to defects in insulin signaling through Ser/Thr phosphorylation of insulin receptor substrate-1 [78].

Some of the PKC isoforms represent such signalling molecules. PKC isoforms are classified as classical (cPKCα, βI, βII, γ), novel (nPKCδ, ε, θ, η) and atypical (aPKCζ, λ). cPKCs are activated by Ca+2 and diacylglycerol (DAG), nPKCs are activated by only DAG and aPKCs respond to neither Ca+2 nor DAG [128]. Among all these PKC isoforms, nPKCs are said to have a modulatory role in insulin signalling. Recent reports also demonstrate a link between nPKCs and FFA induced insulin resistance.

Diacylglycerol is an attractive trigger for fat-induced insulin resistance in skeletal muscle, since it has been shown to increase in muscle during both lipid infusions and fat feeding and it is a known activator of novel protein kinase C (PKC) isoforms [78].

Recent studies have revealed that accumulation of intracellular lipid metabolites activate a serine kinase cascade involving PKC-ε, leading to decreased insulin receptor kinase activity resulting in *1*) lower insulin-stimulated IRS-2 tyrosine phosphorylation, *2*) lower IRS-2–associated PI 3-kinase activity, and 3) lower AKT2 activity [129] . These fat-induced defects in insulin signalling in turn result in reduced insulin stimulation of glycogen synthase activity, resulting in decreased insulin-stimulated hepatic glucose uptake and reduced insulin stimulation of hepatic glucose production. Furthermore, reduced activity of AKT2 results in decreased phosphorylation of forkhead box protein O (FOXO), allowing it to enter the nucleus and activate the transcription of the rate-controlling enzymes of gluconeogenesis (phosphoenolpyruvate carboxykinase, glucose-6-phosphate phosphatase).

Increased gluconeogenesis further exacerbates hepatic insulin resistance and results in fasting hyperglycemia [129- 131]. Mitochondrial glycerol-3-phosphate acyltransferase (mtGPAT) is a key enzyme in de novo fat synthesis in liver, and recent studies in mtGPAT knockout mice have clearly implicated intracellular accumulation of diacylglycerol in triggering fat-induced insulin resistance in liver through activation of PKC-ε [132]. These data have important implications for the development of novel therapeutic agents to reverse and prevent hepatic insulin resistance associated with non-alcoholic fatty liver and type 2 diabetes [133].

Lipid infusion in rats and humans impaired insulin-stimulated glucose disposal into the muscle and concomitant activation of PKCθ and PKCδ [134, 135]. PKCδ has been shown to be a possible candidate for phosphorylation of the IR on serine residues [136]. These result in defects in the insulin signalling pathway imposing insulin resistance.

Recently, the PPARγ co-activator-1 (PGC-1) has been recognized as playing a major role in glucose homeostasis of the organism. Work mainly by Spiegelman's group demonstrated a crucial role of PGC-1 in the regulation of GLUT4 in muscle cells [137]. (PGC)-1α and PGC-1 β are transcriptional factor co-activators that regulate mitochondrial biogenesis. In addition AMP kinase, which is activated during exercise and ischemia by a reduction in the ATP/AMP ratio, has been shown to be an important regulator of mitochondrial biogenesis, mediating its effects through MEF2- and CREB-mediated increased PGC-1α expression [138-141]. Extracellular stimuli such as cold, thyroid hormone, and exercise stimulate mitochondrial biogenesis through PGC-1 in brown fat and skeletal muscle. Increased PGC-1 protein expression leads to increases in the target genes, including nuclear respiratory factor (NRF)-1. NRF-1 is a transcription factor stimulating many nuclear-encoded mitochondrial genes such as OXPHOS genes and also mitochondrial transcription factor A (mtTFA), a key transcriptional factor for the mitochondrial genome. mtTFA can bind to the D-loop of the mitochondrial genome and increase transcription of mitochondrial genes and replication of mitochondrial DNA [142].

A recent study by Ling et al. [143] demonstrated an age dependent decrease in muscle gene expression of PGC-1 α and PGC-1 β in young and elderly dizygotic and monozygotic twins without known diabetes

Adipose tissue also acts as an endocrine organ producing adipokines which modulate glucose homeostasis [144]. Currently, those most intensely discussed are tumor necrosis factor-α (TNF α), leptin, adiponectin and resistin. At a molecular level, TNF α increases serine phosphorylation of IRS-1 and down-regulates GLUT4 expression, thereby contributing to insulin resistance [38]. Furthermore, mice lacking TNF α function were protected from obesity-induced insulin resistance [145]. The role of leptin in regulating food intake and energy expenditure is well established. Humans with leptin deficiency or leptin receptor mutations are severely obese [146,147]. The adiponectin has insulin-sensitizing effects as it enhances inhibition of hepatic glucose output as well as glucose uptake and utilization in fat and muscle. The expression of adiponectin is decreased in obese humans and mice [148]. Thus, in humans, adiponectin levels correlate with insulin sensitivity. Because of its insulin-antagonistic effects, the adipocytokine resistin has attracted a lot of research interest. This is mainly based on data obtained *in-vitro* and from some animal models. Resistin decreases insulin-dependent glucose transport *in-vitro* and increases fasting blood glucose concentrations and hepatic glucose production *in-vivo* [149, 150].

8. Insulin resistance and Forkhead box protein O (FOXO)

The fasting hyperglycaemia in patients with Type 2 diabetes is the clinical correlate of the increased glucose production by the liver because of insulin resistance. This is as a result of the lack of inhibition of the two key gluconeogenic enzymes, phospho-enolpyruvate carboxykinase (PEPCK) and the glucose-6- phosphatase (G6Pase) catalytic subunit. Studies in hepatoma cells [151,152] suggest that Foxo1 and -3 regulate the transcription of reporter genes containing insulin response elements from the PEPCK and G6Pase promoters. Furthermore, Foxo1 is phosphorylated in an insulin-responsive manner by PIP3-dependent kinases, such as Akt. Reduced activity of AKT2 results in decreased phosphorylation of Foxo protein, allowing it to enter the nucleus and activate the transcription of these rate-controlling enzymes of gluconeogenesis [151,153]. There is increasing evidence that Foxo-proteins are critically involved in the insulin dependent regulation of gluconeogenic gene expression and insulin-resistance*in-vivo* [154, 155]. In addition, the PPARγco-activator-1 (PGC-1), a factor integrating the effects of glucocorticoids and cAMP on gluconeogenic geneexpression in the liver [156, 157] is also regulated by PKB and Foxo1 [158].

9. FFA induced Inhibition of Insulin receptor (IR) gene expression by PKCε

Clearly, the IR is one of the major targets in FFA-induced impairment of insulin activity. Recent studies performed *in-vivo* suggested that glucose uptake rather than intracellular glucose metabolism is the rate-limiting step for fatty acid induced insulin resistance in humans [159]. This indicates a mechanism in which accumulation of intracellular fatty acids or their metabolites results in an impairment of signaling through IRS/PI 3-kinase.

Recent evidence has shown that PDK1 can directly phosphorylate all PKCs including nPKCs [160]. The PKCε isotype has recently been shown to be related to insulin resistance. Insulin stimulation of PDK1 phosphorylation is inhibited by an FFA, i.e. palmitate. PKCε phosphorylation is dependent on PDK1; FFA incubation of skeletal muscle cells and adipocytes inhibited PDK1 phosphorylation but surprisingly increased PKCε

phosphorylation. Inhibition of PDK1 by FFA is reflected in Akt phosphorylation as Akt phosphorylation is also dependent on PDK1 [161]. It has been shown that myristic acid incubation of HEPG2 cells causes myristoylation of PKCε which results in constitutive phosphorylation of PKCεat thr566/ser729 in the kinase domain required for PKCε activity. This phosphorylation was totally independent of PDK1, which the workers demonstrated by using PDK1 knockout cells. In the same way, addition of palmitate to skeletal muscle cells or adipocytes may affect palmitoylation of PKCε resulting in constitutive phosphorylation of PKCε [162, 163]. Taken together, it is clear that FFA causes PDK1-independent phosphorylation of PKCε which in turn translocates to the nucleus, and its time of entry into the nucleus coincides with inhibition of IR gene transcription.

10. Conclusion

In this review, current developments contributing to understanding of insulin resistance and to the pathogenesis of metabolic syndrome has been discussed. Among the many molecules involved in the intracellular processing of the signal provided by insulin, IRS-2, PKB, Foxo protein and p85 regulatory subunit of PI-3 kinase have attracted particular interest, because their dysfunction results in insulin resistance *in-vivo*. It has been well established that FFA are responsible for insulin resistance. This review focuses on the current trends in research in this important domain and throws light on certain possibilities regarding the manner in which FFA inhibits insulin activity.

Author details

Sarika Arora*
Department of Biochemistry, ESI Postgraduate Institute of Medical Sciences & Research, New Delhi, India

11. References

[1] Rosenson RS. New approaches in the intensive management of cardiovascular risk in the metabolic syndrome. Curr Probl Cardiol 2005; 20: 313-317.
[2] Reaven GM. Banting lecture 1988: role of insulin resistance in human disease. Diabetes 1988; 37: 1596-1607.
[3] Ginsberg H. Insulin resistance and cardiovascular disease. J Clin Invest 2000; 106: 453–458.
[4] Enas EA, Mohan V, Deepa M, Farooq S, Pazhoor S, Chennikkara H. The metabolic syndrome and dyslipidemia among Asian Indians : a population with high rates of diabetes and premature coronary artery disease. J Cardiometab Syndr 2007; 2: 267-275.

* Corresponding Author

[5] Nestel P, Lyu R, Low LP, Sheu WH, Nitiyanant W, Saito I etal. Metabolic syndrome: Recent prevalence in East and Southeast Asian populations. Asia Pac J Clin Nutr 2007; 16: 362-367.

[6] Eapen D, Kalra GL, Merchant N, Arora A, Khan BV. Metabolic syndrome and cardiovascular disease in South Asians. Vasc Health Risk Manag 2009; 5: 731- 743.

[7] Borch-Johnsen K. The metabolic syndrome in a global perspective. The public health impact. Dan Med Bull 2007; 54: 157-159.

[8] Shulman GI. Cellular mechanisms of insulin resistance in humans. Am J Cardiol 1999; 84 : 3J–10J.

[9] White MF, Shoelson SE, Keutmann H, Kahn CR. A cascade of tyrosine autophosphorylation in the beta-subunit activates the phosphotransferase of the insulin receptor. J Biol Chem1988; 263: 2969 –2980.

[10] Brunetti A, Manfioletti G, Chiefari E, Goldfine ID, Foti D. Transcriptional regulation of human insulin receptor gene by the high-mobility group protein HMGI(Y). FASEB J.2001; 15: 492–500.

[11] Virkamaki A, Ueki K, Kahn CR. Protein-protein interaction in insulin signaling and the molecular mechanisms of insulin resistance. J Clin. Invest. 1999; 103: 931-943.

[12] Sun XJ, Rothenberg P, Kahn CR, Backer JM, Araki E, Wilden PA, etal. Structure of the insulin receptor substrate IRS-1 defines a unique signal transduction protein. Nature (London) 1991; 352: 73-77.

[13] Sun XJ, Wang LM, Zhang Y, Yenush L, Myers MG, Glasheen E, etal. Role of IRS-2 in insulin and cytokine signalling. Nature (London) 1995; 377: 173-177.

[14] Lavan BE, Lane WS, Lienhard GE. The 60-kDa phosphotyrosine protein in insulin-treated adipocytes is a new member of the insulin receptor substrate family. J Biol Chem 1997; 272: 11439-11443.

[15] Lavan BE, Fantin VR, Chang ET, Lane WS, Keller SR, Lienhard GE. A novel 160-kDa phosphotyrosine protein in insulin-treated embryonic kidney cells is a new member of the insulin receptor substrate family. J. Biol. Chem 1997; 272: 21403-21407.

[16] Farhang-Fallah J, Randhawa VK, Nimnual A, Klip A, Bar-Sagi D, Rozakis-Adcock M. The pleckstrin homology (PH) domain-interacting protein couples the insulin receptor substrate 1 PH domain to insulin signaling pathways leading to mitogenesis and GLUT4 translocation. Mol Cell Biol 2002; 22: 7325–7336.

[17] Greene MW, Sakaue H, Wang L, Alessi DR, Roth RA. Modulation of insulin-stimulated degradation of human insulin receptor substrate-1 by Serine 312 phosphorylation. J Biol Chem 2003; 278: 8199–8211.

[18] Paz K, Voliovitch H, Hadari YR, Roberts CT Jr, LeRoith D, Zick Y. Interaction between the insulin receptor and its downstream effectors. Use of individually expressed receptor domains for structure/function analysis. J Biol Chem 1996; 271: 6998–7003.

[19] Voliovitch H, Schindler DG, Hadari YR, Taylor SI, Accili D, Zick Y. Tyrosine phosphorylation of insulin receptor substrate-1 in vivo depends upon the presence of its pleckstrin homology region. J Biol Chem 1995; 270: 18083–18087.

[20] He W, Craparo A, Zhu Y, O'Neill TJ, Wang LM, Pierce JH, Gustafson TA. Interaction of insulin receptor substrate-2 (IRS-2) with the insulin and insulin-like growth factor I

receptors. Evidence for two distinct phosphotyrosine-dependent interaction domains within IRS-2. J Biol Chem 1996; 271: 11641–11645.

[21] Sawka-Verhelle D, Tartare-Deckert S, White MF, Van Obberghen E. Insulin receptor substrate-2 binds to the insulin receptor through its phosphotyrosine-binding domain and through a newly identified domain comprising amino acids 591–786. J Biol Chem 1996; 271: 5980–5983.

[22] Sawka-Verhelle D, Baron V, Mothe I, Filloux C, White MF, Van Obberghen E. Tyr624 and Tyr628 in insulin receptor substrate-2 mediate its association with the insulin receptor. J Biol Chem 1997; 272: 16414–16420.

[23] Alessi DR, Cohen P. Mechanism of activation and function of protein kinase B. Curr Opin Genet Dev 1998; 8: 55–62.

[24] Le Good J A, Ziegler WH, Parekh D B, Alessi D R, Cohen P, Parker P J. Protein kinase C isotypes controlled by phosphoinositide 3-kinase through the protein kinase PDK1. Science 1998; 281: 2042–2045.

[25] Kotani K, Ogawa W, Matsumoto M, Kitamura T, Sakaue H, Hino Y et al. Requirement of atypical protein kinase clamdafor insulin stimulation of glucose uptake but not for Akt activation in 3T3-L1 adipocytes. Mol Cell Biol 1998; 18: 6971–6982.

[26] Taniguchi CM, Emanuelli B, Kahn CR. Critical nodes in signalling pathways: insights into insulin action. Nat Rev Mol Cell Biol 2006; 7: 85–96.

[27] Pessin J E, Thurmond D C, Elmendorf J S, Coker K J and Okada S. Molecular basis of insulin-stimulated GLUT4 vesicle trafficking. J. Biol. Chem 1999; 274 : 2593–2596.

[28] Kupriyanova TA, Kandror KV. Akt-2 binds to Glut4-containing vesicles and phosphorylates their component proteins in response to insulin. J. Biol. Chem.1999; 274: 1458–1464.

[29] Martin S, Millar CA, Lyttle CT, Meerloo T, Marsh B J, Gould GW, etal. Effects of insulin on intracellular GLUT4 vesicles in adipocytes: evidence for a secretory mode of regulation. J Cell Sci 2000; 113: 3427–3438.

[30] Khan AH, Pessin JE. Insulin regulation of glucose uptake: a complex interplay of intracellular signalling pathways. Diabetologia 2002; 45: 1475–1483.

[31] Cheatham B. Phosphatidylinositol 3-kinase activation is required for insulin stimulation of pp70S6 kinase, DNA synthesis, and glucose transporter translocation. Mol Cell Biol 1994; 14: 4902– 4911.

[32] Shepherd PR, Nave BT, Siddle K. Insulin stimulation of glycogen synthesis and glycogen synthase activity is blocked by wortmannin and rapamycin in 3T3–L1 adipocytes: evidence for the involvement of phosphoinositide 3-kinase and p70 ribosomal protein-S6 kinase. Biochem J 1995; 305: 25–28.

[33] Greene MW, Morrice N, Garofalo RS, Roth RA. Modulation of human receptor substrate 1 tyrosine phosphorylation by protein kinase C δ. Biochem J 2004; 378: 105–116.

[34] Zick Y. Insulin resistance: a phosphorylation-based uncoupling of insulin signalling. Trends Cell Biol 2001; 11: 437–441.

[35] White MF. IRS proteins and the common path to diabetes. Am J Physiol Endocrinol Metab 2002; 283: E413–422.

[36] Cho H, Thorvaldsen JL, Chu Q, Feng F, Birnbaum MJ. Akt1/PKBα is required for normal growth but dispensable for maintenance of glucose homeostasis in mice. J Biol Chem 2001; 276: 38349–38352.

[37] Cho H, Mu J, Kim JK, Thorvaldsen JL, Chu Q, Crenshaw EB 3rd et al. Insulin resistance and a diabetes mellitus-like syndrome in mice lacking the protein kinase Akt2 (PKBα). Science 2001; 292: 1728–1731.

[38] Kahn BB, Flier JS. Obesity and insulin resistance. J Clin Invest 2000; 106: 473– 481.

[39] Pessin JE, Saltiel AR. Signaling pathways in insulin action: molecular targets of insulin resistance. J Clin Invest 2000; 106:165–169.

[40] LeRoith D, Zick Y. Recent advances in our understanding of insulin action and insulin resistance. Diabetes Care 2001; 24: 588 –597.

[41] George S, Rochford J, Wolfrum C, Gray SL, Schinner S, Wilson JC et al. Human insulin resistance and diabetes mellitus due to a missense mutation AKT2. Science 2004; 304: 1325–1328.

[42] Brozinick JT Jr, Roberts BR, Dohm GL. Defective Signaling Through Akt-2 and -3 But Not Akt-1 in Insulin-Resistant Human Skeletal Muscle Potential Role in Insulin Resistance. Diabetes 2003; 52: 935-941.

[43] Whitehead JP, Humphreys P, Krook A, Jackson R, Hayward A, Lewis H et al. Molecular scanning of the insulin receptor substrate 1 gene in subjects with severe insulin resistance: detection and functional analysis of a naturally occurring mutation in a YMXM motif. Diabetes 1998; 47: 837–839.

[44] Yamauchi T, Tobe K, Tamemoto H, Ueki K, Kaburagi Y, Yamamoto-Honda R et al. Insulin signalling and insulin actions in the muscles and livers of insulin-resistant, insulin receptor substrate 1-deficient mice. Mol Cell Biol 1996; 16: 3074–3084.

[45] Almind K, Bjorbaek C, Vestergaard H, Hansen T, Echwald S, Pedersen O. Amino acid polymorphism of insulin receptor substrate-1 in non-insulin-dependent diabetes mellitus. Lancet. 1993; 342: 828–832.

[46] Laakso M, Malkki M, Kekalainen P, Kuusisto J, Deeb SS. Insulin receptor substrate-1 variants in non-insulin-dependent diabetes. J Clin Invest. 1994; 94: 1141–1146.

[47] Imai Y, Fusco A, Suzuki Y, Lesniak MA, D'Alfonso R, Sesti G, etal. Variant sequences of insulin receptor substrate-1 in non-insulin-dependent-diabetes mellitus. J Clin Endocrinol Metab. 1994; 79: 1655–1658.

[48] Hitman GA, Hawrami K, McCarthy MI, Viswanathan M, Snehalatha C, Ramachandran A, etal. Insulin receptor substrate-1 gene mutations in NIDDM: implications for the study of polygenic disease. Diabetologia 1995; 38: 481–486.

[49] Pederson O. Genetics of Insulin resistance. Exp Clin Endocrinol Diabet 1999; 107(2): 113-8.

[50] Almind K, Inoue G, Pedersen O, Kahn CR. A common amino acid polymorphism in insulin receptor substrate-1 causes impaired insulin signaling: evidence from transfection studies. J Clin Invest 1996; 97: 2569–2575.

[51] Clausen JO, Hansen T, Bjorbaek C, Echwald SM, Urhammer SA, Rasmussen S, etal. Insulin resistance: interactions between obesity and a common variant of insulin receptor substrate-1. Lancet 1995; 346: 397–402.

[52] Baroni MG, D'Andrea MP, Montali A, Pannitteri G, Barilla F, Campagna F, etal. A common mutation of the insulin receptor substrate-1 gene is a risk factor for coronary artery disease. Arterioscler Thromb Vasc 1999; 19(12): 2975-80.

[53] Previs SF, Withers DJ, Ren JM, White MF, Shulman GI. Contrasting effects of IRS-1 versus IRS-2 gene disruption on carbohydrate and lipid metabolism in vivo. J Biol Chem 2000; 275: 38990–38994.

[54] Araki E, Shimada F, Uzawa H, Mori M and Ebina Y. Characterization of the promoter region of the human insulin receptor gene. J Biol Chem 1994; 262: 16186–16191.

[55] Kubota N, Tobe K, Terauchi Y, Eto K, Yamauchi T, Suzuki R, etal. Disruption of insulin receptor substrate 2 causes type 2 diabetes because of liver insulin resistance and lack of compensatory β-cell hyperplasia. Diabetes 2000; 49:1880 –1889.

[56] Kido Y, Burks DJ, Withers D, Brunning JC, Kahn CR, White MF, etal. Tissue-specific insulin resistance in mice with combined mutations of the insulin receptor. J Clin Invest 2000; 105: 199 –205.

[57] Valverde AM, Burks DJ, Fabregat I, Fisher TL, Carretero J, White MF,etal. Molecular mechanisms of insulin resistance in IRS-2-deficient hepatocytes. Diabetes 2003; 52: 2239-2248.

[58] Bernal D, Almind K, Yenush L, Ayoub M, Zhang Y, Rosshani L, etal. Insulin receptor substrate-2 amino acid polymorphisms are not associated with random type 2 diabetes among Caucasians. Diabetes 1998; 47: 976 –979.

[59] Wang H, Rissanen J, Miettinen R, Karkkainen P, Kekalainen P, Kuusisto J, etal. New amino acid substitutions in the IRS-2 gene in Finnish and Chinese subjects with late-onset type 2 diabetes. Diabetes 2001; 50: 1949 –1951.

[60] El Mkadem SA, Lautier C, Macari F, Molinari N, Lefebvre P, Renard E, etal. Role of allelic variants Gly972Arg of IRS-1 and Gly1057Asp of IRS-2 in moderate-to-severe insulin resistance of women with polycystic ovary syndrome. Diabetes 2001; 50: 2164 – 2168.

[61] Fritsche A, Madaus A, Renn W, Tschritter O, Teigeler A, Weisser M, etal. The prevalent Gly1057Asp polymorphism in the insulin receptor substrate-2 gene is not associated with impaired insulin secretion. J Clin Endocrinol Metab 2001; 86: 4822 –4825.

[62] Almind K, Frederiksen SK, Bernal D, Hansen T, Ambye L, Urhammer S, etal. Search for variants of the gene-promoter and the potential phosphotyrosine encoding sequence of the insulin receptor substrate-2 gene: evaluation of their relation with alterations in insulin secretion and insulin sensitivity. Diabetologia 1999; 42: 1244 –1249.

[63] Ehrmann DA, Tang X, Yoshiuchi I, Cox NJ, Bell GI. Relationship of insulin receptor substrate-1 and -2 genotypes to phenotypic features of polycystic ovary syndrome. J Clin Endocrinol Metab 2002; 87: 4297 –4300.

[64] White MF. The insulin signaling system and the IRS proteins. Diabetologia 1997; 40: S2-S17.

[65] Sawka-Verhelle D, Tartare-Deckert S, White MF, Van Obberghen E. Insulin receptor substrate-2 binds to the insulin receptor through its phosphotyrosine-binding domain and through a newly identified domain comprising amino acid 591–786. J Biol Chem 1996; 271: 5980-5983.

[66] Giovannone B, Scaldaferri ML, Federici M, Porzio O, Lauro D, Fusco A, etal. Insulin receptor substrate (IRS) transduction system: distinct and overlapping signaling potential. Diabetes Metab. Res. Rev 2000; 16: 434-441.
[67] Sun XJ, Pons S, Wang LM, Zhang Y, Yenush L, Burks D, etal. The IRS-2 gene on murine chromosome 8 encodes a unique signaling adapter for insulin and cytokine action. Mol. Endocrinol 1997; 11: 251-262.
[68] Shuppin GT, Pons S, Hugl S, Aiello LP, King GL, White MF, etal. A specific increased expression of Insulin Receptor Substrate 2 in pancreatic β-cell lines is involved in mediating serum-stimulated-cell growth. Diabetes 1998; 47: 1074-1085.
[69] Inoue G, Cheatham B, Emkey R, Kahn CR. Dynamics of insulin signaling in 3T3–L1 adipocytes. Differential compartmentalization and trafficking of insulin receptor substrate (IRS)-1 and IRS-2. J Biol Chem. 1998; 273: 11548-11555.
[70] Ogihara T, Shin BC, Anai M, Katagiri H, Inukai K, Funaki M, etal. Insulin receptor substrate (IRS)-2 is dephosphorylated more rapidly than IRS-1 via its association with phosphatidylinositol 3-kinase in skeletal muscle cells. J Biol Chem 1997; 272: 12868-12873.
[71] Boura-Halfon S, Zick Y. Phosphorylation of IRS proteins, insulin action, and insulin resistance. AJP - Endo 2009; 296: E581-E591.
[72] Draznin B. Molecular Mechanisms of Insulin Resistance: Serine phosphorylation of insulin receptor substrate-1 and increased expression of p85α: The two sides of a coin. Diabetes 2006; 55: 2392–2397.
[73] Um SH, Frogerio F, Watanabe M, Picard F, Joaquin M, Sticker M, etal. Absence of S6K1 protects against age- and diet-induced obesity while enhancing insulin sensitivity. Nature 2004; 431: 200 –205.
[74] Yu CL, Chen Y, Cline GW, Zhang D, Zong H, Wang Y, etal. Mechanisms by which fatty acids inhibit insulin activation of insulin receptor substrate-1 (IRS-1)-associated phosphatidylinositol 3-kinase activity in muscle. J. Biol Chem 2002; 27: 50230–50236.
[75] Kim JK, Fillmore JJ, Sunshine MJ, Albrecht B, Higashimori T, Kim DW, etal. PKC-theta knockout mice are protected from fat-induced insulin resistance. J Clin Invest 2004; 114: 823 –827.
[76] Furukawa N, Ongusaha P, Jahng WJ, Araki K, Choi CS, Kim HJ, etal. Role of Rho-kinase in regulation of insulin action and glucose homeostasis. Cell Metab 2005; 2:119 – 129.
[77] Morino K, Petersen KF, Dufour S, Befroy D, Frattini J, Shatzkes N, etal. Reduced mitochondrial density and increased IRS-1 serine phosphorylation in muscle of insulin-resistant offspring of type 2 diabetic parents. J Clin Invest 2005; 115: 3587 –3593.
[78] Morino K, Petersen KF, Schulman GI. Molecular mechanisms of insulin resistance in humans and their potential links with mitochondrial dysfunction. Diabetes 2006; 55: S9-S15.
[79] Moeschel K, Beck A, Weigert C, Lammers R, Kalbacher H, Voelter W, etal. Protein kinase C-zeta-induced phosphorylation of Ser(318) in insulin receptor substrate-1 (IRS-1) attenuates the interaction with the insulin receptor and the tyrosine phosphorylation of IRS-1. J Biol Chem 2004; 279: 25157 –25163.

[80] Li JP, Defea K, Roth RA. Modulation of insulin receptor substrate-1 tyrosine phosphorylation by an Akt/phosphatidylinositol 3-kinase pathway. J BiolChem 1999; 274: 9351 –9356.

[81] Egawa K, Nakashima N, Sharma PM, Maegawa H, Nagai Y, Kashiwagi A, etal. Persistent activation of phosphatidylinositol 3-kinase causes insulin resistance due to accelerated insulin-induced insulin receptor substrate-1 degradation in 3T3–L1 adipocytes. Endocrinology 2000; 141: 1930 –1935.

[82] Moeschel K, Beck A, Weigert C, Lammers R, Kalbacher H, Voelter W, etal. Protein kinase C-zeta-induced phosphorylation of Ser318 in insulin receptor substrate-1 (IRS-1) attenuates the interaction with the insulin receptor and the tyrosine phosphorylation of IRS-1. J Biol Chem 2004; 279: 25157–25163.

[83] Mussig K, Fiedler H, Staiger H, Weigert C, Lehmann R, Schleicher ED, etal. Insulin-induced stimulation of JNK and the PI 3-kinase/mTOR pathway leads to phosphorylation of serine 318 of IRS-1 in C2C12 myotubes. Biochem Biophys Res Commun 2005; 335: 819–825.

[84] Argiles JM, Lopez-Soriano J, Almendro V, Busquets S, Lopez-Soriano FJ. Cross-talk between skeletal muscle and adipose tissue: a link with obesity? Med Res Rev 2005; 25: 49–65.

[85] Krebs M, Brunmair B, Brehm A, Artwohl M, Szendroedi J, Nowotny P, etal. The Mammalian target of rapamycin pathway regulates nutrient-sensitive glucose uptake in man. Diabetes 2007; 56: 1600–1607.

[86] Tremblay F, Brule S, Hee Um S, Li Y, Masuda K, Roden M, etal. Identification of IRS-1 Ser-1101 as a target of S6K1 in nutrient- and obesity-induced insulin resistance. Proc Natl Acad Sci USA 2007; 104: 14056–14061.

[87] Bouzakri K, Roques M, Gual P, Espinosa S, Guebre-Egziabher F, Riou JP, etal. Reduced activation of phosphatidylinositol-3 kinase and increased serine 636 phosphorylation of insulin receptor substrate-1 in primary culture of skeletal muscle cells from patients with type 2 diabetes. Diabetes 2003; 52: 1319–1325.

[88] Yi Z, Langlais P, De Filippis EA, Luo M, Flynn CR, Schroeder S, etal. Global assessment of regulation of phosphorylation of insulin receptor substrate-1 by insulin in vivo in human muscle. Diabetes 2007; 56: 1508–1516.

[89] Damsbo P, Vaag A, Hother-Nielsen O, Beck-Nielsen H. Reduced glycogen synthase activity in skeletal muscle from obese patients with and without type 2 (non-insulin-dependent) diabetes mellitus. Diabetologia 1991; 34: 239–245.

[90] Groop LC, Kankuri M, Schalin-Jantti C, Ekstrand A, Nikula-Ijas P, Widen E et al. Association between polymorphism of the glycogen synthase gene and non-insulin-dependent diabetes mellitus. N Engl J Med 1993; 328: 10–14.

[91] Rissanen J, Pihlajamaki J, Heikkinen S, Kekalainen P, Mykkanen L, Kuusisto J et al. New variants in the glycogen synthase gene (Gln71His, Met416Val) in patients with NIDDM from eastern Finland. Diabetologia 1997; 40: 1313–1319.

[92] St-Onge J, Joanisse DR, Simoneau J-A. The stimulation-induced increase in skeletal muscle glycogen synthase content is impaired in carriers of the glycogen synthase XbaI gene polymorphism. Diabetes 2001; 50: 195–198.

[93] Lowell BB, Shulman GI. Mitochondrial dysfunction and type 2 diabetes. Science 2005; 307: 384–387.

[94] Petersen KF, Befroy D, Dufour S, Dziura J, Ariyan C, Rothman DL, etal. Mitochondrial dysfunction in the elderly: possible role in insulin resistance. Science 2003; 300 :1140–1142.

[95] Petersen KF, Dufour S, Befroy D, Garcia R, Shulman GI. Impaired mitochondrial activity in the insulin-resistant offspring of patients with type 2 diabetes. N Engl J Med 2004; 350: 664–671.

[96] DiMauro S, Schon EA. Mechanisms of disease: mitochondrial respiratory-chain diseases. N Engl J Med 2003; 348: 2656 –2668.

[97] Li Y, Soos TJ, Li X, Wu J, Degennaro M, Sun X, etal. Protein kinase θ inhibits insulin signaling by phosphorylating IRS1 at Ser^{1101}. J Biol Chem 2004; 279 :45304–45307.

[98] Bell KS, Shcmitz-Peiffer C, Lim-Fraser M, Biden TJ, Cooney GJ, Kraegen EW. Acute reversal of lipid-induced muscle insulin resistance is associated with rapid alteration in PKC-θ localization. Am J Physiol Endocrinol Metab 2000; 279 :E1196–E1201.

[99] Itani SI, Pories WJ, Macdonald KG, Dohm GL. Increased protein kinase C θ in skeletal muscle of diabetic patients. Metabolism 2001; 50: 553–557.

[100] Bandyopadhyay GK, Yu JG, Ofrecio J, Olefsky JM. Increased p85/55/50 expression and decreased phosphatidylinositol 3-kinase activity in insulin-resistant human skeletal muscle. Diabetes 2005; 54: 2351–2359.

[101] Ueki K, Fruman DA, Brachmann SM, Tseng YH, Cantley LC, Kahn CR. Molecular balance between the regulatory and catalytic subunits of phosphoinositide 3-kinase regulates cell signaling and survival. Mol Cell Biol 2002; 22: 965–977.

[102] Shepherd PR, Withers DJ, Siddle K. Phosphoinositide 3-kinase: the key switch mechanism in insulin signaling. Biochem J 1998; 333: 471– 490.

[103] Inukai, K, Anai M, Van Breda E, Hosaka T, Katagiri H, Funaki M, et al. A novel 55-kDa regulatory subunit for phosphatidylinositol 3-kinase structurally similar to p55PIK is generated by alternative splicing of the p85a gene. J Biol Chem 1996; 271: 5317-5320.

[104] Antonetti DA, Algenstaedt P, Kahn CR. Insulin receptor substrate 1 binds two novel splice variants of the regulatory subunit of phosphatidylinositol 3-kinase in muscle and brain. Mol Cell Biol 1996; 16: 2195-2203.

[105] Fruman DA, Cantley LC, Carpenter CL. Structural organization and alternative splicing of the murine phosphoinositide 3-kinase p85a gene. Genomics 1996; 37: 113-121.

[106] Inukai, K, Funaki M, Ogihara T, Katagiri H, Kanda A, Anai M, et al. p85a gene generates three isoforms of regulatory subunit for phosphatidylinositol 3-kinase (PI 3-kinase), p50a, p55a, and p85a, with different PI 3-kinase activity elevating responses to insulin. J Biol Chem 1997; 272: 7873-7882.

[107] Pons S, Asano T, Glasheen E, Miralpeix M, Zhang Y, Fischer TL, et al. The structure and function of p55PIK reveal a new regulatory subunit for phosphatidylinositol 3-kinase. Mol Cell Biol 1995; 15: 4453-4465.

[108] Terauchi Y, Tsuji Y, Satoh S, Minoura H, Murakami K, Okuno A, etal. Increased insulin sensitivity and hypoglycaemia in mice lacking the p85α subunit of phosphoinositide 3-kinase. Nat Genet 1999; 21: 230–235.

[109] Mauvais-Jarvis F, Ueki K, Fruman DA, Hirshman MF, Sakamoto K, Goodyear LJ, etal. Reduced expression of the murine p85α subunit of phosphoinositide 3-kinase improves insulin signalling and ameliorates diabetes. J Clin Invest 2000; 109: 141–149.

[110] Ueki K, Fruman DA, Yballe CM, Fasshauer M, Klein J, Asano T, etal. Positive and negative roles of p85α and p85β regulatory subunits of phosphoinositide 3-kinase in insulin signaling. J BiolChem 2003; 278: 48453– 48466.

[111] Giorgino F, Pedrini MT, Matera L, Smith RJ. Specific increase in p85α expression in response to dexamethazone is associated with inhibition of insulin-like growth factor-I stimulated phosphatidylinositol 3-kinase activity in cultured muscle cells. J Biol Chem 1997; 272: 7455–7463.

[112] Lee YH, Giraud J, Davis RJ, White MF. C-Jun N-terminal kinase (JNK) mediates feedback inhibition of the insulin signaling cascade. J Biol Chem 2003; 278: 2896–2902.

[113] Ueki K, Yballe CM, Brachmann SM, Vicent D, Watt JM, Kahn CR, etal. Increased insulin sensitivity in mice lacking p85β subunit of phosphoinositide 3-kinase. Proc Natl Acad Sci U S A 2002; 99: 419–424.

[114] Lamia KA, Peroni OD, Kim Y-B, Rameh LE, Kahn BB, Cantley LC. Increased insulin sensitivity and reduced adiposity in phosphatidylinositol 5-phosphate 4-kinase β-/- mice. Mol Cell Biol 2004; 24: 5080–5087.

[115] Barbour LA, Shao J, Qiao L, Leitner W, Anderson M, Friedman JE, etal. Human placental growth hormone increases expression of p85 regulatory unit of phosphatidylinositol 3-kinase and triggers severe insulin resistance in skeletal muscle. Endocrinology 2004; 145: 1144 –1150.

[116] Cornier M-A, Bessesen DH, Gurevich I, Leitner JW, Draznin B. Nutritional up-regulation of p85α expression is an early molecular manifestation of insulin resistance. Diabetologia 2006; 49: 748 –754.

[117] Barbour LA, Rahman SM, Gurevich I, Leitner JW, Fisher S, Roper M, etal. Increased P85alpha is a potent negative regulator of skeletal muscle insulin signaling and induces in vivo insulin resistance associated with growth hormone excess. J BiolChem 2005; 280: 37489 –37494.

[118] Kirwan J, Varastehpour A, Jing M, Presley L, Shao J, Friedman JE, etal. Reversal of insulin resistance post-partum is linked to enhanced skeletal muscle insulin signaling. J ClinEndocrinolMetab 2004; 89: 4678–4684.

[119] Klip A, Paquet MR. Glucose transport and glucose transporters in muscle and their metabolic regulation. Diabetes Care 1990; 13: 228– 243.

[120] Randle PJ, Priestman DA, Mistry SC, Halsall A. Glucose fatty acid interactions and the regulation of glucose disposal. J Cell Biochem 1994]: 1–11.

[121] Saloranta C, Groop L. Interactions between glucose and FFA metabolism in man. Diabetes Metab Rev 1996; 12: 15–36.

[122] Boden G. Role of fatty acids in the pathogenesis of insulin resistance and NIDDM [published erratum appears in Diabetes 1997 Mar;46(3):536]. Diabetes 1997; 46: 3–10.

[123] Foley JE. Rationale and application of fatty acid oxidation inhibitors in treatment of diabetes mellitus. Diabetes Care 1992; 15: 773–784.

[124] Nurjhan N, Consoli A, Gerich J. Increased lipolysis and its consequences on gluconeogenesis in non-insulin-dependent diabetes mellitus. J Clin Invest 1992; 89: 169–175.

[125] McGarry, Banting lecture. Dysregulation of fatty acid metabolism in the etiology of type 2 diabetes. Diabetes 2001; 51: 7–18.

[126] Moller DE .New drug targets for type 2 diabetes and the metabolic syndrome. Nature (London) 2001; 414: 821–827.

[127] Dresner A, Laurent D, Marcucci M, Griffin ME, Dufour S, Cline GW, etal. Effects of free fatty acids on glucose transport and IRS-1–associated phosphatidylinositol 3-kinase activity. J Clin Invest 1999; 103: 253 –259.

[128] Newton AC. Regulation of the ABC kinases by phosphorylation: protein kinase C as a paradigm. Biochem J 2003; 370: 361–371.

[129] Samuel VT, Liu ZX, Qu XQ, Elder BD, Bilz S, Befroy D, etal. Mechanism of hepatic insulin resistance in non-alcoholic fatty liver disease. J Biol Chem 2004; 279: 32345–32353.

[130] Savage DB, Choi CS, Samuel VT, Liu ZX, Zhang DY, Wang A, etal. Reversal of diet-induced hepatic steatosis and hepatic insulin resistance by antisense oligonucleotide inhibitors of acetyl-CoA carboxylases 1 and 2. J Clin Invest 2006; 116: 817– 824.

[131] Accili D, Arden KC. FoxOs at the crossroads of cellular metabolism, differentiation, and transformation. Cell 2004; 117: 421– 426.

[132] Neschen S, Morino K, Hammond LE, Zhang DY, Liu ZX, Romanelli AJ, etal. Prevention of hepatic steatosis and hepatic insulin resistance in mitochondrial acyl-CoA: glycerol-sn-3-phosphate acyltransferase 1 knockout mice. Cell Metab 2005; 2: 55–65.

[133] Petersen KF, Dufour S, Befroy D, Lehrke M, Hendler RE, Shulman GI. Reversal of nonalcoholic hepatic steatosis, hepatic insulin resistance, and hyperglycemia by moderate weight reduction in patients with type 2 diabetes. Diabetes 2005; 54: 603– 608.

[134] Boden G, Shulman G I. Free fatty acids in obesity and type 2 diabetes: defining their role in the development of insulin resistance and beta-cell dysfunction. Eur. J. Clin. Invest.2002; 32:Suppl. 3: 14–23.

[135] Itani S I, Ruderman N B, Frank S, Boden G. Lipid induced insulin resistance in human muscle is associated with changes in diacylglycerol, protein kinase C, and Ikb-α. Diabetes 2002; 51: 2005–2011.

[136] Strack V, Stoyanov B, Bossenmaier B, Mosthaf L, Kellerer M, Haring H U. Impact of mutations at different serine residues on the tyrosine kinase activity of the insulin receptor. Biochem. Biophys. Res. Commun.1997; 239: 235–239.

[137] Michael LF, Wu Z, Cheatham RB, Puigserver P, Adelmant G, Lehman JJ,et al. Restoration of insulin-sensitive glucose transporter (GLUT4) gene expression in muscle cells by the transcriptional coactivator PGC-1. Proc Natl Acad Sci USA 2001; 98: 3820–3825.

[138] Akimoto T, Ribar TJ, Williams RS, Yan Z. Skeletal muscle adaptation in response to voluntary running in Ca2/calmodulin-dependent protein kinase IV-deficient mice. Am J Physiol Cell Physiol 2004; 287: C1311–C1319.

[139] Bergeron R, Ren JM, Cadman KS, Moore IK, Perret P, Pypaert M, etal. Chronic activation of AMP kinase results in NRF-1 activation and mitochondrial biogenesis. Am J Physiol Endocrinol Metab 2001; 281: E1340–E1346.

[140] Zong HH, Ren JM, Young LH, Pypaert M, Mu J, Birnbaum MJ, Shulman GI: AMP kinase is required for mitochondrial biogenesis in skeletal muscle in response to chronic energy deprivation. *Proc Natl Acad Sci U S A*99:15983–15987, 2002.

[141] Winder WW, Holmes BF, Rubink DS, Jensen EB, Chen M, Holloszy JO. Activation of AMP-activated protein kinase increases mitochondrial enzymes in skeletal muscle. J Appl Physiol 2000; 88: 2219 –2226.

[142] Scarpulla RC: Nuclear control of respiratory gene expression in mammalian cells. J Cell Biochem 2006; 97:673– 683.

[143] Ling C, Poulsen P, Carlsson E, Ridderstrale M, Almgren P, Wojtaszewski J, etal. Multiple environmental and genetic factors influence skeletal muscle PGC-1 alpha and PGC-1 beta gene expression in twins. J Clin Invest 2004; 114: 1518 –1526.

[144] Saltiel AR, Kahn CR. Insulin signalling and the regulation of glucose and lipid metabolism. Nature 2001; 414: 799–806.

[145] Uysal KT, Wiesbrock SM, Marino MW, Hotamisligil GS. Protection from obesity-induced insulin resistance in mice lacking TNF-alpha function. Nature 1997; 389: 610–614.

[146] Montague CT, Farooqi IS, Whitehead JP, Soos MA, Rau H, Wareham NJ et al. Congenital leptin deficiency is associated with severe early-onset obesity in humans. Nature 1997; 387: 903–908.

[147] Farooqi IS, Jebb SA, Langmack G, Lawrence E, Cheetham CH, Prentice AM et al. Effects of recombinant leptin therapy in a child with congenital leptin deficiency. N Engl J Med 1999; 341: 879–884.

[148] Stumvoll M, Häring H. Resistin and adiponectin—of mice and men. Obes Res 2002; 10: 1197–1199.

[149] Moon B, Kwan JJ, Duddy N, Sweeney G, Begum N. Resistin inhibits glucose uptake in L6 cells independently of changes in insulin signalling and GLUT4 translocation. Am J PhysiolEndocrinolMetab 2003; 285: E106–115.

[150] Pravenec M, Kazdova L, Landa V, Zidek V, Mlejnek P, Jansa P et al. Transgenic and recombinant resistin impair skeletal muscle glucose metabolism in the spontaneously hypertensive rat. J BiolChem 2003; 278: 45209–45215.

[151] Hall RK, Yamasaki T, Kucera T, Waltner-Law M, O'Brien R, Granner DK. Regulation of phosphoenolpyruvatecarboxykinase and insulin-like growth factor-binding protein-1 gene expression by insulin. J BiolChem 2000; 275: 30169 –30175.

[152] Schmoll D, Walker KS, Alessi D, Grempler R, Burchell A, Guo S, etal. Regulation of glucose-6-phosphatase gene expression by protein kinase B alpha and the forkhead transcription factor FKHR. J BiolChem 2000; 275: 36324 –36333.

[153] Wolfrum C, Besser D, Luca E, Stoffel M. Insulin regulates the activity of forkhead transcription factor Hnf-3/Foxa-2 by Akt-mediated phosphorylation and nuclear/cytosolic localization. Proc Natl Acad Sci USA 2003; 100: 11624–11629.

[154] Nakae J, Biggs WH 3rd, Kitamura T, Cavenee WK, Wright CV, Arden KC et al. Regulation of insulin action and pancreatic β-cell function by mutated alleles of the gene encoding forkhead transcription factor Foxo1. Nat Genet 2002; 32: 245–253.

[155] Zhao X, Gan L, Pan H, Kan D, Majeski M, Adam SA, et al. Multiple elements regulate nuclear/cytoplasmic shuttling of FOXO1: characterization of phosphorylation- and 14-3-3-dependent and -independent mechanisms. Biochem J 2004; 378: 839–849.

[156] Yoon JC, Puigserver P, Chen G, Donovan J, Wu Z, Rhee J et al. Control of hepatic gluconeogenesis through the transcriptional coactivator PGC-1. Nature 2001; 413: 131–138.

[157] Herzig S, Long F, Jhala US, Hedrick S, Quinn R, Bauer A, et al. CREB regulates hepatic gluconeogenesis through the co-activator PGC- 1. Nature 2001; 413: 179–183.

[158] Puigserver P, Rhee J, Donovan J, Walkey CJ, Yoon JC, Oriente F, et al. Insulin-regulated hepatic gluconeogenesis through FOXO1–PGC-1α interaction. Nature 2003; 423: 550–555.

[159] Shulman GI. Cellular mechanisms of insulin resistance. J Clin Invest 2000; 106: 171–176.

[160] Toker A, Newton AC. Cellular signaling: pivoting around PDK-1.Cell 2000; 103: 185–188.

[161] Bhattacharya S, Dey D, Roy SS. Molecular mechanisms of insulin resistance. J. Biosci. 2007; 32: 405–413.

[162] Dey D, Basu D, Roy S S, Bandyopadhyay A, Bhattacharya S. Involvement of novel PKC isoforms in FFA induced defects in insulin signalling. Mol. Cell. Endocrinol.2006; 26: 60–64.

[163] Dey D, Mukherjee M, Basu D, Datta M, Roy S S, Bandyopadhyay A, etal. Inhibition of insulin receptor gene expression and insulin signaling by fatty acid: interplay of PKC isoforms therein. Cell. Physiol. Biochem.2005; 16: 217–228.

Chapter 2

Mitochondrial Dysfunction in Insulin Insensitivity and Type 2 Diabetes and New Insights for Their Prevention and Management

Chih-Hao Wang, Kun-Ting Chi, and Yau-Huei Wei

Additional information is available at the end of the chapter

http://dx.doi.org/10.5772/52320

1. Introduction

There are two major types of diabetes mellitus. Type 1 diabetes is caused by the loss of insulin-secreting β cells of the pancreas, which leads to a deficiency of insulin in the human body. Type 2 diabetes, known as non-insulin-dependent diabetes mellitus (NIDDM), is characterized by insulin resistance of insulin-responsive tissues, such as the muscle and adipose tissues. Inability of glucose disposal in these tissues after a meal leads to the elevation of glucose level in the blood circulation of the patients. Subsequently, the long-term effect of hyperglycemia may induce inflammation and oxidative damage to other organs and result in many complications such as cardiovascular disease, blindness, amputations and renal failure [1]. Unfortunately, type 2 diabetes has high prevalence compared to type 1 diabetes in modern societies because the pathogenesis of this disease is quite complicated, multi-factorial, and is strongly associated with lifestyle, dietary habits, and environmental toxins. In light of these findings, many biomedical researchers and clinicians have made great efforts to better understand the pathophysiology of insulin resistance and to explore new avenues for the therapy of type 2 diabetes [2].

2. Mitochondrial role in the regulation of cellular metabolism

2.1. Overview of mitochondria

Mitochondria play important roles in energy metabolism, apoptosis and biosynthesis of heme and pyrimidine nucleotides because many vital biochemical reactions take place in the organelles. They are also called the powerhouse of mammalian cells because they generate a majority of ATP required by the cells. Mitochondria contain key enzymes involved in the tricarboxylic acid (TCA) cycle, β oxidation of fatty acids and the electron carriers of the respiratory chain. Metabolic intermediates generated from catabolism of carbohydrates and lipids by TCA cycle and β oxidation provide reducing equivalents (NADH and $FADH_2$), which are funneled into the electron transport chain that consists of a series of respiratory enzyme complexes I, II, III and IV. The proton gradient generated from the electron transport chain across the inner membrane is then utilized by Complex V to drive the phosphorylation of ADP to produce ATP in mitochondria to meet the energy need of the cell [3]. Mitochondrion has its own genome, mtDNA, which is a 16.6 kb circular double-stranded DNA. Mammalian mtDNA encodes 2 rRNAs, 22 tRNAs and 13 polypeptides required for the assembly of respiratory enzymes. Each mammalian cell contains several hundreds to more than a thousand of mitochondria, and each mitochondrion contains 2-10 copies of mtDNA to meet different energy needs of the cells. Most importantly, mtDNA is naked, compact, and has no efficient DNA repair systems, which renders it prone to free radical attack and oxidative damage, and thereby increases its risk of acquiring DNA mutations. More than one hundred mutations in mtDNA have been reported to be associated with human diseases [4].

2.2. Regulation of mitochondrial biogenesis

The mitochondrial biogenesis of the human cells is controlled by extracellular stimuli such as low temperature, thyroid hormone, fasting, and exercise through up-regulation of the master control, peroxisome proliferator-activated receptor gamma co-activator 1α◎(PGC-1α). PGC-1α can promote nuclear respiratory factor 1 (NRF-1) and NRF-2 to transcribe their target genes that produce many nuclear DNA-encoded mitochondrial proteins and mitochondrial transcription factor A (mtTFA), which is a key transcriptional factor for the expression of genes encoded by the mitochondrial genome. A great majority of the nuclear DNA-encoded proteins are translocated from the cytosol to mitochondria and are assembled with mtDNA-encoded proteins to form functional respiratory enzyme complexes on the inner membrane. Because mitochondrial biogenesis is a complicated process involved with the expression of genes in the two genomes, the communication between mitochondria and the nucleus is essential for the proper functioning of mitochondria under different physiological conditions [5, 6].

2.3. ROS and antioxidant enzyme system in mitochondria

Mitochondria are also the major source of intracellular reactive oxygen species (ROS). Within mitochondria, the superoxide anions ($O_2^{\cdot-}$) are produced in the reaction between O_2 and the electrons leaked out from Complex I and III of the respiratory chain. Subsequently, the $O_2^{\cdot-}$ can be converted to lipid-permeable hydrogen peroxide (H_2O_2) by the Mn-dependent superoxide dismutase (MnSOD), and further changes to more reactive hydroxyl radicals ($OH^{\cdot-}$) via Fenton reaction. There is a set of enzymatic and non-enzymatic ROS-scavenging system to protect cells from the assault by ROS. The H_2O_2 can be reduced to H_2O by catalase (CAT), glutathione peroxidase (GPx) or a group of small cysteine-containing proteins such as thioredoxins (Trx) and peroxiredoxins (Prx) [7-9]. Nevertheless, overproduction of ROS by defective mitochondria and inefficient antioxidant enzyme system may cause oxidative damage to cellular components such as DNA, especially mtDNA, proteins, and lipids of target tissues in aging and age-related diseases [10]. It has been reported that mitochondrial defects caused by mtDNA mutation or oxidative stress also play a role in insulin resistance or diabetes [11-13].

3. Mitochondrial dysfunction contributes to insulin resistance and type 2 diabetes

In the early 1990s, diabetes has been discovered to be one of the symptoms associated with some of the mitochondrial diseases such as mitochondrial encephalopathy, lactic acidosis and stroke-like episodes (MELAS) and maternally inherited diabetes and deafness (MIDD) syndrome, and patients with these syndromes frequently harbor an A to G transition at nucleotide position 3243 of mtDNA [11]. However, until recent years diabetes has been usually thought as a secondary effect of aging or age-related diseases in patients with an mtDNA mutation. Several recent studies provided the linkage between mitochondrial dysfunction or defects in mitochondrial biogenesis and the pathogenesis of insulin resistance or type 2 diabetes [12-22]. These studies showed that the tissues of mice and human subjects with insulin insensitivity or type 2 diabetes displayed lower expression levels of the genes encoding subunits constituting respiratory enzymes, decrease in the activities of respiratory enzyme complexes, decreased expression of genes involved in mitochondrial biogenesis, mutation or deletion of mtDNA, decrease in the bioenergetic capacity, or defects in β oxidation of fatty acids. In summary, impairment in the mitochondrial OXPHOS function was a common observation in insulin-responsive muscle and adipose tissues of diabetic mice or patients. Most importantly, the amplitude of the decline of mitochondrial function was found to be related to the severity of diabetic symptoms and insulin resistance. These findings support the notion that mitochondrial dysfunction is one of the major etiological factors for insulin resistance and type 2 diabetes.

4. Mitochondrial DNA alteration causes insulin resistance and type 2 diabetes

In order to prove the concept that mitochondrial dysfunction is involved in the development of insulin resistance, chemical treatments and genetic manipulation have been used to impair mitochondria by alteration of the quantity or quality of mtDNA. Park and Lee [23] observed a decrease of insulin sensitivity and impaired activation of insulin signaling in mtDNA-depleted muscle cells after chronic treatment with a low dose of ethidium bromide (EtBr). Moreover, repletion of mtDNA by removal of EtBr revealed that the defects in insulin response could be recovered [23]. Besides, Pravenec et al. [24] demonstrated that sequence variations in mtDNA could directly lead to metabolic dysregulation that includes glucose intolerance and insulin insensitivity in the conplastic strains of rats. In addition, defects in oxidative phosphorylation caused by treatment of oligomycin A, an inhibitor of Complex V, also resulted in a decline of insulin-stimulated glucose uptake and inactivation of Akt and IRS-1 in the insulin signaling pathway in murine C2C12 myotube cells [25]. The above two lines of experiments clearly demonstrated a relationship between mtDNA alteration-induced mitochondrial dysfunction and insulin insensitivity.

4.1. Overproduction of ROS impairs insulin signaling

Excess ROS production from defective mitochondria has been considered as one of the possible unifying factors leading to insulin resistance. Increased concentration of glucose in the culture medium was found to significantly increase the ROS level and led to insulin resistance in mouse adipocytes and rat primary adipocytes and this effect could be prevented by pre-treatment of the adipocytes with the antioxidant N-acetylcysteine [26, 27]. After administration with ROS-scavenging enzymes, the insulin sensitivity of muscle cells was found to be improved in diabetic mice [28]. Recent studies also demonstrated that the amount of superoxide anions generated by mitochondria was increased in four different animal models of insulin resistance. Furthermore, it was reported that by addition of mitochondria-targeting superoxide dismutase mimetics to decrease the level of ROS could alleviate insulin resistance in the insulin-insensitive animals [29]. The mechanisms underlying the disruption of insulin signaling by overproduction of ROS have been extensively investigated in the past decade. It was demonstrated that, at a certain concentration range, ROS could cause an increase in the activity of multiple stress-sensitive serine/threonine kinases such as p38 MAPK, JNK, ERK, and NFκB and elicit subsequent phosphorylation of IRS1 and downstream signaling proteins, which may culminate in the compromise of insulin sensitivity [30].

4.2. Accumulation of fatty acids impairs insulin signaling

It is thought that impaired lipid metabolism resulted from defects in β oxidation of fatty acids is involved in the disturbance of insulin signaling. Accumulation of intracellular lipids by the decreased activities of carnitine palmitoyl transferase (CPT), which transports long-chain fatty acids into mitochondria, and long-chain acyl-CoA dehydrogenase (LCAD), an enzyme involved in β oxidation of fatty acids, led to insulin resistance in insulin-targeting cells [31]. It has been demonstrated that an accumulation of fatty acid metabolites, such as diacylglycerol, fatty acyl-CoA and ceramides, could induce activation of serine/threonine protein kinases such as PKCβ and PKCδ in human tissues [32]. In turn, the activation of PKCs phosphorylates IRS-1 and IRS-2 on serine/threonine residues to inhibit their enzymatic function and activate the downstream PI3K/Akt signaling pathway. The above-mentioned observations suggest that ROS overproduction and lipid accumulation elicited by mitochondrial dysfunction may play a role in the dysregulation of insulin signaling pathway, which then leads to an attenuation of insulin response in affected tissues.

4.3. Loss of mild stress-induced AMPKα activation may lead to insulin resistance

Low concentration of ROS is a normal byproduct of cellular functions and is known as the secondary messenger in the regulation of intracellular signaling to adapt to the extracellular environment. But prolong exposure to oxidative environment may lead to oxidative damage to tissue cells and development of diseases. Recent studies revealed that activation of AMPK by low dose of ROS is involved in the activation of antioxidant defense system, the influx of glycolysis and lipid metabolism [33, 34]. The activation of the downstream targets of AMPK, including GLUT4, PFK2, and ACC, enhances the β oxidation of fatty acids and the basal and insulin-stimulated glucose uptake. Besides, activated AMPK can directly phosphorylate the forkhead transcription factor 3a (FOXO3a) to promote its nuclear translocation and formation of a transcription complex, which in turn up-regulates the expression of thioredoxin and peroxiredoxin [35]. It has been shown that activation of the AMPK-FOXO3a pathway via AICAR or metformin, an antidiabetic drug, can decrease the intracellular ROS level to improve insulin sensitivity in epithelial cells [35, 36]. These findings indicate that mild oxidative stress-elicited activation of AMPK and FOXO3a may safeguard glucose homeostatsis and redox status in healthy subjects. Taken together, the decrease in the sensitivity and capacity of the response to low-level oxidative stress may play a role in insulin insensitivity and type 2 diabetes.

5. The roles of sirtuins in the maintenance of glucose homeostasis and their defects in insulin resistance and type 2 diabetes

5.1. Introduction of sirtuins

Sirtuins are a highly conserved family of proteins that exhibit NAD+-dependent protein deacetylase and ADP-ribosyltransferase activities. Mammals contain seven sirtuins that are confined in different subcellular compartments and regulate diverse functions, such as intermediary metabolism, energy homeostasis, and oxidative stress. SIRT1, SIRT6 and SIRT7 are primarily localized to the nucleus, SIRT2 is a cytosolic protein, and SIRT3, SIRT4 and SIRT5 are all located in mitochondria. Sirtuins can regulate the function of enzymes or transcription factors by deacetylation of target proteins to cope with nutrient deprivation or metabolic stress. In addition to getting involved in the regulation of aging and longevity, some of the sirtuins have emerged as important regulators of glucose homeostasis. Sirtuins may regulate the activities of some of the regulatory proteins or enzymes involved in the insulin-mediated signaling pathways and regulation of mitochondrial function, which in turn determine the sensitivity and acuity of biochemical response to high blood glucose of the muscle and other peripheral tissues in the human body.

5.2. SIRT1 and type 2 diabetes

Accumulating evidence has established that SIRT1 contributes to the pathogenesis of type 2 diabetes through its effect on oxidative metabolism of the liver, skeletal muscle, adipose tissue, and pancreatic β cells, which indicate that mammalian sirtuins play an essential role in the pathogenesis of diabetes and aging-associated metabolic diseases [37]. Increasing evidence has suggested that SIRT1 provides overall protection against type 2 diabetes. SIRT1-overexpressing transgenic mice showed significant protection from the adverse effects of high-fat diet, including hepatic inflammation and impaired insulin sensitivity [38, 39]. In addition, administration of resveratrol and SIRT1-activating compounds was found to improve glucose homeostasis and insulin sensitivity in diet-induced and genetically-predisposed type 2 diabetic mice [40, 41]. It has been reported that certain sequence variations of the SIRT1 gene is strongly associated with type 2 diabetes and obesity in a Dutch population [42]. Taken together, these findings suggest that SIRT1 plays a role in the pathogenesis of type 2 diabetes and its manipulation has great potential in the prevention and treatment of type 2 diabetes in animals and the human.

5.3. SIRT3 and type 2 diabetes

In recent years, it has become increasingly clear that reversible lysine acetylation is an important posttranslational modification of mitochondrial proteins for the regulation of their proper function [43]. A number of proteomics studies have revealed that many key metabolic enzymes are acetylated in mitochondria and that their enzymatic activities are regulated by changes in acetylation in response to environmental stimuli [44]. Among seven members of the sirtuin family, three sirtuins (SIRT3, SIRT4 and SIRT5) are primarily located and exert functions in mitochondria. It is a remarkable fact that SIRT3 is the most important one regarding the regulation of mitochondrial function because it is responsible for deacetylation of the majority of mitochondrial proteins [45]. SIRT3 has been shown to control multiple key metabolic pathways through its deacetylase activity in response to nutrient deprivation. For example, SIRT3 can deacetylate and activate the mitochondrial enzyme acetyl-CoA synthetase 2 (AceCS2). The oxidation of acetate is required for the generation of ATP and heat under low-glucose or ketogenic condition [46, 47]. Besides, SIRT3 has been shown to deacetylate long-chain acyl-CoA dehydrogenase (LCAD) during fasting and thereby promotes β-oxidation of fatty acids in the liver mitochondria [48]. Recently, some studies provide critical insights into the connection between SIRT3 and the pathogenesis of type 2 diabetes and metabolic syndrome. It has been demonstrated that the SIRT3 expression in skeletal muscle is reduced in animal models of type 1 and type 2 diabetes and that results in the decrease of mitochondrial bioenergetic function and over-production of ROS, which in turn disturbs insulin signaling pathway leading to insulin insensitivity [49]. These findings suggest that decreased SIRT3 expression and activity could contribute to the metabolic abnormalities in skeletal muscle and pathogenesis of diabetes mellitus. On the other hand, mitochondrial dysfunction induced by SIRT3 deficiency in pancreatic β cells might contribute to the defects in insulin secretion upon stimulation with various insulin secretagogues [50]. In a recent study, Hirschey and coworkers [51] showed that loss of SIRT3 and resultant mitochondrial protein hyperacetylation contribute to obesity, hyperlipidemia, insulin resistance, and steatohepatitis. In addition, they identified a single nucleotide polymorphism in the human SIRT3 gene, which causes a loss of the enzyme activity of SIRT3 and is highly associated with the prevalence of metabolic syndrome. Abundant evidence has been accumulated to show the importance of reversible acetylation/deacetylation of mitochondrial proteins through the action of SIRT3 and its potential role in the development of insulin resistance and metabolic disorders. Thus, site-specific acetylation of mitochondrial proteins and the development of new SIRT3-targeted drugs may serve as therapeutic tools to regain normal cellular redox status and energy homeostasis in the patients with diabetes and insulin resistance, as well as some of the mitochondrial diseases.

6. Defects in the secretion or function of adipokines as an important contributor to insulin resistance or type 2 diabetes

6.1. Regulation of glucose homeostasis by adipocyte-derived adipokines

The adipose tissue has traditionally been considered as the site for lipid storage in the human body. In recent years, a growing number of studies have revealed that adipose tissues can perform endocrine function in secreting several adipokines, which can modulate the intermediary metabolism and glucose homeostasis in the peripheral tissues. Adipocyte-derived adipokines can be divided into two groups according to their action in the regulation of glucose metabolism in the mammals. One group is called as "anti-hyperglycemic adipokines", which include leptin, adiponectin, omentin, and visfatin. They enhance insulin sensitivity in the peripheral tissues to increase glucose utilization and decrease the glucose level in blood circulation. Another group of adipokines is termed "pro-hyperglycemic adipokines" or "pro-inflammatory adipokines", which include resistin, TNF-α, and RBP4 since they tend to result in an increase of blood glucose and systemic inflammation. The imbalance of these two groups of adipokines in blood has been frequently observed in patients with insulin resistance [52, 53].

6.2. Adiponectin improves insulin sensitivity

Adiponectin has been considered the most important adipokine due to its higher concentration in blood than the others and a decrease in its level is highly correlated with type 2 diabetes [54]. Several clinical studies demonstrated that the plasma level of adiponectin in obese subjects or patients with type 2 diabetes was significantly lower compared with those of normal subjects, and that blood glucose was higher and insulin sensitivity was largely decreased in mice with adiponectin deficiency [55, 56]. Besides, administration or overexpression of adiponectin in mice can enhance insulin sensitivity and glucose utilization to ameliorate the symptoms of insulin resistance [57-59]. This indicates that dysregulation of secretion of adipokines from adipose tissues is an important contributor for the pathogenesis of type 2 diabetes. Thus, adiponectin has become the most attractive adipokine and its function has been gradually unraveled. The underlying mechanism of adiponectin in improvement of insulin sensitivity and fatty acid β oxidation in skeletal muscle has been demonstrated by Yamauchi and his colleagues [60]. They showed that the phosphorylation and activation of AMPK is stimulated when adiponectin binds to adiponectin receptor 1 (AdipoR1), which is a seven-transmembrane receptor specifically expressed in the skeletal muscle. In turn, AMPK can induce GLUT4 translocation to the plasma membrane for the increase of glucose uptake. On the other hand, the phosphorylated AMPK also activates acetyl-CoA carboxylase to increase the oxidation of fatty acids through independent pathways.

6.3. Bi-directional regulation of the biogenesis and function of mitochondria by adiponectin

Because the decrease of adiponectin expression and the biogenesis and function of mitochondria have been observed concurrently in adipose tissues of diabetic mice and human subjects [22], some researchers made an effort to elucidate the connection between these two cellular events. Koh and coworkers demonstrated that the biogenesis and function of mitochondria are important for the maintenance of the adiponectin level in adipocytes [61]. They found that adiponectin expression and the mitochondrial content in adipose tissues were both reduced in obese mice, and these changes could be reversed by the administration of rosiglitazone, a mainstay drug used for treatment of diabetes. Induction of mitochondrial biogenesis via adenoviral overexpression of nuclear respiratory factor-1 (NRF-1) in cultured adipocytes increased the expression of adiponectin. Besides, they found that inhibition of mitochondrial function by a respiratory inhibitor or uncoupler decreased the level of adiponectin in plasma through activation of ROS-dependent kinase such as JNK. This finding suggests that mitochondrial function is linked to adiponectin synthesis in adipocytes, and explain the observation that mitochondrial dysfunction is associated with the defects of secretion and function of adiponectin, which may lead to systemic insulin resistance in obesity and type 2 diabetes.

On the other hand, a recent study also showed that adiponectin can increase the activity of PGC-1α and enhance the biogenesis and respiratory function of mitochondria in muscle cells [62]. The study provided evidence that adiponectin induces extracellular Ca2+ influx through binding to AdipoR1, which is essential for subsequent activation of Ca2+/calmodulin-dependent protein kinase kinase β (CaMKKβ), AMPK and SIRT1. Adiponectin ultimately causes an increase in the expression of PGC-1α by CaMK, a downstream target of CaMKK, and increase in the activity of PGC-1α by deacetylation of SIRT1. These events may in turn elevate the biogenesis and function of mitochondria in muscle cells. This new insight into the up-regulation of mitochondrial function by adiponectin signaling accounts for the long-term effect of adiponectin on the gene expression and provides a biochemical mechanism by which adiponectin improves insulin sensitivity of the muscle.

7. Environmental toxins in mitochondrial dysfunction and insulin insensitivity

Because of the increasing prevalence of type 2 diabetes and metabolic syndrome in westernized and industrialized countries, type 2 diabetes is thought as an "epidemic disease". With this consideration in mind, scientists conjectured that one of the causative factors for type 2 diabetes is probably related to the environmental impact of industrialization. A growing body of evidence has indicated that the cause of type 2 diabetes and metabolic syndrome is strongly associated with some environmental pollutants and mitochondrial toxins. Persistent organic pollutants (POPs), which are organic compounds present in many herbicides, insecticides, rodenticides, industrial products and wastes, are resistant to photolytic degradation and other chemical or biological destruction processes. Owning to these chemical characteristics, POPs can be present for a long time in our environment and are accumulated in the human body. Thus, POPs are potential environmental risk factors that may affect the human health [63].

7.1. POPs cause insulin insensitivity

By analysis of the results from National Health and Nutrition Examination Survey in 1999-2000, Lee and colleagues found that the prevalence rate of type 2 diabetes was highly correlated with the serum concentration of POPs of the American population [64, 65]. Contamination of POPs in the human diets might be a contributor to the pathogenesis of metabolic diseases including the diabetes. For example, atrazine (ATZ, 2-chloro-4-ethylamine-6-isopropylamino-S-triazine), one of the herbicides, has been extensively used in the corn fields of the United States since the early 1960s. Interestingly, the time and areas of ATZ usage are matched with the timing of increase in the incidence of obesity and other metabolic syndromes [66, 67]. In addition, long-term exposure of Australian outdoor workers to pesticides was found to associate with the disturbance of glucose homeostasis, including higher blood glucose and insulin resistance in these subjects [68]. It was demonstrated that mice fed with a high-fat diet with POPs-contaminated farmed salmon fillet would exaggerate insulin resistance, visceral obesity, and glucose intolerance [69]. However, remission of the above symptoms was observed in the mice fed with farmed salmon fillet containing low level of POPs [69]. Furthermore, the mortality rate of diabetes was positively correlated with the concentration of exposed pesticides [70]. In order to establish a cause and effect relationship in humans, Lee et al. [71, 72] approached the Nested case control study to measure the serum levels of POPs in certain population before the development of metabolic disease phenotypes. The results revealed that increased serum levels of some POPs were highly associated with the incidence of adiposity, dyslipidemia, and insulin resistance in a healthy population. This finding indicates that exposure to low dose of POP may contribute to excess adiposity and other features of metabolic syndrome.

7.2. Impairment of mitochondrial dysfunction by POPs

Several studies have demonstrated that environmental toxins could cause oxidative damage to mitochondria, the organelles are most susceptible to extrinsic toxins including POPs. It has been shown that 2,3,7,8-tetrachlorodibenzo-p-dioxin (TCDD), one of the POPs, caused a loss of mitochondrial membrane potential and increase of ROS production in mammalian cells. The oxygen consumption rate was increased, due to the uncoupling of respiration, and the intracellular ATP content and ADP/O ratio were decreased due to defects in F_oF_1-ATPase in the affected tissues of TCDD-treated mice [73]. Recently, some animal studies revealed that POPs could result in insulin insensitivity by impairment of mitochondrial function. It was found that chronic exposure to POPs led to mitochondrial dysfunction, morphological disruption of mitochondria, decreased activities of respiratory enzymes and decreased oxygen consumption rate in the liver and skeletal muscle of mice [74]. Besides, POPs were found to down-regulate the expression of leptin in adipose tissues and inactivated insulin signaling pathway in the skeletal muscle [75]. These subsequently resulted in insulin resistance, hyperlipidemia, abdominal obesity, and hepatosteatosis in mice and the severity of these symptoms was more pronounced in the mice fed on high-fat diets. Moreover, mitochondria could be the primary organelles involved in the initiation of inflammation, leading to chronic damage in the affected cells or organs. High level of polychlorinated biphenyls (PCBs) could promote accumulation of lipids and expression of pro-inflammatory adipokines, which decreased the expression of adiponectin and the insulin-stimulated glucose uptake in the adipose tissue, leading to systemic obesity and obesity-associated atherosclerosis [76]. Taken the findings from the epidemiological survey and the above observations together, we suggest that the mitochondrial dysfunction resulted from environmental pollutants or toxins play a role in the pathogenesis and prevalence of type 2 diabetes and insulin resistance.

8. Improvement of the biogenesis and function of mitochondria by exercise and pharmaceutical agents for treatment of insulin resistance and type 2 diabetes

In light of the observations of mitochondrial impairment and increased oxidative stress in the patients with type 2 diabetes, it has been thought that an increase of mitochondrial function or scavengers of ROS may be effective therapies for these patients. Biomedical researchers and clinicians have made considerable efforts in looking for possible ways to improve insulin sensitivity in target tissues through up-regulation of the mitochondrial function or antioxidant defense system. In this section, we provide experimental evidence to demonstrate increase of mitochondrial function and enhancement of the antioxidant defense by exercise, treatment of natural products or pharmaceutical agents that can effectively ameliorate the symptoms of insulin resistance and type 2 diabetes.

8.1. Anti-diabetic drugs

Clinically, the thiazolidinediones (TZDs) have been commonly used to treat patients with type 2 diabetes by increasing insulin sensitivity of the muscle and adipose tissues. These drugs include pioglitazone, rosiglitazone, and troglitazone, which belong to the group of PPARγ agonists and can up-regulate the expression of PGC-1α, a master control of mitochondrial biogenesis, and a set of genes involved in the regulation of oxidative metabolism [77]. Recent studies revealed that these drugs not only increase insulin sensitivity of cells, but also significantly improve the mitochondrial biogenesis, function and morphology *in vitro* and *in vivo* [78, 79]. New insights in improving mitochondrial function by these anti-diabetic drugs further substantiate the idea that manipulation of mitochondrial gene expression is a feasible therapy for the patients with insulin insensitivity or type 2 diabetes.

8.2. Regular exercise

It is worth mentioning that mitochondrial biogenesis can be up-regulated by regular exercise through the activation of PGC-1α and its downstream targets including mtTFA and nuclear respiratory factors NRF1 and NRF2 [80, 81], which regulate the expression of a number of polypeptides constituting the respiratory enzyme complexes. These molecular events culminate in the increase of the bioenergetic function of mitochondria and thereby improve the insulin sensitivity of the animals or human subjects doing regular exercise [82]. In light of these laboratory findings and the documentation that exercise can alleviate the symptoms of patients with type 2 diabetes [83], we suggest that the increase of the biogenesis and function of mitochondria is one of the key underlying mechanisms by which exercise improves the insulin sensitivity of patients with type 2 diabetes.

8.3. Natural products and chemicals

Resveratrol (3,5,4'-trihydroxystilbene), a polyphenol and a well-known antioxidant, has been demonstrated to be able to promote mitochondrial biogenesis and fatty acid β oxidation as well as insulin sensitivity in a mouse model [84]. Resveratrol treatment was found to lead to the decrease of PGC-1α acetylation through activation of SIRT1 and thereby increased the activity of PGC-1α. In turn, an array of oxidative metabolism-related genes was up-regulated and mitochondrial OXPHOS was also elevated in the muscle tissues of the mice that had been treated with resveratrol. Moreover, resveratrol increased insulin sensitivity in the muscle and protected mice from obesity or insulin resistance when fed on a high-fat diet [40]. Additionally, epigallocatechin-3-gallate (EGCG), which is the most effective and abundant catechin in green tea, has been reported to have the antioxidant, anti-obesity and anti-cancer activities [85]. Several studies on cultured adipocytes and animal models demonstrated that EGCG decreased intracellular levels of ROS and inhibited extracellular signal-related kinases (ERK) activation. Moreover, EGCG was found to activate the AMPK to elevate mitochondrial function and β-oxidation of fatty acids to decrease the accumulation of lipids [86]. All of these downstream effects of EGCG would be of great use to improve insulin sensitivity of the target tissue cells.

On the other hand, attention should be paid to the therapeutic potential of pyruvate in the treatment of diabetes. Pyruvate, an intermediate located at the key position of glucose metabolism, has been involved in anaerobic glycolysis and aerobic respiration. Some beneficial effects were reported about the administration of pyruvate to patients harboring with A3243 or A8344G mutation of mtDNA [87]. Pyruvate can not only improve the intracellular redox status by elimination of hydrogen peroxide via non-enzymatic reaction, but also increases ATP production by oxidation of NADH to NAD^+ by lactate dehydrogenease (LDH). The high level of NAD^+ may also enhance the activity of SIRT3, an NAD^+-dependent deacetylase. In addition, it was found that through the inhibition of TNFα production and NFκB signaling pathways pyruvate could ameliorate the inflammatory symptom of insulin resistance [88].

8.4. Increase of antioxidant defense

Treatment of lipoic acid, an antioxidant, could not only decrease the intracellular ROS but also enhance insulin-stimulated glucose utilization in skeletal muscle of diabetic animals with insulin resistance. Yaworsky et al. [89] demonstrated that lipoic acid significantly increased insulin-stimulated glucose uptake of adipocytes through rapid translocation of Glut1 and Glut4 to the plasma membrane *via* the activation of insulin signaling pathway, which includes an increase in tyrosine phosphorylation of IR and IRS-1 as well as activation of PI3K and Akt. In addition to its antioxidant activity, lipoic acid was found to significantly increase mitochondrial biogenesis and function, including oxygen consumption rate and β-oxidation of fatty acids in adipocytes [90]. All of these effects of lipoic acid were enhanced by co-treatment of cells with acetyl L-carnitine (ALCAR), another mitochondrial nutrient [91]. These findings suggest that lipoic acid improves insulin sensitivity of adipocytes through its ability to elevate the antioxidant capacity and to enhance mitochondrial function. In addition, several studies have demonstrated that increasing antioxidant capacities by addition of cell- permeabilized MnSOD [29, 30] or overexpression of catalase [92, 93] and GPx3 [94] to reduce intracellular ROS could improve insulin sensitivity in cultured cells or mice. Taken together, the above-mentioned observations clearly indicate that therapeutic agents targeting to mitochondria or antioxidant defense system could ameliorate the symptoms or insulin insensitivity in cultured cells and animals, and perhaps also in the patients. These findings also support the notion that mitochondrial function is essential for the maintenance of insulin sensitivity and glucose homeostasis in the human body.

9. Concluding remarks

This chapter has provided an overview of recent advances in the understanding of mitochondrial role in the insulin insensitivity and type 2 diabetes, including the clinical observations and possible mechanisms of the insulin insensitivity induced by mitochondrial dysfunction in the insulin-responsive tissues. Mitochondrial defects resulted from inheritable A3243G or A8344G mutation of mtDNA or environmental pollutants and toxins or dysregulated acetylation status of metabolic enzymes may lead to an overproduction of intracellular ROS and lipids. These events culminate in the inactivation of the insulin signaling pathway and result in insulin insensitivity in muscle and adipocytes. Improvement of insulin sensitivity and glucose homeostasis may be achieved by the strategy to up-regulate mitochondrial biogenesis, function and antioxidant defense through exercise, therapeutic agents, and dietary supplement of antioxidants or natural products

(Figure 1). These recent advances not only provide novel information for us to better understand the connection between mitochondrial dysfunction and metabolic diseases but also lead us to a new avenue in the prevention and treatment of type 2 diabetes or metabolic syndrome by the mitochondria-targeting medicine.

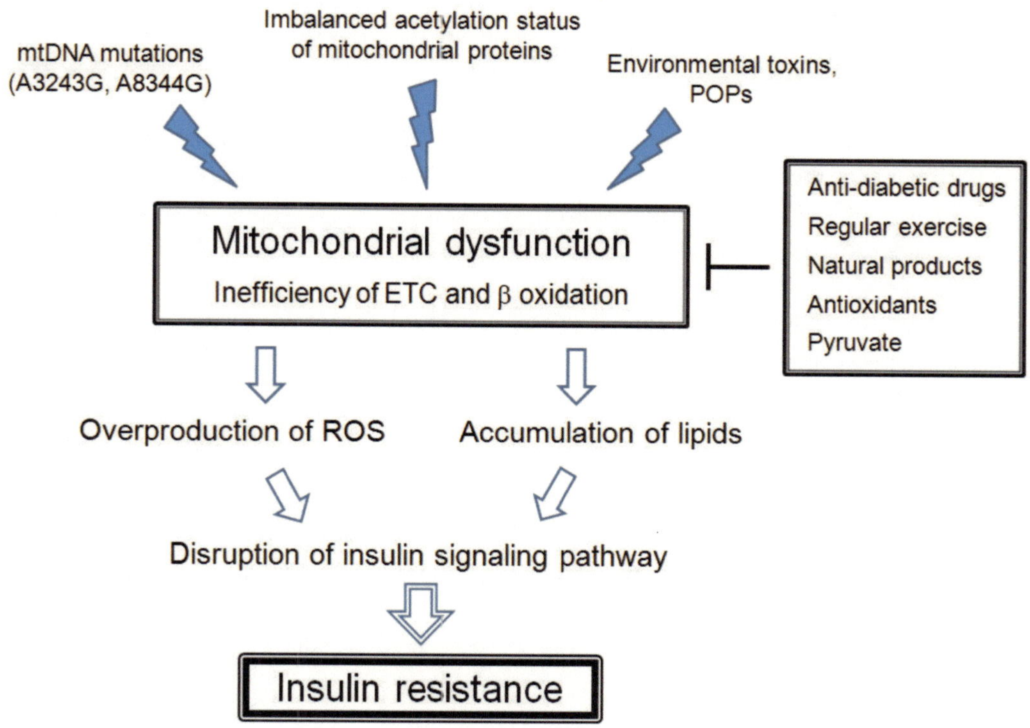

Figure 1. The scheme illustrating the role of mitochondria in the pathogenesis and therapeutic target of insulin resistance

Author details

Chih-Hao Wang and Kun-Ting Chi

Institute of Biochemistry and Molecular Biology, National Yang-Ming University, Taipei 112, Taiwan

Yau-Huei Wei*

Institute of Biochemistry and Molecular Biology, National Yang-Ming University, Taipei 112, Taiwan

Department of Medicine, Mackay Medical College, Sanjhih, New Taipei City 252, Taiwan

* Corresponding Author

Acknowledgement

We would like to thank the National Science Council of Taiwan for a research grant (NSC101-2321-B-010-015) and the long-term support of the studies on mitochondrial dysfunction in the pathogenesis of insulin insensitivity and type 2 diabetes.

10. References

[1] Rother KI (2007) Diabetes Treatment--Bridging the Divide. N. Engl. J. Med. 356: 1499-1501.

[2] Wild S, Roglic G, Green A, Sicree R, King H (2004) Global Prevalence of Diabetes: Estimates for the Year 2000 and Projections for 2030. Diabetes Care 27: 1047-1053.

[3] Wallace DC (2005) A Mitochondrial Paradigm of Metabolic and Degenerative Diseases, Aging, and Cancer: a Dawn for Evolutionary Medicine. Annu. Rev. Genet. 39: 359-407.

[4] Wiesner RJ, Rüegg JC, Morano I (1992) Counting Target Molecules by Exponential Polymerase Chain Reaction: Copy Number of Mitochondrial DNA in Rat Tissues. Biochem. Biophys. Res. Commun. 183: 553-559.

[5] Wu Z, Puigserver P, Andersson U, Zhang C, Adelmant G, Mootha V, Troy A, Cinti S, Lowell B, Scarpulla RC, Spiegelman BM (1999) Mechanisms Controlling Mitochondrial Biogenesis and Respiration through the Thermogenic Coactivator PGC-1. Cell 98: 115-124.

[6] St-Pierre J, Lin J, Krauss S, Tarr PT, Yang R, Newgard CB, Spiegelman BM (2003) Bioenergetic Analysis of Peroxisome Proliferator-Activated Receptor Gamma Coactivators 1α and 1β (PGC-1α and PGC-1β) in Muscle Cells. J. Biol. Chem. 278: 26597-26603.

[7] Valko M, Leibfritz D, Moncol J, Cronin MT, Mazur M, Telser J (2007) Free Radicals and Antioxidants in Normal Physiological Functions and Human Disease. Int. J. Biochem. Cell Biol. 39: 44-84.

[8] Cadenas E, Davies KJ (2000) Mitochondrial Free Radical Generation, Oxidative Stress, and Aging. Free Radic. Biol. Med. 29: 222-230

[9] Balaban RS, Nemoto S, Finkel T (2005) Mitochondria, Oxidants, and Aging. Cell 120: 483-495.

[10] Turrens JF (2003) Mitochondrial Formation of Reactive Oxygen Species. J. Physiol. 552: 335-344

[11] van den Ouweland JM, Lemkes HH, Ruitenbeek W, Sandkuijl LA, de Vijlder MF, Struyvenberg PA, van de Kamp JJ, Maassen JA (1992) Mutation in Mitochondrial tRNA(Leu)(UUR) Gene in a Large Pedigree with Maternally Transmitted Type II Diabetes Mellitus and Deafness. Nat. Genet.1: 368-371.

[12] Mootha VK, Lindgren CM, Eriksson KF, Subramanian A, Sihag S, Lehar J, Puigserver P, Carlsson E, Ridderstråle M, Laurila E, Houstis N, Daly MJ, Patterson N, Mesirov JP,

Golub TR, Tamayo P, Spiegelman B, Lander ES, Hirschhorn JN, Altshuler D, Groop LC (2003) PGC-1alpha-Responsive Genes Involved in Oxidative Phosphorylation are Coordinately Downregulated in Human Diabetes. Nat. Genet. 34: 267-273.

[13] Kelley DE, He J, Menshikova EV, Ritov VB (2002) Dysfunction of Mitochondria in Human Skeletal Muscle in Type 2 Diabetes. Diabetes 51: 2944-2950.

[14] Patti ME, Butte AJ, Crunkhorn S, Cusi K, Berria R, Kashyap S, Miyazaki Y, Kohane I, Costello M, Saccone R, Landaker EJ, Goldfine AB, Mun E, DeFronzo R, Finlayson J, Kahn CR, Mandarino LJ (2003) Coordinated Reduction of Genes of Oxidative Metabolism in Humans with Insulin Resistance and Diabetes: Potential Role of PGC1 and NRF1. Proc. Natl. Acad. Sci. USA 100: 8466-8471.

[15] Pagel-Langenickel I, Bao J, Joseph JJ, Schwartz DR, Mantell BS, Xu X, Raghavachari N, Sack MN (2008) PGC-1alpha Integrates Insulin Signaling, Mitochondrial Regulation, and Bioenergetic Function in Skeletal Muscle. J. Biol. Chem. 283: 22464-22472.

[16] Maassen JA, Jahangir Tafrechi RS, Janssen GM, Raap AK, Lemkes HH, 't Hart LM (2006) New Insights in the Molecular Pathogenesis of the Maternally Inherited Diabetes and Deafness Syndrome. Endocrinol. Metab. Clin. North Am. 35: 385-396.

[17] Liang P, Hughes V, Fukagawa NK (1997) Increased Prevalence of Mitochondrial DNA Deletions in Skeletal Muscle of Older Individuals with Impaired Glucose Tolerance: Possible Marker of Glycemic Stress. Diabetes 46: 920-923.

[18] Scheuermann-Freestone M, Madsen PL, Manners D, Blamire AM, Buckingham RE, Styles P, Radda GK, Neubauer S, Clarke K (2003) Abnormal Cardiac and Skeletal Muscle Energy Metabolism in Patients with Type 2 Diabetes. Circulation 107: 3040-3046.

[19] Mogensen M, Sahlin K, Fernström M, Glintborg D, Vind BF, Beck-Nielsen H, Højlund K (2007) Mitochondrial Respiration is Decreased in Skeletal Muscle of Patients with Type 2 Diabetes. Diabetes 56: 1592-1599.

[20] Petersen KF, Dufour S, Befroy D, Garcia R, Shulman GI (2004) Impaired Mitochondrial Activity in the Insulin-Resistant Offspring of Patients with Type 2 Diabetes. N. Engl. J. Med. 350: 664-671.

[21] Gaster M, Rustan AC, Aas V, Beck-Nielsen H (2004) Reduced Lipid Oxidation in Skeletal Muscle from Type 2 Diabetic Subjects May be of Genetic Origin: Evidence from Cultured Myotubes. Diabetes 53: 542-548

[22] Choo HJ, Kim JH, Kwon OB, Lee CS, Mun JY, Han SS, Yoon YS, Yoon G, Choi KM, Ko YG (2006) Mitochondria are Impaired in the Adipocytes of Type 2 Diabetic Mice. Diabetologia 49: 784-791.

[23] Park SY, Lee W (2007) The Depletion of Cellular Mitochondrial DNA Causes Insulin Resistance through the Alteration of Insulin Receptor Substrate-1 in Rat Myocytes. Diabetes Res. Clin. Pract. 77 Suppl 1: S165-S171.

[24] Pravenec M, Hyakukoku M, Houstek J, Zidek V, Landa V, Mlejnek P, Miksik I, Dudová-Mothejzikova K, Pecina P, Vrbacky M, Drahota Z, Vojtiskova A, Mracek T, Kazdova L, Oliyarnyk O, Wang J, Ho C, Qi N, Sugimoto K, Kurtz T (2007) Direct Linkage of

Mitochondrial Genome Variation to Risk Factors for Type 2 Diabetes in Conplastic Strains. Genome Res. 17: 1319-1326

[25] Lim JH, Lee JI, Suh YH, Kim W, Song JH, Jung MH (2006) Mitochondrial Dysfunction Induces Aberrant Insulin Signalling and Glucose Utilisation in Murine C2C12 Myotube Cells. Diabetologia 49: 1924-1936.

[26] Talior I, Yarkoni M, Bashan N, Eldar-Finkelman H (2003) Increased Glucose Uptake Promotes Oxidative Stress and PKC-delta Activation in Adipocytes of Obese, Insulin Resistant Mice. Am. J. Physiol. Endocrinol. Metab. 285: E295-E302.

[27] Lu B, Ennis D, Lai R, Bogdanovic E, Nikolov R, Salamon L, Fantus C, Le-Tien H, Fantus IG (2001) Enhanced Sensitivity of Insulin-Resistant Adipocytes to Vanadate is Associated with Oxidative Stress and Decreased Reduction of Vanadate (+5) to Vanadyl (+4). J. Biol. Chem. 276: 35589-35598.

[28] Houstis N, Rosen ED, Lander ES (2006) Reactive Oxygen Species Have a Causal Role in Multiple Forms of Insulin Resistance. Nature 440: 944-948.

[29] Hoehn KL, Salmon AB, Hohnen-Behrens C, Turner N, Hoy AJ, Maghzal GJ, Stocker R, Van Remmen H, Kraegen EW, Cooney GJ, Richardson AR, James DE (2009) Insulin Resistance is a Cellular Antioxidant Defense Mechanism. Proc. Natl. Acad. Sci. USA 106: 17787-17792.

[30] Erol A (2007) Insulin Resistance is an Evolutionarily Conserved Physiological Mechanism at the Cellular Level for Protection against Increased Oxidative Stress. BioEssays 29: 811-818.

[31] Zhang D, Liu ZX, Choi CS, Tian L, Kibbey R, Dong J, Cline GW, Wood PA, Shulman GI (2007) Mitochondrial Dysfunction due to Long-Chain Acyl-CoA Dehydrogenase Deficiency Causes Hepatic Steatosis and Hepatic Insulin Resistance. Proc. Natl. Acad. Sci. USA 104: 17075-17080.

[32] Itani SI, Pories WJ, Macdonald KG, Dohm GL (2001) Increased Protein Kinase C Theta in Skeletal Muscle of Diabetic Patients. Metabolism 50: 553-557.

[33] Mu J, Brozinick JT Jr, Valladares O, Bucan M, Birnbaum MJ (2001) A Role for AMP-Activated Protein Kinase in Contraction- and Hypoxia-Regulated Glucose Transport in Skeletal Muscle. Mol. Cell 7: 1085-1094.

[34] Mihaylova MM, Shaw RJ (2011) The AMPK Signalling Pathway Coordinates Cell Growth, Autophagy and Metabolism. Nat. Cell Biol. 13: 1016-1023

[35] Li XN, Song J, Zhang L, LeMaire SA, Hou X, Zhang C, Coselli JS, Chen L, Wang XL, Zhang Y, Shen YH (2009) Activation of the AMPK-FOXO3 Pathway Reduces Fatty Acid-Induced Increase in Intracellular Reactive Oxygen Species by Upregulating Thioredoxin. Diabetes 58: 2246-2257.

[36] Hou X, Song J, Li XN, Zhang L, Wang X, Chen L, Shen YH (2010) Metformin Reduces Intracellular Reactive Oxygen Species Levels by Upregulating Expression of the Antioxidant Thioredoxin via the AMPK-FOXO3 Pathway. Biochem. Biophys. Res. Commun. 396: 199-205.

[37] Imai S, Guarente L (2010) Ten Years of NAD-Dependent SIR2 Family Deacetylases: Implications for Metabolic Diseases. Trends Pharmacol. Sci. 31: 212-220

[38] Banks AS, Kon N, Knight C, Matsumoto M, Gutiérrez-Juárez R, Rossetti L, Gu W, Accili D (2008) Sirt1 Gain of Function Increases Energy Efficiency and Prevents Diabetes in Mice. Cell Metab. 8: 333-341.

[39] Pfluger PT, Herranz D, Velasco-Miguel S, Serrano M, Tschöp MH (2008) Sirt1 Protects Against High-Fat Diet-Induced Metabolic Damage. Proc. Natl. Acad. Sci. USA 105: 9793-9798.

[40] Lagouge M, Argmann C, Gerhart-Hines Z, Meziane H, Lerin C, Daussin F, Messadeq N, Milne J, Lambert P, Elliott P, Geny B, Laakso M, Puigserver P, Auwerx J (2006) Resveratrol Improves Mitochondrial Function and Protects against Metabolic Disease by Activating SIRT1 and PGC-1alpha. Cell127: 1109-1122.

[41] Milne JC, Lambert PD, Schenk S, Carney DP, Smith JJ, Gagne DJ, Jin L, Boss O, Perni RB, Vu CB, Bemis JE, Xie R, Disch JS, Ng PY, Nunes JJ, Lynch AV, Yang H, Galonek H, Israelian K, Choy W, Iffland A, Lavu S, Medvedik O, Sinclair DA, Olefsky JM, Jirousek MR, Elliott PJ, Westphal CH (2007) Small Molecule Activators of SIRT1 as Therapeutics for the Treatment of Type 2 Diabetes. Nature 450: 712-716.

[42] Zillikens MC, van Meurs JB, Rivadeneira F, Amin N, Hofman A, Oostra BA, Sijbrands EJ, Witteman JC, Pols HA, van Duijn CM, Uitterlinden AG (2009) SIRT1 Genetic Variation is Related to BMI and Risk of Obesity. Diabetes 58: 2828-2834

[43] Kim SC, Sprung R, Chen Y, Xu Y, Ball H, Pei J, Cheng T, Kho Y, Xiao H, Xiao L, Grishin NV, White M, Yang XJ, Zhao Y (2006) Substrate and Functional Diversity of Lysine Acetylation Revealed by a Proteomics Survey. Mol. Cell 23: 607-618.

[44] Guan KL, Xiong Y (2011) Regulation of Intermediary Metabolism by Protein Acetylation. Trends Biochem. Sci. 36: 108-116.

[45] Lombard DB, Alt FW, Cheng HL, Bunkenborg J, Streeper RS, Mostoslavsky R, Kim J, Yancopoulos G, Valenzuela D, Murphy A, Yang Y, Chen Y, Hirschey MD, Bronson RT, Haigis M, Guarente LP, Farese RV Jr, Weissman S, Verdin E, Schwer B (2007) Mammalian Sir2 homolog SIRT3 Regulates Global Mitochondrial Lysine Acetylation. Mol. Cell Biol. 27: 8807-8814.

[46] Schwer B, Bunkenborg J, Verdin RO, Andersen JS, Verdin E (2006) Reversible Lysine Acetylation Controls the Activity of the Mitochondrial Enzyme Acetyl-CoA Synthetase 2. Proc. Natl. Acad. Sci. USA 103: 10224-10229.

[47] Sakakibara I, Fujino T, Ishii M, Tanaka T, Shimosawa T, Miura S, Zhang W, Tokutake Y, Yamamoto J, Awano M, Iwasaki S, Motoike T, Okamura M, Inagaki T, Kita K, Ezaki O, Naito M, Kuwaki T, Chohnan S, Yamamoto TT, Hammer RE, Kodama T, Yanagisawa M, Sakai J (2009) Fasting-Induced Hypothermia and Reduced Energy Production in Mice Lacking Acetyl-CoA Synthetase 2. Cell Metab. 9: 191-202.

[48] Hirschey MD, Shimazu T, Goetzman E, Jing E, Schwer B, Lombard DB, Grueter CA, Harris C, Biddinger S, Ilkayeva OR, Stevens RD, Li Y, Saha AK, Ruderman NB, Bain JR, Newgard CB, Farese RV Jr, Alt FW, Kahn CR, Verdin E (2010) SIRT3 Regulates

Mitochondrial Fatty-Acid Oxidation by Reversible Enzyme Deacetylation. Nature 464: 121-125.

[49] Jing E, Emanuelli B, Hirschey MD, Boucher J, Lee KY, Lombard D, Verdin EM, Kahn CR (2011) Sirtuin-3 (Sirt3) Regulates Skeletal Muscle Metabolism and Insulin Signaling via Altered Mitochondrial Oxidation and Reactive Oxygen Species Production. Proc. Natl. Acad. Sci. USA 108: 14608-14613.

[50] Jitrapakdee S, Wutthisathapornchai A, Wallace JC, MacDonald MJ (2010) Regulation of Insulin Secretion: Role of Mitochondrial Signalling. Diabetologia 53: 1019-1032.

[51] Hirschey MD, Shimazu T, Jing E, Grueter CA, Collins AM, Aouizerat B, Stančáková A, Goetzman E, Lam MM, Schwer B, Stevens RD, Muehlbauer MJ, Kakar S, Bass NM, Kuusisto J, Laakso M, Alt FW, Newgard CB, Farese RV Jr, Kahn CR, Verdin E (2011) SIRT3 Deficiency and Mitochondrial Protein Hyperacetylation Accelerate the Development of the Metabolic Syndrome. Mol. Cell 44: 177-190.

[52] Rosen ED, Spiegelman BM (2006) Adipocytes as Regulators of Energy Balance and Glucose Homeostasis. Nature 444: 847-853.

[53] Tilg H, Moschen AR (2008) Adipocytokines: Mediators Linking Adipose Tissue, Inflammation and Immunity. Nat. Rev. Immunol. 6: 772-783.

[54] Dyck DJ (2009) Adipokines as Regulators of Muscle Metabolism and Insulin Sensitivity. Appl. Physiol. Nutr. Metab. 34: 396-402.

[55] Hotta K, Funahashi T, Arita Y, Takahashi M, Matsuda M, Okamoto Y, Iwahashi H, Kuriyama H, Ouchi N, Maeda K, Nishida M, Kihara S, Sakai N, Nakajima T, Hasegawa K, Muraguchi M, Ohmoto Y, Nakamura T, Yamashita S, Hanafusa T, Matsuzawa Y (2000) Plasma Concentrations of a Novel, Adipose-Specific Protein, Adiponectin, In Type 2 Diabetic Patients. Arterioscler. Thromb. Vasc. Biol. 20: 1595-1599.

[56] Li K, Li L, Yang GY, Liu H, Li SB, Boden G (2010) Effect of Short Hairpin RNA-Mediated Adiponectin/Acrp30 Down-Regulation on Insulin Signaling and Glucose Uptake in the 3T3-L1 Adipocytes. J. Endocrinol. Invest. 33: 96-102.

[57] Fruebis J, Tsao TS, Javorschi S, Ebbets-Reed D, Erickson MR, Yen FT, Bihain BE, Lodish HF (2001) Proteolytic Cleavage Product of 30-kDa Adipocyte Complement-Related Protein Increases Fatty Acid Oxidation in Muscle and Causes Weight Loss in Mice. Proc. Natl. Acad. Sci. USA 98: 2005-2010.

[58] Yamauchi T, Kamon J, Waki H, Terauchi Y, Kubota N, Hara K, Mori Y, Ide T, Murakami K, Tsuboyama-Kasaoka N, Ezaki O, Akanuma Y, Gavrilova O, Vinson C, Reitman ML, Kagechika H, Shudo K, Yoda M, Nakano Y, Tobe K, Nagai R, Kimura S, Tomita M, Froguel P, Kadowaki T (2001) The Fat-Derived Hormone Adiponectin Reverses Insulin Resistance Associated with both Lipoatrophy and Obesity. Nat. Med. 7: 941-946.

[59] Combs TP, Pajvani UB, Berg AH, Lin Y, Jelicks LA, Laplante M, Nawrocki AR, Rajala MW, Parlow AF, Cheeseboro L, Ding YY, Russell RG, Lindemann D, Hartley A, Baker GR, Obici S, Deshaies Y, Ludgate M, Rossetti L, Scherer PE (2004) A Transgenic Mouse with a Deletion in the Collagenous Domain of Adiponectin Displays Elevated

Circulating Adiponectin and Improved Insulin Sensitivity. Endocrinology 145: 367-383

[60] Yamauchi T, Kamon J, Minokoshi Y, Ito Y, Waki H, Uchida S, Yamashita S, Noda M, Kita S, Ueki K, Eto K, Akanuma Y, Froguel P, Foufelle F, Ferre P, Carling D, Kimura S, Nagai R, Kahn BB, Kadowaki T (2002) Adiponectin Stimulates Glucose Utilization and Fatty-Acid Oxidation by Activating AMP-Activated Protein Kinase. Nat. Med. 8: 1288-1295.

[61] Koh EH, Park JY, Park HS, Jeon MJ, Ryu JW, Kim M, Kim SY, Kim MS, Kim SW, Park IS, Youn JH, Lee KU (2007) Essential Role of Mitochondrial Function in Adiponectin Synthesis in Adipocytes. Diabetes 56: 2973-2981.

[62] Iwabu M, Yamauchi T, Okada-Iwabu M, Sato K, Nakagawa T, Funata M, Yamaguchi M, Namiki S, Nakayama R, Tabata M, Ogata H, Kubota N, Takamoto I, Hayashi YK, Yamauchi N, Waki H, Fukayama M, Nishino I, Tokuyama K, Ueki K, Oike Y, Ishii S, Hirose K, Shimizu T, Touhara K, Kadowaki T (2010) Adiponectin and AdipoR1 Regulate PGC-1alpha and Mitochondria by Ca(2+) and AMPK/SIRT1. Nature 464: 1313-1319.

[63] Kallenborn R (2006) Persistent Organic Pollutants (POPs) as Environmental Risk Factors in Remote High-Altitude Ecosystems. Ecotoxicol. Environ. Saf. 63: 100-107.

[64] Lee DH, Lee IK, Song K, Steffes M, Toscano W, Baker BA, Jacobs DR Jr (2006) A Strong Dose-Response Relation between Serum Concentrations of Persistent Organic Pollutants and Diabetes: Results from the National Health and Examination Survey 1999-2002. Diabetes Care 29: 1638-1644.

[65] Lee DH, Lee IK, Porta M, Steffes M, Jacobs DR Jr (2007) Relationship between Serum Concentrations of Persistent Organic Pollutants and the Prevalence of Metabolic Syndrome among Non-Diabetic Adults: Results from the National Health and Nutrition Examination Survey 1999-2002. Diabetologia 50: 1841-1851.

[66] Mokdad AH, Bowman BA, Ford ES, Vinicor F, Marks JS, Koplan JP (2001) The Continuing Epidemics of Obesity and Diabetes in The United States. JAMA. 286: 1195-1200.

[67] Solomon KR, Baker DB, Richards RP, Dixon KR, Klaine SJ, La Point TW, Kendall RJ, Weisskopf CP, Giddings JM, Giesy JP, Hall LW Jr, Williams WM (1996) Ecological Risk Assessment of Atrazine in North American Surface Waters. Environ. Toxicol. Chem. 15: 31–76.

[68] Beard J, Sladden T, Morgan G, Berry G, Brooks L, McMichael A (2003) Health Impacts of Pesticide Exposure in a Cohort of Outdoor Workers. Environ. Health Perspect. 111: 724-730.

[69] Ibrahim MM, Fjære E, Lock EJ, Naville D, Amlund H, Meugnier E, Le Magueresse Battistoni B, Frøyland L, Madsen L, Jessen N, Lund S, Vidal H, Ruzzin J (2011) Chronic Consumption of Farmed Salmon Containing Persistent Organic Pollutants Causes Insulin Resistance and Obesity in Mice. PLoS One 6: e25170.

[70] Beard J, Sladden T, Morgan G, Berry G, Brooks L, McMichael A (2003) Health Impacts of Pesticide Exposure in a Cohort of Outdoor Workers. Environ. Health Perspect. 111: 724-730.

[71] Lee DH, Steffes MW, Sjödin A, Jones RS, Needham LL, Jacobs DR Jr (2011) Low Dose Organochlorine Pesticides and Polychlorinated Biphenyls Predict Obesity, Dyslipidemia, and Insulin Resistance among People Free of Diabetes. PLoS One 6: e15977.

[72] Lee DH, Steffes MW, Sjödin A, Jones RS, Needham LL, Jacobs DR Jr (2010) Low Dose of Some Persistent Organic Pollutants Predicts Type 2 Diabetes: a Nested Case-Control Study. Environ. Health Perspect. 118: 1235-1242

[73] Shertzer HG, Genter MB, Shen D, Nebert DW, Chen Y, Dalton TP (2006) TCDD Decreases ATP Levels and Increases Reactive Oxygen Production through Changes in Mitochondrial FoF1-ATP Synthase and Ubiquinone. Toxicol. Appl. Pharmacol. 217: 363-374.

[74] Lim S, Ahn SY, Song IC, Chung MH, Jang HC, Park KS, Lee KU, Pak YK, Lee HK (2009) Chronic Exposure to the Herbicide, Atrazine, Causes Mitochondrial Dysfunction and Insulin Resistance. PLoS One 4: e5186.

[75] Ruzzin J, Petersen R, Meugnier E, Madsen L, Lock EJ, Lillefosse H, Ma T, Pesenti S, Sonne SB, Marstrand TT, Malde MK, Du ZY, Chavey C, Fajas L, Lundebye AK, Brand CL, Vidal H, Kristiansen K, Frøyland L (2010) Persistent Organic Pollutant Exposure Leads to Insulin Resistance Syndrome. Environ. Health Perspect. 118: 465-471.

[76] Arsenescu V, Arsenescu RI, King V, Swanson H, Cassis LA (2008) Polychlorinated Biphenyl-77 Induces Adipocyte Differentiation and Proinflammatory Adipokines and Promotes Obesity and Atherosclerosis. Environ. Health Perspect. 116: 761-768.

[77] Wilson-Fritch L, Nicoloro S, Chouinard M, Lazar MA, Chui PC, Leszyk J, Straubhaar J, Czech MP, Corvera S (2004) Mitochondrial Remodeling in Adipose Tissue Associated with Obesity and Treatment with Rosiglitazone. J. Clin. Invest. 114: 1281-1289.

[78] Wilson-Fritch L, Burkart A, Bell G, Mendelson K, Leszyk J, Nicoloro S, Czech M, Corvera S (2003) Mitochondrial Biogenesis and Remodeling during Adipogenesis and in Response to the Insulin Sensitizer Rosiglitazone. Mol. Cell Biol. 23: 1085-1094.

[79] Mensink M, Hesselink MK, Russell AP, Schaart G, Sels JP, Schrauwen P (2007) Improved Skeletal Muscle Oxidative Enzyme Activity and Restoration of PGC-1 alpha and PPAR beta/delta Gene Expression upon Rosiglitazone Treatment in Obese Patients with Type 2 Diabetes Mellitus. Int. J. Obes. (London) 31: 1302-1310.

[80] Lira VA, Benton CR, Yan Z, Bonen A (2010) PGC-1alpha Regulation by Exercise Training and Its Influences on Muscle Function and Insulin Sensitivity. Am. J. Physiol. Endocrinol. Metab. 299: E145-E161.

[81] Li L, Pan R, Li R, Niemann B, Aurich AC, Chen Y, Rohrbach S (2011) Mitochondrial Biogenesis and Peroxisome Proliferator-Activated Receptor-γ Coactivator-1α (PGC-1α)

Deacetylation by Physical Activity: Intact Adipocytokine Signaling is Required. Diabetes 60: 157-167.

[82] Hernández-Alvarez MI, Thabit H, Burns N, Shah S, Brema I, Hatunic M, Finucane F, Liesa M, Chiellini C, Naon D, Zorzano A, Nolan JJ (2010) Subjects with Early-Onset Type 2 Diabetes Show Defective Activation of the Skeletal Muscle PGC-1 Alpha/Mitofusin-2 Regulatory Pathway in Response to Physical Activity. Diabetes Care 33: 645-651

[83] Phielix E, Meex R, Moonen-Kornips E, Hesselink MK, Schrauwen P (2010) Exercise Training Increases Mitochondrial Content and ex vivo Mitochondrial Function Similarly in Patients with Type 2 Diabetes and in Control Individuals. Diabetologia 53: 1714-1721.

[84] Chen LL, Zhang HH, Zheng J, Hu X, Kong W, Hu D, Wang SX, Zhang P (2011) Resveratrol Attenuates High-Fat Diet-Induced Insulin Resistance by Influencing Skeletal Muscle Lipid Transport and Subsarcolemmal Mitochondrial β-Oxidation. Metabolism 60: 1598-1609.

[85] Moon HS, Lee HG, Choi YJ, Kim TG, Cho CS (2007) Proposed Mechanisms of (-)-Epigallocatechin-3-Gallate for Anti-Obesity. Chem. Biol. Interact. 167: 85-98.

[86] Hwang JT, Park IJ, Shin JI, Lee YK, Lee SK, Baik HW, Ha J, Park OJ (2005) Genistein, EGCG, and Capsaicin Inhibit Adipocyte Differentiation Process via Activating AMP-Activated Protein Kinase. Biochem. Biophys. Res. Commun. 338: 694-699.

[87] Tanaka M, Nishigaki Y, Fuku N, Ibi T, Sahashi K, Koga Y (2007) Therapeutic Potential of Pyruvate Therapy for Mitochondrial Diseases. Mitochondrion 7: 399-401.

[88] Das UN (2006) Is Pyruvate an Endogenous Anti-Inflammatory Molecule? Nutrition 22: 965-972.

[89] Yaworsky K, Somwar R, Ramlal T, Tritschler HJ, Klip A (2000) Engagement of the Insulin-Sensitive Pathway in the Stimulation of Glucose Transport by Alpha-Lipoic Acid in 3T3-L1 Adipocytes. Diabetologia 43:294-303.

[90] Shen W, Hao J, Feng Z, Tian C, Chen W, Packer L, Shi X, Zang W, Liu J (2011) Lipoamide or Lipoic Acid Stimulates Mitochondrial Biogenesis in 3T3-L1 Adipocytes via the Endothelial NO Synthase-cGMP-Protein Kinase G Signalling Pathway. Br. J. Pharmacol. 162: 1213-1224.

[91] Shen W, Liu K, Tian C, Yang L, Li X, Ren J, Packer L, Cotman CW, Liu J (2008) R-Alpha-Lipoic Acid and Acetyl-L-Carnitine Complementarily Promote Mitochondrial Biogenesis in Murine 3T3-L1 Adipocytes. Diabetologia 51: 165-174.

[92] Ikemura M, Nishikawa M, Hyoudou K, Kobayashi Y, Yamashita F, Hashida M (2010) Improvement of Insulin Resistance by Removal of Systemic Hydrogen Peroxide by PEGylated Catalase in Obese Mice. Mol. Pharm. 7: 2069-2076.

[93] Lee HY, Choi CS, Birkenfeld AL, Alves TC, Jornayvaz FR, Jurczak MJ, Zhang D, Woo DK, Shadel GS, Ladiges W, Rabinovitch PS, Santos JH, Petersen KF, Samuel VT, Shulman GI (2010) Targeted Expression of Catalase to Mitochondria Prevents Age-

Associated Reductions in Mitochondrial Function and Insulin Resistance. Cell Metab. 12: 668-674.

[94] Chung SS, Kim M, Youn BS, Lee NS, Park JW, Lee IK, Lee YS, Kim JB, Cho YM, Lee HK, Park KS (2009) Glutathione Peroxidase 3 Mediates the Antioxidant Effect of Peroxisome Proliferator-Activated Receptor Gamma in Human Skeletal Muscle Cells. Mol. Cell Biol. 29: 20-30.

Chapter 3

Impact of Genetic Polymorphisms on Insulin Resistance

Evrim Komurcu-Bayrak

Additional information is available at the end of the chapter

http://dx.doi.org/10.5772/51595

1. Introduction

The identification of DNA polymorphisms in human populations is an important step towards understanding the contribution of functional genetic variants to predisposition of diseases or clinical phenotypes. Approach to the determination of the predisposition uses polymorphisms as marker for a disease in an affected DNA population compared to a control DNA population. Subsequently, the polymorphisms statistically associated with the disease group may be directly informative or linked to the probable causative variant. There are currently over 10 million single nucleotide polymorphisms (SNPs) including insertion/deletion variants in public databases that potentially provide a marker set for disease-gene association studies. This large variant set might not represent the variants causative of disease because it was performed in genomes of only a limited number of individuals. For this reason, the discovery genetic variation in regions of functional DNA sequence in the genomes of individuals with disease is important for disease-gene association studies. However, this situation is not practicable for complex polygenic disease. Therefore, recently, genome-wide association (GWA) or candidate gene approaches are used in the understanding of the molecular genetic background of complex polygenic disease.

Insulin resistance has a complex and heterogeneous genetic background. Insulin resistance is caused by the reduced ability of peripheral target tissues to respond properly to insulin stimulation. Insulin resistance predates beta cell dysfunction and plays the crucial role in the pathogenesis of type 2 diabetes. In addition, insulin resistance is considered the core factor in the pathogenesis of atherosclerosis and the metabolic syndrome, and is often associated with obesity, hypertension and also a dyslipidemic profile characterized by high plasma triacylglycerol concentrations and low HDL-C (Reaven, 1988; Filippi et al., 2004). Until now, many hypotheses have been proposed to explain the molecular mechanisms of insulin resistance such as insulin signaling cascade, the role of free fatty acids, adipocytokines, and inflammation (Perseghin et al., 2003; Bhattacharya et al. 2007; Choi & Kim, 2010; Erion & Shulman, 2010; Muoio &, Newgard, 2008). Given the crucial roles of pathways in the pathogenesis of liver and muscle insulin resistance, understanding the molecular mechanism of insulin resistance is vital for the development of new and more effective therapies for metabolic disorders. The homeostasis model assessment (HOMA) index for insulin resistance was calculated as the product of fasting plasma insulin (in microunits per milliliter) and fasting plasma glucose (in millimoles per liter), divided by 22.5 (Matthews et al. 1985). Higher HOMA values indicate higher insulin resistance.

Genetic and epidemiological studies strongly suggest that insulin resistance is, at least in part, genetically determined. However, the involved genes and their effective variants are mostly unknown. The numerous genes have been suggested as a potential candidate gene for insulin resistance, but the findings of these studies were controversial. This chapter is to provide an overview of our recent understanding of genetic predisposition to insulin resistance. It is aimed to summarize the results of the recent studies about the genetics of insulin resistance.

2. Genes related to the lipid homeostasis

2.1. The polymorphisms of the FABP genes

Fatty acid-binding proteins (FABPs) are members of a superfamily of lipid-binding proteins. These tissue specific proteins (FABP1-4) play the physiological role in the uptake, intracellular metabolism and excretion of long-chain fatty acids (LCFA) (Zimmerman & Veerkamp, 2002). The polymorphisms of these genes have been studied in several metabolic phenotypes such as obesity, metabolic syndrome, hypertriglyceridemia and insulin sensitivity (Mansego et al. 2012).

The liver FABP (FABP1) is an abundant cytosolic lipid-binding protein that regulates lipid transport and metabolism. The c.334-135G>A polymorphism (rs2197076) located in the 3 prime untranslated region (UTR) of the FABP1 gene was associated with the risk of type 2 diabetes and HOMA index in the Spanish population. In this study, it has been shown that carriers of the allele A of this polymophism had HOMA index values higher than homozygotes GG. However, none of the other analyzed variants in FABP2, FABP3 and FABP4 genes were associated with type 2 diabetes and insulin resistance in this study (Mansego et al. 2012).

The intestinal FABP (FABP2) plays a key role in the absorption and intracellular transport of dietary LCFA (Weiss, 2002). Therefore, the FABP2 gene has been suggested as a possible candidate gene for type 2 diabetes and insulin resistance. In vitro experiments have shown that Ala54Thr polymorphism increases the affinity of FABP2 for LCFA and is associated with increased triglyceride transport in human intestinal cells (Baier et al., 1996; Prochazka et al., 1993). Previous studies have reported significant associations between the FABP2 gene and increased prevalence of insulin resistance (Baier et al., 1995; Mitchell et al., 1995; Yamada et al. 1997; Chiu et al., 2001; Kim et al., 2001) as well as no association was found in

Finnish individuals (Sipiläinen et al., 1997) and Spanish population (Mansego et al. 2012). Baier et al. reported the significant associations between the common FABP2 Ala54Thr polymorphism (rs1799883) and increased fasting insulin concentration, fasting fatty acid oxidation, and decreased insulin sensitivity in Pima Indians, a population with a high prevalence of obesity and type 2 diabetes (Baier et al., 1995). Furthermore, the linkage analysis of the FABP2 locus with insulin resistance was also found in a study in Mexican Americans who were of a mixed American-Indian and -European ancestry (Mitchell et al., 1995). However, sib-pair analysis failed to detect any linkage of the FABP2 locus or the Ala54Thr polymorphism with diabetes-related phenotypes in other ethnic groups. The homozygous Thr54/Thr54 genotype has found the associations with higher fasting insulin levels and also TNF-α levels in 33 adult obese women (Albala et al., 2004). However, the findings of this study would need to be confirmed in studies involving a larger number of subjects. A number of conflicting and inconclusive studies have investigated the possible association of the FABP2 Ala54Thr polymorphism with insulin resistance. A meta-analysis of these published studies has suggested that the Thr54 allele of the FABP2 Ala54Thr is weakly associated with a higher degree of insulin resistance, higher fasting insulin and blood glucose level. As gender and ethnicity probably were important variables in determining associative risk with insulin resistance and type 2 diabetes, Zhao et al. have performed subgroup analyses of gender and ethnicity. These weak effects of Ala54Thr polymorphism on insulin resistance and fasting insulin have been particularly established in East Asians (Zhao et al., 2010).

2.2. The polymorphisms of the ELOVL6 gene

Elongase of long chain fatty acids family 6 (ELOVL6) is expressed in lipogenic tissues. This enzyme specifically catalyze the elongation of saturated and monounsaturated fatty acids with 12, 14 and 16 carbons. A population-based study has suggested that the genetic variations in the ELOVL6 gene are related with insulin resistance. In this study, five SNPs of the ELOVL6 gene and their haplotypes were analyzed. In this population from southern Spain, carriers of the minor alleles of the rs9997926 and rs6824447 polymorphisms had a lower risk of having high HOMA index, whereas carriers of the minor allele rs17041272 had a higher risk of being insulin resistant. Finally, Morcillo et al. has suggested that the ELOVL6 gene could be a future therapeutic target in the treatment of diabetes and related disorders (Morcillo et al., 2011). However, the validation of associations between this novel candidate gene and insulin resistance should be performed in different and large populations.

2.3. The polymorphisms of the APOE gene

Apolipoprotein E (ApoE) is primarily involved in plasma lipid homeostasis. However, a number of studies with experimental mouse models have shown that apoE also has an important role in the development of obesity and insulin resistance (Kypreos et al., 2009; Gao et al., 2007). ApoE is involved in excess fat accumulation and energy metabolism, including the regulation of food intake and energy expenditure. Therefore, excess fat accumulation via an apoE-dependent pathway might play a role in the development of insulin resistance (Kypreos et al., 2006). Some studies have suggested that the APOE ε2/ε3/ε4 polymorphism may modify the effect of insulin on CHD or some CHD risk factors, including obesity and lipid profile levels (Després et al., 1993; Valdez et al., 1995; Elosua et al., 2003), whereas the Framingham Offspring Study and Turkish Adult Risk Factor (TARF) Study found that this polymorphism was not associated with insulin resistance (Meigs et al., 2000; Komurcu-Bayrak et al., 2011). Two other of the functional SNPs, i.e., -219G>T (rs405509) and +113G>C (rs440446) in APOE gene had shown association with plasma apoE concentrations (Lambert et al., 2000; Moreno et al., 2003), insulin resistance (Viitanen et al., 2001), insulin sensitivity in response to a diet rich in satured fats (Moreno et al., 2005). In a cross-sectional study, the impacts of these polymorphisms have been analyzed on lipid, apolipoprotein, glucose, and serum insulin concentrations in the TARF cohort, a representative of Turkish adults. In this study, the -219G>T and +113G>C genotypes and diplotypes of haplotype 2 (TCε3) showed negative correlation to serum fasting insulin and the HOMA index, but not to serum lipids. The significant associations between these functional polymorphisms and fasting insulin levels and the HOMA index were found only in the apoE3 group (ε3ε3 genotypes of the APOE ε2/ε3/ε4 polymorphism) without type 2 diabetes (Komurcu-Bayrak et al., 2011). On the other hand, a large population-based family study related with type 2 diabetes found a relationship for the polymorphisms of the APOE gene and the nearby muscle glycogen synthase (GYS1) gene on chromosome 19 with cardiovascular mortality, independently of each other (Fredriksson et al., 2007). Other functional polymorphisms in the GYS1 gene may relate to developing insulin resistance.

3. Genes related to the energy metabolism

3.1. The polymorphisms of the UCP genes

Uncoupling protein 2 and 3 (UCP2 and UCP3) play an important role in human energy homeostasis (Brand et al., 200 4) and have been considered candidate genes for obesity, type 2 diabetes and insulin resistance. Thus, UCP2 and UCP3 are involved in regulating ATP synthesis, generation of reactive oxygen species and glucose-stimulated insulin secretion by pancreatic β cells. The -866G>A (rs659366) polymorphism of UCP2 gene was located in a region with putative binding sites for two β-cell transcription factors (Dalgaard et al., 2003). A number of studies have been performed seeking for an association between genetic variants in this gene cluster with type 2 diabetes and/or insulin resistance. These studies have demonstrated association of the -866A-allele with increased (D'Adamo et al., 2004; Krempler et al., 2002; Gable et al., 2006) and decreased (Wang et al., 2004; Bulotta et al., 2005; Lyssenko et al., 2005; Rai et al., 2007) risk of type 2 diabetes as well as no association at all (Kovacs et al., 2005; Reis et al., 2004; Zee et al., 2011). Finally, the two recent meta-analysis on the association of type 2 diabetes with -866G>A polymorphism concluded that this variant does not confer increased risk of type 2 diabetes (Xu et al., 2011; 40, Andersen et al., 2012). However, Andersen et al has found an association between this variant and obesity in

Danish individuals and established case-control studies. This study has shown that the -866G-allele was associated with elevated fasting serum insulin levels and insulin resistance (HOMA index) and decreased insulin sensitivity in Danish subjects (Andersen et al., 2012). Furthermore, in a study performed with a Spanish group of 193 obese children and adolescents and 170 controls, Ochoa et al. reported that the -55C>T (rs1800849) polymorphism of the UCP3 gene directly associated with higher fasting insulin levels and insulin resistance in heterozygous subjects from the control group. In addition, they found that the individual polymorphisms were not associated with obesity, but the (-866G) - (Del; 45 bp) - (-55T) haplotype was significantly associated with obesity and its presence in the control group increased about nine times the insulin resistance risk (Ochoa et al., 2007). Recently, a study has demonstrated that morbidly obese patients with –55CT genotype (n=15) had higher weight, fat mass, and insulin resistance (HOMA index) than the individuals with –55CC genotype (n=32) (de Luis Roman et al., 2010).

3.2. The polymorphisms of the ADRB genes

β-adrenoceptors (ADRB1, ADRB2, ADRB3) in the sympathetic nervous system play a role in regulating energy expenditure and lipolysis. ADRBs gene variation is an intense area of investigation because β-adrenoceptors are well described in organ system distribution, catecholamine-mediated physiological processes, disease states and treatment targets (Eisenach & Wittwer, 2010). One of the most studied polymorphism (rs1801253) in the ADRB1 gene encode for arginine or glycine in amino acid 389 (Arg389Gly). In 238 healthy young Caucasians and African-Americans, Gly389 carriers had a higher level of insulin and insulin resistance than non-carriers, and this allele was more prevalent in the subjects with higher body mass index (BMI; Lima et al. 2007). In previous studies, it has been found that this polymorphism was associated with serum insulin levels and insulin resistance (HOMA index) but, no association with obesity among Swedish women (Mottagui-Tabar et al., 2008). However, there are limited number of studies evaluating the association between these genes and insulin resistance. In larger scale studies with different populations should be performed for these genes to support the association between genotype and phenotype.

4. Genes encoding hormones and hormone receptors

4.1. The polymorphisms of the APM1, ADIPOR1, and ADIPOR2 genes

Adiponection is an adipokine secreted by adipocytes. The polymorphisms in adiponectin (APM1,ADIPOQ, ACRP30) gene, and its receptors (ADIPOR1 and ADIPOR2) are strongly associated with metabolic syndrome, obesity, type 2 diabetes and, insulin resistance. High adiponectin predicts increased insulin sensitivity (Tschritter et al. 2003). There is evidence indicating that insulin directly affects plasma adiponectin (Möhlig et al., 2002; Hung et al., 2008; Brame et al., 2005). In recent studies, plasma adiponectin concentrations were reduced in type 2 diabetes and obesity (Arita et al., 1999; Lindsay et al. 2002; Spranger et al., 2003). Furthermore, administration of thiazolidinediones (TZD), an insulin-sensitising class of drugs, to insulin-resistant subjects significantly increased the plasma adiponectin levels, and this effect was correlated with the amelioration of insulin resistance in these subjects (Maeda et al., 2001). Many studies have, in fact, reported the association between polymorphisms of the APM1, ADIPOR1, and ADIPOR2 and adiponectin concentrations, insulin resistance, type 2 diabetes and metabolic syndrome phenotypes (Kondo et al., 2002; Hara et al., 2002; Menzaghi et al., 2002; Stumvoll et al., 2002; Hivert et al., 2008; Menzaghi et al.,2007; Sheng et al., 2008; Ferguson et al., 2010). While, in the study from Stumvoll et al, the +45T>G (rs2241766) polymorphism was associated with obesity and derangement of insulin sensitivity (Stumvoll et al., 2002), in the study from Melistas et al, this polymorphism was associated with lower insulin levels in Greek women without diabetes (Melistas et al., 2009). In a study from Menzaghi et al, a haplotype of the adiponectin gene was associated with several features of insulin resistance in nondiabetic individuals, including low serum adiponectin levels (Menzaghi et al., 2002). In addition, the +276G>T (rs1501299) polymorphism in the adiponectin gene was associated with higher insulin levels and insulin resistance (HOMA index) in Italian population from the Lazio region (diabetes and/or the metabolic syndrome was excluded) (Filippi et al., 2004) and in Greek female population without diabetes (Melistas et al., 2009). The association of the -11391G>A (rs17300539) polymorphism with plasma insulin and HOMA index was independent of plasma adiponectin in another study, which implies a direct effect of this polymorphism on plasma insulin and insulin sensitivity (Henneman et al., 2010). Recently, Vasseur et al have reported on the association of a haplotype G-G (including -11391G>A and -11377C>G polymorphisms located in the APM1 proximal promoter) with plasma adiponectin levels and type 2 diabetes, although no association with HOMA index was observed (Vasseur et al., 2002). The reasons for partially discrepant results between polymorphisms in these genes and metabolic measures could be due to the different genetic background of the studied populations or environmental interactions, particularly dietary factors. Gene-nutrient interactions can modulate in the development of metabolic phenotypes. Although, so far, there has been little focus on gene-nutrient interactions with adiponectin and its receptors, two studies found that there was an interaction between the rs266729 polymorphism of APM1 and the percentage of dietary-derived energy from fat with the development of obesity in women (Santos et al., 2006) and an association between this polymorphism and also the rs10920533 polymorphism of ADIPOR1 and plasma saturated fatty acids with the insulin resistance (Ferguson et al., 2010).

4.2. The polymorphisms of the D2 and TSHR genes

Thyroid hormones are known to upregulate the expression of glucose transporter type 4 (GLUT4) in skeletal muscle, and consequently increase glucose uptake (Weinstein et al., 1994). Thyroxine (T4), a major secretory product of the thyroid gland, needs to be converted to triiodothyronine (T3) to exert its biological activity. Type 2 deiodinase (D2) catalyzes T4 to T3 conversion, and plays a critical role in maintaining intracellular T3 levels in specialized tissues, such as the anterior pituitary and brown adipose tissue (Bianco et al., 2005). Thr92Ala polymorphism of D2 gene showed an association with lower glucose disposal rate in nondiabetic subjects and also a higher prevalence of insulin resistance in Pima Indians and Mexican–Americans (Mentuccia et al., 2002). Furthermore, D2 Ala/Ala genotype was also associated in previous studies with increased insulin levels and increased insulin resistance (increased HOMA index) and also worse glycemic control (increased HbA1c levels) in a cohort of patients with type 2 diabetes (Grozovsky et al., 2009; Dora et al., 2010). In addition, this polymorphism was associated with greater insulin resistance in type 2 diabetes patients and with lower enzyme activity in thyroid tissue samples (Canani et al., 2005). However, some population-based studies failed to demonstrate an association between the D2 Thr92Ala polymorphism and increased risk for type 2 diabetes (Mentuccia et al., 2005; Maia et al., 2007; Grarup et al. 2007). Thyroid hormone interacts with the TSH receptor (TSHR) in the thyroid gland. A previous study has investigated the association between serum thyroid parameters and the TSHR Asp727Glu polymorphism in nondiabetic elderly men. Peeters et al. reported that this polymorphism was associated with relative insulin resistance. Carriers of the Glu727 allele had also a significantly higher glucose, insulin, HOMA index and leptin levels, but no association with serum TSH levels (Peeters et al., 2007). Peeters et al. have suggested that this association was studied in one cohort only, and as the mechanism remains to be elucidated, replication of results in an independent cohort (of healthy elderly subjects) was essential.

4.3. The polymorphisms of the SHBG gene

Some studies have suggested that the polymorphisms in genes encoding sex hormones may be effective on the development of insulin resistance. Previous studies have shown that androgen supplementation in the presence of central obesity and low testosterone levels increases insulin sensitivity in men (Mårin et al., 1992; Simon et al., 2001; Boyanov et al., 2003). Moreover, polycystic ovarian syndrome was associated with higher risk of type 2 diabetes and insulin resistance in women (Dunaif, 1995). Recent studies have demonstrated that higher levels of circulating sex hormone binding protein (SHBG) were associated with reduce risk of type 2 diabetes (Ding et al., 2009; Perry et al., 2010). In addition, rs6259, rs6257 and rs1799941 polymorphisms in the SHBG gene were strongly associated with SHBG levels and type 2 diabetes (Zeggini et al., 2008; Perry et al., 2010). However, there was no evidence that this variant is associated with diabetes-related intermediate traits, including several measures of insulin secretion and resistance (Perry et al., 2010).

4.4. The polymorphisms of the LEP and LEPR genes

Leptin (LEP), a hormone secreted by adipocytes, and its receptor (LEPR) are other candidate genes for insulin resistance. Common variants in the LEPR gene have been associated with hyperinsulinemia (Lakka et al., 2000; Wauters et al., 2002), type 2 diabetes (Lakka et al., 2000), obesity, and leptin levels (Chagnon et al., 1999; Chagnon et al., 2000; Chagnon et al., 2001; de Luis Roman et al., 2006). However, the roles of leptin and its receptor in the development of metabolic traits in the general population are less clear. A few studies have, in fact, reported the association between polymorphisms of the LEP and LEPR genes and insulin resistance (Wauters et al., 2001; de Luis et al., 2008; Gu et al., 2012; Takahashi-Yasuno et al., 2004; Ren et al., 2004). While, in the study from Wauters et al, Lys109Arg, Gln223Arg, and Lys656Asn polymorphisms in LEPR gene were associated with insulin and glucose metabolism in postmenopausal obese women with impaired glucose homeostasis (Wauters et al., 2001), in the study from de Luis et al, Lys656Asn polymorphism was associated with higher levels of insulin, HOMA, and leptin in men without diabetes (de Luis et al., 2008) , in the study from Gu et al, Lys109Arg was associated with waist-to-hip ratio, oral glucose tolerance test (OGTT)-2h glucose, and HOMA index in Chinese subjects with essential hypertension, but no correlation between Lys109Arg polymorphism and hypertension were found (Gu et al., 2012). Also' -2549C>A polymorphism in the promoter region of the LEP gene is related to fasting plasma leptin level (Mammès et al., 1998; Le Stunff et al., 2000; Gu et al., 2012), obesity phenotypes (Mammès et al., 1998; Mammès et al., 2000; Le Stunff et al., 2000), and also fasting serum insulin level and HOMA index in Chinese patient with type 2 diabetes (Ren et al., 2004). However, the findings of the study from Ren et al. should be confirmed with studies involving larger number of subjects and different populations.

4.5. The polymorphisms of the RBP4 gene

Retinol-binding protein 4 (RBP4) is an adipokine with potential contribution to systemic insulin resistance (Yang et al., 2005). The -803G>A promoter polymorphism (rs3758539) of RBP4 gene is associated with increased risk for obesity and type 2 diabetes in adults (Munkhtulga et al., 2010 ; Munkhtulga et al., 2007; van Hoek et al., 2008). Munkhtulga et al. have reported in 2010 that the -803A allele of this polymorphism was associated with higher BMI in Japanese men and women and in Mongolian women (Munkhtulga et al., 2010) and also in 2007 they found that the rare alleles of four SNPs (-803G>A, +5169C>T, +6969G>C, +7542T>del) were associated with increased risk of diabetes in Mongolian case-control study (Munkhtulga et al., 2007). van Hoek et al. have shown that homozygosity for the −803A allele was associated with increased risk of type 2 diabetes in the Rotterdam population (van Hoek et al., 2008). More recent studies failed to confirm an association of this variant with circulating RBP4 levels, type 2 diabetes susceptibility, adiposity or metabolic parameters (Friebe et al., 2011; Kovacs et al., 2007; Shea et al., 2010; Wu et al., 2009; Craig et al., 2007). Shea et al. have analyzed five SNPs including -803G>A polymorphism within RBP4 gene and they have found a significant association between the minor allele of rs10882280 (C>A intron) and rs11187545 (A>G intron) polymorphisms and higher serum HDL-C levels in Newfoundland population, but not between insulin resistance and any polymorphism (Shea et al., 2010). Craig et al. have found that only a haplotype (-804G, 390G, 406T, 759G, 6969G, 9476T, 10670G, and 11881C) in RBP4 gene showed an association with type 2 diabetes in African Americans and Caucasians. Furthermore, -803G>A and +9476T>G (rs34571439) polymorphisms were associated with reduced insulin secretion, and +390C>G (novel) with reduced insulin sensitivity in Caucasians (Craig et al., 2007). The discrepancy among previous publications about insulin resistance may be resolved by analyzing a larger number of samples.

4.6. The polymorphisms of the RETN gene

Resistin (RETN), a hormone secreted by adipocytes, has been examined as candidate gene for obesity and type 2 diabetes and insulin resistance. However, there are many conflicting findings about these metabolic phenotypes. Osawa et al. have reported that the GG genotype of RETN -420C>G promoter polymorphism (rs1862513), increased type 2 diabetes susceptibility (Osawa et al., 2004) and fasting plasma resistin (Osawa et al., 2007; Azuma et al., 2004) in the Japanese population. Silha et al. and Osawa et al. have found correlation between resistin levels and insulin resistance (Silha et al.,2003; Osawa et al., 2007), but not Lee et al. (Lee et al., 2003). Some genetic association studies have found an association between certain resistin gene variants and insulin resistance in Finnish nondiabetic individuals (Conneely et al., 2004), in nondiabetic Caucasians from Sicily and Gargano areas of Italy (Pizzuti et al., 2002), and in 20 nondiabetic Caucasians (Wang et al., 2002), while others report no such association in 60 Japanese obese nondiabetic individuals (Azuma et al., 2004) and in 258 families with 323 affected with polycystic ovary syndrome offspring (Urbanek et al., 2003). These conflicting findings have made it difficult to determine a role for resistin in insulin resistance. The reasons for discrepant results are not known, and may reside in the different genetic background of the studied populations or the different-designed studies.

5. Genes related to the renin-angiotensin system

The renin-angiotensin system (RAS) plays a central role in the regulation of insulin sensitivity (Reaven, 1995; Higashiura et al., 2000; Ura et al., 1999). Many studies have examined the genetic effect of homozygous deletion polymorphism (DD) in exon 16 of the angiotensin-converting enzyme gene (ACE) in insulin resistance, but their results have been controversial (Katsuya et al., 1995; Perticone et al., 2001; Yamamoto et al., 1999). Hypertension is related to insulin resistance and a number of studies have reported an association between RAS gene polymorphisms and hypertension (Sugimoto et al. 2004; Jin et al., 2003; Kikuya et al., 2003; Ono et al., 2003). Akasaka et al., 2006; The insertion/deletion (I/D) polymorphism of the angiotensin-converting enzyme gene (ACE), the Met235Thr polymorphism of the angiotensinogen gene (AGT), and the 1166A>C polymorphism of the angiotensin II type 1 receptor gene (AGTR1) were not associated with HOMA index, whereas borderline association was found between the 1166A>C polymorphism and dichotomous categorization of insulin resistance (defined as HOMA index ≥1.73). However, further studies are required to confirm the impact of these candidate gene polymorphisms in the larger and different populations.

6. Genes related to the inflammation

6.1. The polymorphisms of the TNF-α gene

Tumor necrosis factor alpha (TNF-α) is a multifunctional proinflammatory cytokine and also an adipokine produced in adipocytes. Increased levels of the TNF-α have been shown to elevate the risk of insulin resistance by impairing β cell function and glucose homeostasis (Hotamisligil et al., 1993; Hotamisligil et al., 1994; Katsuki et al., 1998). In addition, the TNF-α affects lipid metabolism and may lead to hypertriglyceridemia by decreasing hepatic lipoprotein lipase activity and by increasing hepatic de novo fatty acid synthesis (Zinman et al., 1999). Circulating levels of TNF-α have also been reported to correlate with insulin resistance and type 2 diabetes (Hotamisligil & Spiegelman, 1994; Hu et al., 2004). Previous studies have shown that TNF-α -308G>A polymorphism is associated with insulin resistance (Fernandez-Real et al., 1997), obesity (Hoffstedt et al., 2000), type 2 diabetes (Vendrell et al., 2003; Kubaszek et al., 2003) and metabolic syndrome (Gupta et al., 2012). However, many other studies have reported conflicting results, with no association between this variant and insulin resistance (Gupta et al., 2012; Ranjith et al., 2008). A meta-analysis of many published studies including different populations has suggested that -308A TNF-α gene variant is associated with increased risk of developing obesity compared with controls and significantly higher systolic arterial blood pressure and plasma insulin levels (Sookoian et al., 2005). On the other hand, another recent meta-analyses has reported that TNF-α -238G>A and -308G>A polymorphisms were not associated with type 2 diabetes mellitus; however, -308G>A polymorphism was positively associated with type 1 diabetes (Feng et al., 2009a; Feng et al., 2009b; Feng et al., 2011). TNF-α -857C>T polymorphism is also associated with obese type 2 diabetes (Kamizono et al. 2000) and insulin resistance in Japanese diabetic subjects with adiponectin +276GG genotype (Ohara et al., 2012). The study of Ohara et al has shown interaction of TNF-α and adiponectin genes with insulin resistance and fatty liver (Ohara et al., 2012).

6.2. The polymorphisms of the IL-6 gene

Interleukin-6 (IL-6) is a proinflammatory cytokine that is associated with type 2 diabetes and insulin resistance (Di Renzo et al., 2008; Wannamethee et al., 2007; Hu et al., 2004). Recent studies has demonstrated that the association between -174G>C polymorphism (rs1800795) in the promoter region of the IL-6 gene and insulin resistance is modified by body mass index (BMI), with the -174C allele associated with higher insulin resistance and type 2 diabetes in individuals with obesity (Herbert et al., 2006; Mohlig et al., 2004; Goyenechea et al., 2007; Di Renzo et al., 2008; Underwood et al., 2012). However, in meta-analysis including 5383 diabetes cases and 12 069 controls, it has been found that -174G>C polymorphism was not associated with the risk of type 2 diabetes (Qi et al., 2006). The reasons underlying the discrepancy among studies are unclear. Other genetic or environmental factors may play important roles in modulating the relationships.

7. Conclusion

The insulin resistance is highly heritable and originates from the interactions of multiple genes and environmental factors. Figure 1 shows the main factors contributing to the development of insulin resistance and type 2 diabetes. However, the molecular mechanism of insulin resistance is not clear yet. Until now, goal of many studies was to use a candidate gene approach to identify genes associated with insulin resistance and several genes have been investigated in many association-based studies. However, most of the time, results of these studies reveal conflicting findings. These discrepant results might be due to differences in the study populations and design of these studies. In addition, the candidate gene polymorphisms have been searched in a number of small-scale studies with variable results. Limited number meta-analyses have been done to demonstrate the effect of several candidate gene polymorphisms on insulin resistance. But, the larger, well-characterized and independent association studies will be needed. On the other hand, the use of genome-wide association (GWA) studies will identify novel polymorphisms related to insulin resistance. This knowledge will allow the determination of the genetic predisposition to the insulin resistance and new approaches to treatment and prevention of the clinical phenotypes such as type 2 diabetes, obesity, hypertension and metabolic syndrome.

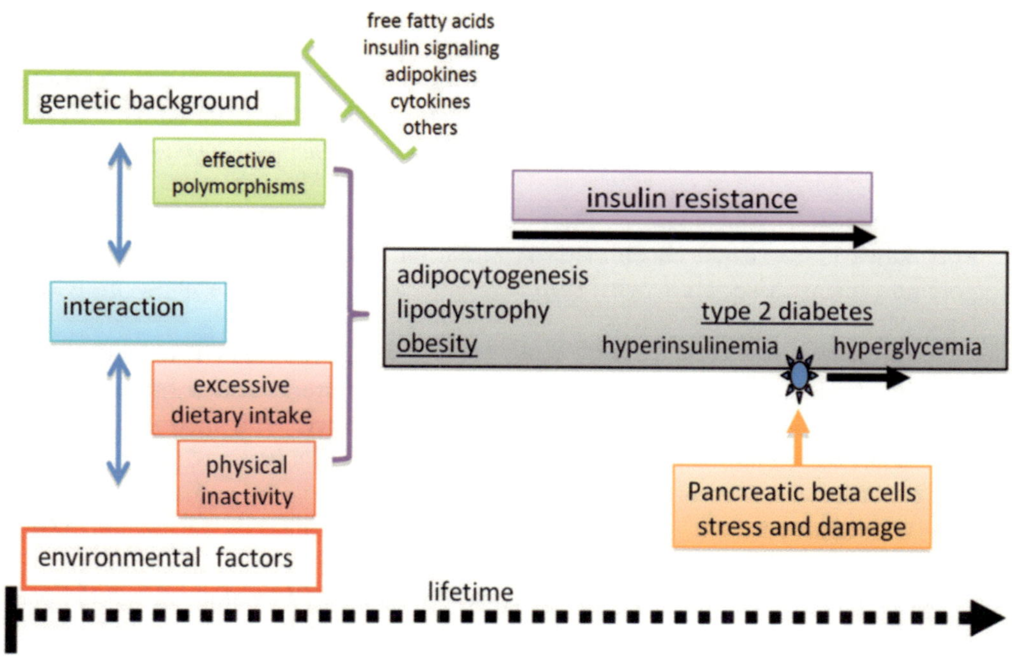

Figure 1. General overview of genetic and environmental factors contributing to the development of insulin resistance and type 2 diabetes. The combination of genetic predisposition (genetic polymorphisms effecting free fatty acid metabolism, insulin signalling, adipokines and cytokines) and some environmental factors such as excessive dietary intake and physical inactivity results with the occurrence of adipocytogenesis, lipodystrophy and obesity which increase the development risk of insulin resistance. Insulin resistance predates pancreatic beta cell dysfunction and plays the crucial role in the pathogenesis of type 2 diabetes.

Author details

Evrim Komurcu-Bayrak
Department of Genetics, Institute for Experimental Medicine, Istanbul University, Turkey

8. References

Akasaka H, Katsuya T, Saitoh S, Sugimoto K, Fu Y, Takagi S, Ohnishi H, Rakugi H, Ura N, Shimamoto K & Ogihara T. (2006). Effects of angiotensin II type 1 receptor gene polymorphisms on insulin resistance in a Japanese general population: the Tanno-Sobetsu study. *Hypertens Res.* 29(12), pp. 961-7.

Albala C, Santos JL, Cifuentes M, Villarroel AC, Lera L, Liberman C, Angel B & Pérez-Bravo F. (2004). Intestinal FABP2 A54T polymorphism: association with insulin resistance and obesity in women. *Obes Res.* 12(2), pp. 340-5.

Andersen G, Dalgaard LT, Justesen JM, Anthonsen S, Nielsen T, Thørner LW, Witte D, Jørgensen T, Clausen JO, Lauritzen T, Holmkvist J, Hansen T & Pedersen O. (2012). The frequent UCP2 -866G>A polymorphism protects against insulin resistance and is associated with obesity: a study of obesity and related metabolic traits among 17636 Danes. *Int J Obes* (Lond). doi: 10.1038/ijo.2012.22.

Arita Y, Kihara S, Ouchi N, Takahashi M, Maeda K, Miyagawa J, Hotta K, Shimomura I, Nakamura T, Miyaoka K, Kuriyama H, Nishida M, Yamashita S, Okubo K, Matsubara K, Muraguchi M, Ohmoto Y, Funahashi T & Matsuzawa Y. (1999). Paradoxical decrease of an adipose-specific protein, adiponectin, in obesity. *Biochem Biophys Res Commun.* 257(1), pp. 79-83.

Azuma K, Oguchi S, Matsubara Y, Mamizuka T, Murata M, Kikuchi H, Watanabe K, Katsukawa F, Yamazaki H, Shimada A & Saruta T. (2004). Novel resistin promoter polymorphisms: association with serum resistin level in Japanese obese individuals. *Horm Metab Res.* 36(8), pp. 564-70.

Baier LJ, Sacchettini JC, Knowler WC, Eads J, Paolisso G, Tataranni PA, Mochizuki H, Bennett PH, Bogardus C & Prochazka M. (1995). An amino acid substitution in the human intestinal fatty acid binding protein is associated with increased fatty acid binding, increased fat oxidation, and insulin resistance. *J Clin Invest.* 95(3), pp. 1281-7.

Baier LJ, Bogardus C & Sacchettini JC. (1996). A polymorphism in the human intestinal fatty acid binding proteins alters fatty acid transport across Caco-2 cells. *J Biol Chem.* 271, pp. 10892–6.

Bhattacharya S, Dey D & Roy SS. (2007). Molecular mechanism of insulin resistance. *J Biosci.* 32(2):405-13.

Bianco AC, Maia AL, da Silva WS, Christoffolete MA. (2005). Adaptive activation of thyroid hormone and energy expenditure. *Biosci Rep.* 25(3-4), pp. 191-208.

Boyanov MA, Boneva Z & Christov VG. (2003). Testosterone supplementation in men with type 2 diabetes, visceral obesity and partial androgen deficiency. *Aging Male.* 6(1), pp. 1-7.

Brame LA, Considine RV, Yamauchi M, Baron AD & Mather KJ. (2005). Insulin and endothelin in the acute regulation of adiponectin in vivo in humans. *Obes Res* 13, pp. 582–588

Brand MD, Affourtit C, Esteves TC, Green K, Lambert AJ, Miwa S, Pakay JL & Parker N. (2004). Mitochondrial superoxide: production, biological effects, and activation of uncoupling proteins. *Free Radic Biol Med.* 37(6), pp. 755-67.

Bulotta A, Ludovico O, Coco A, Di Paola R, Quattrone A, Carella M, Pellegrini F, Prudente S & Trischitta V. (2005). The common -866G/A polymorphism in the promoter region of the UCP-2 gene is associated with reduced risk of type 2 diabetes in Caucasians from Italy. *J Clin Endocrinol Metab.* 90(2), pp. 1176-80.

Canani LH, Capp C, Dora JM, Meyer EL, Wagner MS, Harney JW, Larsen PR, Gross JL, Bianco AC & Maia AL. (2005). The type 2 deiodinase A/G (Thr92Ala) polymorphism is associated with decreased enzyme velocity and increased insulin resistance in patients with type 2 diabetes mellitus. *J Clin Endocrinol Metab.* 90(6), pp. 3472-8.

Chagnon YC, Chung WK, Pérusse L, Chagnon M, Leibel RL & Bouchard C. (1999). Linkages and associations between the leptin receptor (LEPR) gene and human body composition in the Québec Family Study. *Int J Obes Relat Metab Disord.* 23(3), pp. 278-86.

Chagnon YC, Wilmore JH, Borecki IB, Gagnon J, Pérusse L, Chagnon M, Collier GR, Leon AS, Skinner JS, Rao DC & Bouchard C. (2000). Associations between the leptin receptor gene and adiposity in middle-aged Caucasian males from the HERITAGE family study. *J Clin Endocrinol Metab.* 85(1), pp. 29-34.

Chiu KC, Chuang LM &Yoon C. (2001). The A54T polymorphism at the intestinal fatty acid binding protein 2 is associated with insulin resistance in glucose tolerant Caucasians. *BMC Genet.* 2, pp. 7–13.

Choi K & Kim YB. (2010). Molecular mechanism of insulin resistance in obesity and type 2 diabetes. *Korean J Intern Med.* 25(2), pp. 119-29.

Conneely KN, Silander K, Scott LJ, Mohlke KL, Lazaridis KN, Valle TT, Tuomilehto J, Bergman RN, Watanabe RM, Buchanan TA, Collins FS & Boehnke M. (2004). Variation in the resistin gene is associated with obesity and insulin-related phenotypes in Finnish subjects. *Diabetologia.* 47(10), pp. 1782-8.

Craig RL, Chu WS & Elbein SC. (2007). Retinol binding protein 4 as a candidate gene for type 2 diabetes and prediabetic intermediate traits. *Mol Genet Metab.* 90(3), pp. 338-44.

D'Adamo M, Perego L, Cardellini M, Marini MA, Frontoni S, Andreozzi F, Sciacqua A, Lauro D, Sbraccia P, Federici M, Paganelli M, Pontiroli AE, Lauro R, Perticone F, Folli F & Sesti G. (2004). The -866A/A genotype in the promoter of the human uncoupling protein 2 gene is associated with insulin resistance and increased risk of type 2 diabetes. *Diabetes.* 53(7), pp. 1905-10.

Dalgaard LT, Andersen G, Larsen LH, Sørensen TI, Andersen T, Drivsholm T, Borch-Johnsen K, Fleckner J, Hansen T, Din N & Pedersen O. (2003). Mutational analysis of the UCP2 core promoter and relationships of variants with obesity. *Obes Res.* 11(11), pp. 1420-7.

de Luis DA, Gonzalez Sagrado M, Aller R, Izaola O & Conde R.(2008). Influence of Lys656Asn polymorphism of the leptin receptor gene on insulin resistance in nondiabetic obese patients. *J Diabetes Complications.* 22(3), pp. 199-204.

de Luis Roman D, de la Fuente RA, Sagrado MG, Izaola O & Vicente RC. (2006). Leptin receptor Lys656Asn polymorphism is associated with decreased leptin response and weight loss secondary to a lifestyle modification in obese patients. *Arch Med Res.* 37(7), pp. 854-9.

de Luis Roman DA, Aller R, Izaola Jauregui O, Gonzalez Sagrado M, Conde Vicente R, de la Fuente Salvador B & Romero Bobillo E. (2010). Relation of -55CT polymorphism of uncoupling protein 3 gene with fat mass and insulin resistance in morbidly obese patients. *Metabolism.* 59(4), pp. 608-12.

Després JP, Verdon MF, Moorjani S, Pouliot MC, Nadeau A, Bouchard C, Tremblay A & Lupien PJ. (1993). Apolipoprotein E polymorphism modifies relation of hyperinsulinemia to hypertriglyceridemia. *Diabetes.* 42, pp. 1474-81.

Ding EL, Song Y, Manson JE, Hunter DJ, Lee CC, Rifai N, Buring JE, Gaziano JM & Liu S. (2009). Sex hormone-binding globulin and risk of type 2 diabetes in women and men. *N Engl J Med.* 361(12), pp. 1152-63.

Di Renzo L, Bertoli A, Bigioni M, Del Gobbo V, Premrov MG, Calabrese V, Di Daniele N & De Lorenzo A. (2008). Body composition and -174G/C interleukin-6 promoter gene polymorphism: association with progression of insulin resistance in normal weight obese syndrome. *Curr Pharm Des.* 14(26), pp. 2699-706.

Dora JM, Machado WE, Rheinheimer J, Crispim D & Maia AL. (2010). Association of the type 2 deiodinase Thr92Ala polymorphism with type 2 diabetes: case-control study and meta-analysis. *Eur J Endocrinol.* 163(3), pp. 427-34.

Dunaif A. (1995). Hyperandrogenic anovulation (PCOS): a unique disorder of insulin action associated with an increased risk of non-insulin-dependent diabetes mellitus. *Am J Med.* 98(1A), pp. 33S-39S.

Eisenach JH & Wittwer ED. (2010). {beta}-Adrenoceptor gene variation and intermediate physiological traits: prediction of distant phenotype. *Exp Physiol.* 95(7), pp. 757-64.

Elosua R, Demissie S, Cupples LA, Meigs JB, Wilson PW, Schaefer EJ, Corella D & Ordovas JM. (2003). Obesity modulates the association among APOE genotype, insulin, and glucose in men. *Obes Res.* 11:1502-8.

Erion DM & Shulman GI. (2010). Diacylglycerol-mediated insulin resistance. *Nat Med.* 16(4), pp. 400-2.

Feng RN, Li Y & Sun CH (2009a) TNF 308 G/A polymorphism and type 1 diabetes: a meta-analysis. *Diab Res Clin Pract* 85, pp. e4–e7.

Feng R, Li Y, Zhao D, Wang C, Niu Y & Sun C. (2009b). Lack of association between TNF 238 G/A polymorphism and type 2 diabetes: a meta-analysis. *Acta Diabetol* 46, pp. 339–343.

Feng RN, Zhao C, Sun CH & Li Y. (2011). Meta-Analysis of TNF 308 G/A Polymorphism and Type 2 Diabetes Mellitus. *PLoS One* 6, pp. e18480.

Ferguson JF, Phillips CM, Tierney AC, Pérez-Martínez P, Defoort C, Helal O, Lairon D, Planells R, Shaw DI, Lovegrove JA, Gjelstad IM, Drevon CA, Blaak EE, Saris WH, Leszczynska-Golabek I, Kiec-Wilk B, Risérus U, Karlström B, Miranda JL & Roche HM. (2010). Gene-nutrient interactions in the metabolic syndrome: single nucleotide polymorphisms in ADIPOQ and ADIPOR1 interact with plasma saturated fatty acids to modulate insulin resistance. *Am J Clin Nutr.* 91(3), pp. 794-801.

Fernández-Real JM, Gutierrez C, Ricart W, Casamitjana R, Fernández-Castañer M, Vendrell J, Richart C & Soler J. (1997). The TNF-alpha gene Nco I polymorphism influences the relationship among insulin resistance, percent body fat, and increased serum leptin levels. *Diabetes.* 46(9), pp. 1468-72.

Filippi E, Sentinelli F, Trischitta V, Romeo S, Arca M, Leonetti F, Di Mario U & Baroni MG. (2004). Association of the human adiponectin gene and insulin resistance. *Eur J Hum Genet.* 12(3), pp. 199-205.

Fredriksson J, Anevski D, Almgren P, Sjögren M, Lyssenko V, Carlson J, Isomaa B, Taskinen MR, Groop L, Orho-Melander M & Botnia Study Group. (2007). Variation in GYS1 interacts with exercise and gender to predict cardiovascular mortality. *PLoS One.* 2, pp. e285.

Friebe D, Kovacs P, Neef M, Blüher S, Schleinitz D, Kiess W & Körner A. (2011). The promoter variant -803G>A in the RBP4 gene is not associated with BMI, metabolic parameters or blood pressure in Caucasian children. *Exp Clin Endocrinol Diabetes.* 119(10), pp. 628-32.

Gable DR, Stephens JW, Cooper JA, Miller GJ & Humphries SE. (2006). Variation in the UCP2-UCP3 gene cluster predicts the development of type 2 diabetes in healthy middle-aged men. *Diabetes* 55, pp. 1504- 1511.

Gao J, Katagiri H, Ishigaki Y, Yamada T, Ogihara T, Imai J, Uno K, Hasegawa Y, Kanzaki M, Yamamoto TT, Ishibashi S & Oka Y. (2007). Involvement of apolipoprotein E in excess fat accumulation and insulin resistance. *Diabetes.* 56, pp. 24-33.

Goyenechea E, Parra D & Martínez JA. (2007). Impact of interleukin 6 -174G>C polymorphism on obesity-related metabolic disorders in people with excess in body weight. *Metabolism.* 56(12), pp. 1643-8.

Grarup N, Andersen MK, Andreasen CH, Albrechtsen A, Borch-Johnsen K, Jørgensen T, Auwerx J, Schmitz O, Hansen T & Pedersen O. (2007). Studies of the common DIO2 Thr92Ala polymorphism and metabolic phenotypes in 7342 Danish white subjects. *J Clin Endocrinol Metab.* 92(1), pp. 363-6.

Grozovsky R, Ribich S, Rosene ML, Mulcahey MA, Huang SA, Patti ME, Bianco AC & Kim BW. (2009). Type 2 deiodinase expression is induced by peroxisomal proliferator-activated receptor-gamma agonists in skeletal myocytes. *Endocrinology.* 150(4), pp. 1976-83.

Gu P, Jiang W, Chen M, Lu B, Shao J, Du H & Jiang S. (2012). Association of leptin receptor gene polymorphisms and essential hypertension in a Chinese population. *J Endocrinol Invest.*

Gupta V, Gupta A, Jafar T, Gupta V, Agrawal S, Srivastava N, Kumar S, Singh AK, Natu SM, Agarwal CG & Agarwal GG. (2012). Association of TNF-α promoter gene G-308A polymorphism with metabolic syndrome, insulin resistance, serum TNF-α and leptin levels in Indian adult women. *Cytokine.* 57(1), pp. 32-6.

Hara K, Boutin P, Mori Y, Tobe K, Dina C, Yasuda K, Yamauchi T, Otabe S, Okada T, Eto K, Kadowaki H, Hagura R, Akanuma Y, Yazaki Y, Nagai R, Taniyama M, Matsubara K, Yoda M, Nakano Y, Tomita M, Kimura S, Ito C, Froguel P & Kadowaki T. (2002). Genetic variation in the gene encoding adiponectin is associated with an increased risk of type 2 diabetes in the Japanese population. *Diabetes.* 51(2), pp. 536-40.

Henneman P, Aulchenko YS, Frants RR, Zorkoltseva IV, Zillikens MC, Frolich M, Oostra BA, van Dijk KW & van Duijn CM. (2010). Genetic architecture of plasma adiponectin overlaps with the genetics of metabolic syndrome-related traits. *Diabetes Care.* 33(4), pp. 908-13.

Herbert A, Liu C, Karamohamed S, Liu J, Manning A, Fox CS, Meigs JB & Cupples LA. (2006). BMI modifies associations of IL-6 genotypes with insulin resistance: the Framingham Study. *Obesity* (Silver Spring). 14(8), pp. 1454-61.

Higashiura K, Ura N, Takada T, Li Y, Torii T, Togashi N, Takada M, Takizawa H & Shimamoto K. (2000). The effects of an angiotensin-converting enzyme inhibitor and an angiotensin II receptor antagonist on insulin resistance in fructose-fed rats. *Am J Hypertens.* 13(3), pp. 290-7.

Hivert MF, Manning AK, McAteer JB, Florez JC, Dupuis J, Fox CS, O'Donnell CJ, Cupples LA & Meigs JB. (2008). Common variants in the adiponectin gene (ADIPOQ) associated with plasma adiponectin levels, type 2 diabetes, and diabetes-related quantitative traits: the Framingham Offspring Study. *Diabetes* 57, pp. 3353–3359.

Hoffstedt J, Eriksson P, Hellström L, Rössner S, Rydén M & Arner P. (2000). Excessive fat accumulation is associated with the TNF alpha-308 G/A promoter polymorphism in women but not in men. *Diabetologia.* 43(1), pp. 117-20.

Hotamisligil GS, Shargill NS & Spiegelman BM. (1993). Adipose expression of tumour necrosis factor-alpha: direct role in obesity-linked insulin resistance. *Science.* 259, pp. 87–91.

Hotamisligil GS & Spiegelman BM. (1994). Tumour necrosis factor alpha: a key component of the obesity-diabetes link. *Diabetes.* 43, pp. 1271–8.

Hotamisligil GS, Murray DL, Choy LN & Spiegelman BM. (1994). Tumor necrosis factor alpha inhibits signaling from the insulin receptor. *Proc Natl Acad Sci U S A.* 91, pp. 4854–8.

Hu FB, Meigs JB, Li TY, Rifai N & Manson JE. (2004). Inflammatory markers and risk of developing type 2 diabetes in women. *Diabetes.* 53, pp. 693–700.

Hung J, McQuillan BM, Thompson PL & Beilby JP. (2008). Circulating adiponectin levels associate with inflammatory markers, insulin resistance and metabolic syndrome independent of obesity. *Int J Obes* (Lond) 32, pp. 772–779

Jin JJ, Nakura J, Wu Z, Yamamoto M, Abe M, Chen Y, Tabara Y, Yamamoto Y, Igase M, Bo X, Kohara K & Miki T. (2003). Association of angiotensin II type 2 receptor gene variant with hypertension. *Hypertens Res.* 26(7), pp. 547-52.

Kamizono S, Yamada K, Seki N, Higuchi T, Kimura A, Nonaka K & Itoh K. (2000). Susceptible locus for obese type 2 diabetes mellitus in the 5'-flanking region of the tumor necrosis factor-alpha gene. *Tissue Antigens.* 55(5), pp. 449-52.

Katsuki A, Sumida Y, Murashima S, Murata K, Takarada Y, Ito K, Fujii M, Tsuchihashi K, Goto H, Nakatani K & Yano Y. (1998). Serum levels of tumor necrosis factor-alpha are increased in obese patients with noninsulin-dependent diabetes mellitus. *J Clin Endocrinol Metab.* 83(3), pp. 859-62.

Katsuya T, Horiuchi M, Chen YD, Koike G, Pratt RE, Dzau VJ & Reaven GM. (1995). Relations between deletion polymorphism of the angiotensin-converting enzyme gene and insulin resistance, glucose intolerance, hyperinsulinemia, and dyslipidemia. *Arterioscler Thromb Vasc Biol.* 15(6), pp. 779-82.

Kikuya M, Sugimoto K, Katsuya T, Suzuki M, Sato T, Funahashi J, Katoh R, Kazama I, Michimata M, Araki T, Hozawa A, Tsuji I, Ogihara T, Yanagisawa T, Imai Y & Matsubara M. (2003). A/C1166 gene polymorphism of the angiotensin II type 1 receptor (AT1) and ambulatory blood pressure: the Ohasama Study. *Hypertens Res.* 26(2), pp. 141-5.

Kim CH, Yun SK, Byun DW, Yoo MH, Lee KU & Suh KI. (2001). Codon 54 polymorphism of the fatty acid binding protein 2 gene is associated with increased fat oxidation and hyperinsulinemia, but not with intestinal fatty acid absorption in Korean men. *Metabolism.* 50(4), pp. 473-6.

Komurcu-Bayrak E, Onat A, Yuzbasiogullari B, Mononen N, Laaksonen R, Kähönen M, Hergenc G, Lehtimäki T & Erginel-Unaltuna N. (2011). The APOE -219G/T and +113G/C polymorphisms affect insulin resistance among Turks. *Metabolism.* 60(5), pp. 655-63.

Kondo H, Shimomura I, Matsukawa Y, Kumada M, Takahashi M, Matsuda M, Ouchi N, Kihara S, Kawamoto T, Sumitsuji S, Funahashi T & Matsuzawa Y. (2002). Association of adiponectin mutation with type 2 diabetes: a candidate gene for the insulin resistance syndrome. *Diabetes.* 51(7), pp. 2325-8.

Kovacs P, Ma L, Hanson RL, Franks P, Stumvoll M, Bogardus C & Baier LJ. (2005). Genetic variation in UCP2 (uncoupling protein-2) is associated with energy metabolism in Pima Indians. *Diabetologia.* 48(11), pp. 2292-5.

Kovacs P, Geyer M, Berndt J, Klöting N, Graham TE, Böttcher Y, Enigk B, Tönjes A, Schleinitz D, Schön MR, Kahn BB, Blüher M & Stumvoll M. (2007). Effects of genetic variation in the human retinol binding protein-4 gene (RBP4) on insulin resistance and fat depot-specific mRNA expression. *Diabetes.* 56(12), pp. 3095-100.

Krempler F, Esterbauer H, Weitgasser R, Ebenbichler C, Patsch JR, Miller K, Xie M, Linnemayr V, Oberkofler H & Patsch W. (2002). A functional polymorphism in the promoter of UCP2 enhances obesity risk but reduces type 2 diabetes risk in obese middle-aged humans. *Diabetes.* 51(11), pp. 3331-5.

Kubaszek A, Pihlajamäki J, Komarovski V, Lindi V, Lindström J, Eriksson J, Valle TT, Hämäläinen H, Ilanne-Parikka P, Keinänen-Kiukaanniemi S, Tuomilehto J, Uusitupa M, Laakso M & Finnish Diabetes Prevention Study. (2003). Promoter polymorphisms of the TNF-alpha (G-308A) and IL-6 (C-174G) genes predict the conversion from impaired glucose tolerance to type 2 diabetes: the Finnish Diabetes Prevention Study. *Diabetes.* 52(7), pp. 1872-6.

Kypreos KE, Karagiannides I, Fotiadou EH, Karavia EA, Brinkmeier MS, Giakoumi SM & Tsompanidi EM. (2009). Mechanisms of obesity and related pathologies: role of apolipoprotein E in the development of obesity. *FEBS J.* 276, pp. 5720-8.

Lakka HM, Oksanen L, Tuomainen TP, Kontula K & Salonen JT. (2000). The common pent-nucleotide polymorphism of the 3- untranslated region of the leptin receptor gene is associated with serum insulin levels and the risk of type 2 diabetes in non-diabetic men: a prospective case-control study. *J Intern Med* 248, pp. 77-83.

Lambert JC, Brousseau T, Defosse V, Evans A, Arveiler D, Ruidavets JB, Haas B, Cambou JP, Luc G, Ducimetière P, Cambien F, Chartier-Harlin MC & Amouyel P. (2000). Independent association of an APOE gene promoter polymorphism with increased risk of myocardial infarction and decreased APOE plasma concentrations-the ECTIM study. *Hum Mol Genet.* 9, pp. 57-61.

Lee JH, Chan JL, Yiannakouris N, Kontogianni M, Estrada E, Seip R, Orlova C & Mantzoros CS. (2003). Circulating resistin levels are not associated with obesity or insulin resistance in humans and are not regulated by fasting or leptin administration: cross-sectional and interventional studies in normal, insulin-resistant, and diabetic subjects. *J Clin Endocrinol Metab.* 88(10), pp. 4848-56.

Le Stunff C, Le Bihan C, Schork NJ & Bougnères P. (2000). A common promoter variant of the leptin gene is associated with changes in the relationship between serum leptin and fat mass in obese girls. *Diabetes*. 49(12), pp. 2196-200.

Lima JJ, Feng H, Duckworth L, Wang J, Sylvester JE, Kissoon N & Garg H. (2007). Association analyses of adrenergic receptor polymorphisms with obesity and metabolic alterations. *Metabolism*. 56(6), pp. 757-65.

Lindsay RS, Funahashi T, Hanson RL, Matsuzawa Y, Tanaka S, Tataranni PA, Knowler WC, Krakoff J. (2002). Adiponectin and development of type 2 diabetes in the Pima Indian population. *Lancet*. 6;360(9326):57-8.

Lyssenko V, Almgren P, Anevski D, Orho-Melander M, Sjögren M, Saloranta C, Tuomi T, Groop L & Botnia Study Group. (2005). Genetic prediction of future type 2 diabetes. *PLoS Med.* 2(12), pp. e345.

Maeda N, Takahashi M, Funahashi T, Kihara S, Nishizawa H, Kishida K, Nagaretani H, Matsuda M, Komuro R, Ouchi N, Kuriyama H, Hotta K, Nakamura T, Shimomura I & Matsuzawa Y. (2001). PPARgamma ligands increase expression and plasma concentrations of adiponectin, an adipose-derived protein. *Diabetes.* 50(9), pp. 2094-9.

Maia AL, Dupuis J, Manning A, Liu C, Meigs JB, Cupples LA, Larsen PR & Fox CS. (2007). The type 2 deiodinase (DIO2) A/G polymorphism is not associated with glycemic traits: the Framingham Heart Study. *Thyroid.* 17(3), pp. 199-202.

Mammès O, Betoulle D, Aubert R, Giraud V, Tuzet S, Petiet A, Colas-Linhart N & Fumeron F. (1998). Novel polymorphisms in the 5' region of the LEP gene: association with leptin levels and response to low-calorie diet in human obesity. *Diabetes*. 47(3) pp. 487-9.

Mammès O, Betoulle D, Aubert R, Herbeth B, Siest G & Fumeron F. (2000). Association of the G-2548A polymorphism in the 5' region of the LEP gene with overweight. *Ann Hum Genet*. 64(Pt 5), pp.391-4.

Mansego ML, Martínez F, Martínez-Larrad MT, Zabena C, Rojo G, Morcillo S, Soriguer F, Martín-Escudero JC, Serrano-Ríos M, Redon J & Chaves FJ. (2012). Common variants of the liver Fatty Acid binding protein gene influence the risk of type 2 diabetes and insulin resistance in spanish population. *PLoS One.* 7(3), pp. e31853.

Mårin P, Holmäng S, Jönsson L, Sjöström L, Kvist H, Holm G, Lindstedt G & Björntorp P. (1992). The effects of testosterone treatment on body composition and metabolism in middle-aged obese men. *Int J Obes Relat Metab Disord.* 16(12), pp. 991-7.

Matthews DR, Hosker JP, Rudenski AS, Naylor BA, Treacher DF, Turner RC. (1985). Homeostasis model assessment: insulin resistance and beta-cell function from fasting plasma glucose and insulin concentrations in man. *Diabetologia* 28, pp. 412– 9.

Meigs JB, Ordovas JM, Cupples LA, Singer DE, Nathan DM, Schaefer EJ & Wilson PW. (2000). Apolipoprotein E isoform polymorphisms are not associated with insulin resistance: the Framingham Offspring Study. *Diabetes Care.* 23, pp. 669-74.

Melistas L, Mantzoros CS, Kontogianni M, Antonopoulou S, Ordovas JM & Yiannakouris N. (2009). Association of the +45T>G and +276G>T polymorphisms in the adiponectin gene with insulin resistance in nondiabetic Greek women. *Eur J Endocrinol.* 161(6), pp. 845-52.

Mentuccia D, Proietti-Pannunzi L, Tanner K, Bacci V, Pollin TI, Poehlman ET, Shuldiner AR & Celi FS. (2002). Association between a novel variant of the human type 2 deiodinase gene Thr92Ala and insulin resistance: evidence of interaction with the Trp64Arg variant of the beta-3-adrenergic receptor. *Diabetes.* 51(3), pp. 880-3.

Mentuccia D, Thomas MJ, Coppotelli G, Reinhart LJ, Mitchell BD, Shuldiner AR & Celi FS. (2005). The Thr92Ala deiodinase type 2 (DIO2) variant is not associated with type 2 diabetes or indices of insulin resistance in the old order of Amish. *Thyroid.* 15(11), pp. 1223-7.

Menzaghi C, Ercolino T, Di Paola R, Berg AH, Warram JH, Scherer PE, Trischitta V & Doria A. (2002). A haplotype at the adiponectin locus is associated with obesity and other features of the insulin resistance syndrome. *Diabetes.* 51(7), pp. 2306-12.

Menzaghi C, Trischitta V & Doria A.(2007). Genetic influences of adiponectin on insulin resistance, type 2 diabetes, and cardiovascular disease. *Diabetes* 56, pp. 1198–209.

Mitchell BD, Kammerer CM, O'Connell P, Harrison CR, Manire M, Shipman P, Moyer MP, Stern MP & Frazier ML. (1995). Evidence for linkage of postchallenge insulin levels with intestinal fatty acid-binding protein (FABP2) in Mexican-Americans. *Diabetes.* 44(9), pp. 1046-53.

Möhlig M, Wegewitz U, Osterhoff M, Isken F, Ristow M, Pfeiffer AF & Spranger J. (2002). Insulin decreases human adiponectin plasma levels. *Horm Metab Res* 34, pp. 655–658.

Möhlig M, Boeing H, Spranger J, Osterhoff M, Kroke A, Fisher E, Bergmann MM, Ristow M, Hoffmann K & Pfeiffer AF. (2004). Body mass index and C-174G interleukin-6 promoter polymorphism interact in predicting type 2 diabetes. *J Clin Endocrinol Metab.* 89(4), pp. 1885-90.

Morcillo S, Martín-Núñez GM, Rojo-Martínez G, Almaraz MC, García-Escobar E, Mansego ML, de Marco G, Chaves FJ & Soriguer F. (2011). ELOVL6 genetic variation is related to insulin sensitivity: a new candidate gene in energy metabolism. *PLoS One.* 6(6), pp. e21198.

Moreno JA, López-Miranda J, Marín C, Gómez P, Pérez-Martínez P, Fuentes F, Fernández de la Puebla RA, Paniagua JA, Ordovas JM & Pérez-Jiménez F.(2003). The influence of the apolipoprotein E gene promoter (-219G/ T) polymorphism on postprandial lipoprotein metabolism in young normolipemic males. *J Lipid Res.* 44, pp. 2059-64.

Moreno JA, Pérez-Jiménez F, Marín C, Pérez-Martínez P, Moreno R, Gómez P, Jiménez-Gómez Y, Paniagua JA, Lairon D & López-Miranda J. (2005). The apolipoprotein E gene promoter (-219G/T) polymorphism determines insulin sensitivity in response to dietary fat in healthy young adults. *J Nutr.* 135, pp. 2535-40.

Mottagui-Tabar S, Hoffstedt J, Brookes AJ, Jiao H, Arner P & Dahlman I. (2008). Association of ADRB1 and UCP3 gene polymorphisms with insulin sensitivity but not obesity. *Horm Res.* 69(1), pp. 31-6.

Munkhtulga L, Nakayama K, Utsumi N, Yanagisawa Y, Gotoh T, Omi T, Kumada M, Erdenebulgan B, Zolzaya K, Lkhagvasuren T & Iwamoto S. (2007). Identification of a regulatory SNP in the retinol binding protein 4 gene associated with type 2 diabetes in Mongolia. *Hum Genet.* 120(6), pp. 879-88.

Munkhtulga L, Nagashima S, Nakayama K, Utsumi N, Yanagisawa Y, Gotoh T, Omi T, Kumada M, Zolzaya K, Lkhagvasuren T, Kagawa Y, Fujiwara H, Hosoya Y, Hyodo M,

Horie H, Kojima M, Ishibashi S & Iwamoto S. (2010). Regulatory SNP in the RBP4 gene modified the expression in adipocytes and associated with BMI. *Obesity* (Silver Spring). 18(5), pp. 1006-14.

Muoio DM & Newgard CB. (2008). Mechanisms of disease: molecular and metabolic mechanisms of insulin resistance and beta-cell failure in type 2 diabetes. *Nat Rev Mol Cell Biol.* 9(3), pp. 193-205.

Ochoa MC, Santos JL, Azcona C, Moreno-Aliaga MJ, Martínez-González MA, Martínez JA, Marti A & GENOI Members. (2007). Association between obesity and insulin resistance with UCP2-UCP3 gene variants in Spanish children and adolescents. *Mol Genet Metab.* 92(4), pp. 351-8.

Ohara M, Maesawa C, Takebe N, Takahashi T, Yamashina M, Ono M, Matsui M, Sasai T, Honma H, Nagasawa K, Fujiwara F, Kajiwara T, Taneichi H, Takahashi K & Satoh J. (2012). Different susceptibility to insulin resistance and fatty liver depending on the combination of TNF-α C-857T and adiponectin G+276T gene polymorphisms in Japanese subjects with type 2 diabetes. *Tohoku J Exp Med.* 226(2), pp. 161-9.

Ono K, Mannami T, Baba S, Yasui N, Ogihara T & Iwai N. (2003). Lack of association between angiotensin II type 1 receptor gene polymorphism and hypertension in Japanese. *Hypertens Res* 26, pp. 131–134.

Osawa H, Yamada K, Onuma H, Murakami A, Ochi M, Kawata H, Nishimiya T, Niiya T, Shimizu I, Nishida W, Hashiramoto M, Kanatsuka A, Fujii Y, Ohashi J & Makino H. (2004). The G/G genotype of a resistin single-nucleotide polymorphism at -420 increases type 2 diabetes mellitus susceptibility by inducing promoter activity through specific binding of Sp1/3. *Am J Hum Genet.* 75(4), pp. 678-86.

Osawa H, Tabara Y, Kawamoto R, Ohashi J, Ochi M, Onuma H, Nishida W, Yamada K, Nakura J, Kohara K, Miki T & Makino H. (2007). Plasma resistin, associated with single nucleotide polymorphism -420, is correlated with insulin resistance, lower HDL cholesterol, and high-sensitivity C-reactive protein in the Japanese general, pp.population. *Diabetes Care.* 30(6):1501-6.

Peeters RP, van der Deure WM, van den Beld AW, van Toor H, Lamberts SW, Janssen JA, Uitterlinden AG &Visser TJ. (2007). The Asp727Glu polymorphism in the TSH receptor is associated with insulin resistance in healthy elderly men. *Clin Endocrinol* (Oxf). 66(6), pp. 808-15.

Perry JR, Weedon MN, Langenberg C, Jackson AU, Lyssenko V, Sparsø T, Thorleifsson G, Grallert H, Ferrucci L, Maggio M, Paolisso G, Walker M, Palmer CN, Payne F, Young E, Herder C, Narisu N, Morken MA, Bonnycastle LL, Owen KR, Shields B, Knight B, Bennett A, Groves CJ, Ruokonen A, Jarvelin MR, Pearson E, Pascoe L, Ferrannini E, Bornstein SR, Stringham HM, Scott LJ, Kuusisto J, Nilsson P, Neptin M, Gjesing AP, Pisinger C, Lauritzen T, Sandbaek A, Sampson M; MAGIC, Zeggini E, Lindgren CM, Steinthorsdottir V, Thorsteinsdottir U, Hansen T, Schwarz P, Illig T, Laakso M, Stefansson K, Morris AD, Groop L, Pedersen O, Boehnke M, Barroso I, Wareham NJ, Hattersley AT, McCarthy MI & Frayling TM. (2010). Genetic evidence that raised sex hormone binding globulin (SHBG) levels reduce the risk of type 2 diabetes. *Hum Mol Genet.* 19(3), pp. 535-44.

Perseghin G, Petersen K & Shulman GI. (2003). Cellular mechanism of insulin resistance: potential links with inflammation. *Int J Obes Relat Metab Disord.* 27 Suppl 3, pp. S6-11.

Perticone F, Ceravolo R, Iacopino S, Cloro C, Ventura G, Maio R, Gulletta E, Perrotti N & Mattioli PL. (2001). Relationship between angiotensin-converting enzyme gene polymorphism and insulin resistance in never-treated hypertensive patients. *J Clin Endocrinol Metab.* 86(1), pp. 172-8.

Pizzuti A, Argiolas A, Di Paola R, Baratta R, Rauseo A, Bozzali M, Vigneri R, Dallapiccola B, Trischitta V & Frittitta L. (2002). An ATG repeat in the 3'-untranslated region of the human resistin gene is associated with a decreased risk of insulin resistance. *J Clin Endocrinol Metab.* 87(9), pp. 4403-6.

Prochazka M, Lillioja S, Tait JF, Knowler WC, Mott DM, Spraul M, Bennett PH & Bogardus C. (1993). Linkage of chromosomal markers on 4q with a putative gene determining maximal insulin action in Pima Indians. *Diabetes.* 42(4), pp. 514-9.

Qi L, van Dam RM, Meigs JB, Manson JE, Hunter D & Hu FB. (2006). Genetic variation in IL6 gene and type 2 diabetes: tagging-SNP haplotype analysis in large-scale case-control study and meta-analysis. *Hum Mol Genet.* 15(11), pp. 1914-20.

Quinton ND, Lee AJ, Ross RJ, Eastell R & Blakemore AI. (2001). A single nucleotide polymorphism (SNP) in the leptin receptor is associated with BMI, fat mass and leptin levels in postmenopausal Caucasian women. *Hum Genet* 108, pp. 233-6.

Rai E, Sharma S, Koul A, Bhat AK, Bhanwer AJ & Bamezai RN. (2007). Interaction between the UCP2-866G/A, mtDNA 10398G/A and PGC1alpha p.Thr394Thr and p.Gly482- Ser polymorphisms in type 2 diabetes susceptibility in North Indian population. *Hum Genet* 122, pp. 535-40.

Ranjith N, Pegoraro RJ, Naidoo DP, Shanmugam R & Rom L. (2008). Genetic variants associated with insulin resistance and metabolic syndrome in young Asian Indians with myocardial infarction. *Metab Syndr Relat Disord* 6(3), pp. 209–14.

Reaven GM. (1988). Banting lecture 1988. Role of insulin resistance in human disease. *Diabetes.* 37, pp. 1595-607.

Reaven GM. (1995). Pathophysiology of insulin resistance in human disease. *Physiol Rev* 75, pp. 473–86.

Reis AF, Dubois-Laforgue D, Bellanne-Chantelot C, Timsit J & Velho G. (2004). A polymorphism in the promoter of UCP2 gene modulates lipid levels in patients with type 2 diabetes. *Mol Genet Metab* 82: 339- 344.

Ren W, Zhang SH, Wu J & Ni YX. (2004). Polymorphism of the leptin gene promoter in pedigrees of type 2 diabetes mellitus in Chongqing, China. *Chin Med J* (Engl). 117(4), pp. 558-61

Santos JL, Boutin P, Verdich C, Holst C, Larsen LH, Toubro S, Dina C, Saris WH, Blaak EE, Hoffstedt J, Taylor MA, Polak J, Clement K, Langin D, Astrup A, Froguel P, Pedersen O, Sorensen TI, Martinez JA & NUGENOB* consortium.(2006). Genotype-by-nutrient interactions assessed in European obese women. A case-only study. *Eur J Nutr.* 45(8), pp. 454-62.

Shea JL, Loredo-Osti JC & Sun G. (2010). Association of RBP4 gene variants and serum HDL cholesterol levels in the Newfoundland population. *Obesity* (Silver Spring). 18(7), pp. 1393-7.

Sheng T & Yang K. (2008). Adiponectin and its association with insulin resistance and type 2 diabetes. J Genet *Genomics* 35, pp. 321–6.
Silha JV, Krsek M, Skrha JV, Sucharda P, Nyomba BL & Murphy LJ. (2003). Plasma resistin, adiponectin and leptin levels in lean and obese subjects: correlations with insulin resistance. *Eur J Endocrinol.* 149(4), pp. 331-5.
Simon D, Charles MA, Lahlou N, Nahoul K, Oppert JM, Gouault-Heilmann M, Lemort N, Thibult N, Joubert E, Balkau B & Eschwege E. (2001). Androgen therapy improves insulin sensitivity and decreases leptin level in healthy adult men with low plasma total testosterone: a 3-month randomized placebo-controlled trial. *Diabetes Care.* 24(12), pp. 2149-51.
Sipiläinen R, Uusitupa M, Heikkinen S, Rissanen A & Laakso M. (1997). Variants in the human intestinal fatty acid binding protein 2 gene in obese subjects. *J Clin Endocrinol Metab.* 82(8), pp. 2629-32.
Sookoian SC, González C & Pirola CJ. (2005). Meta-analysis on the G-308A tumor necrosis factor alpha gene variant and phenotypes associated with the metabolic syndrome. *Obes Res.* 13(12), pp. 2122-31
Spranger J, Kroke A, Möhlig M, Bergmann MM, Ristow M, Boeing H & Pfeiffer AF. (2003). Adiponectin and protection against type 2 diabetes mellitus. *Lancet.* 361(9353), pp. 226-8.
Stumvoll M, Tschritter O, Fritsche A, Staiger H, Renn W, Weisser M, Machicao F & Häring H. (2002). Association of the T-G polymorphism in adiponectin (exon 2) with obesity and insulin sensitivity: interaction with family history of type 2 diabetes. *Diabetes.* 51(1), pp. 37-41.
Sugimoto K, Katsuya T, Ohkubo T, Hozawa A, Yamamoto K, Matsuo A, Rakugi H, Tsuji I, Imai Y & Ogihara T. (2004). Association between angiotensin II type 1 receptor gene polymorphism and essential hypertension: the Ohasama Study. *Hypertens Res.* 27(8), pp. 551-6.
Takahashi-Yasuno A, Masuzaki H, Miyawaki T, Matsuoka N, Ogawa Y, Hayashi T, Hosoda K, Yoshimasa Y, Inoue G & Nakao K. (2004). Association of Ob-R gene polymorphism and insulin resistance in Japanese men. *Metabolism.* 53(5), pp. 650-4.
Tschritter O, Fritsche A, Thamer C, Haap M, Shirkavand F, Rahe S, Staiger H, Maerker E, Häring H & Stumvoll M. (2003). Plasma adiponectin concentrations predict insulin sensitivity of both glucose and lipid metabolism. *Diabetes.* 52(2), pp. 239-43.
Underwood PC, Chamarthi B, Williams JS, Sun B, Vaidya A, Raby BA, Lasky-Su J, Hopkins PN, Adler GK & Williams GH. (2012). Replication and meta-analysis of the gene-environment interaction between body mass index and the interleukin-6 promoter polymorphism with higher insulin resistance. *Metabolism.* 61, pp. 667-671.
Ura N, Higashiura K & Shimamoto K. (1999). The mechanisms of insulin sensitivity improving effects of angiotensin converting enzyme inhibitor. *Immunopharmacology* 44, pp. 153–159.
Urbanek M, Du Y, Silander K, Collins FS, Steppan CM, Strauss JF 3rd, Dunaif A, Spielman RS & Legro RS. (2003). Variation in resistin gene promoter not associated with polycystic ovary syndrome. *Diabetes.* 52(1), pp. 214-7

Valdez R, Howard BV, Stern MP & Haffner SM. (1995). Apolipoprotein E polymorphism and insulin levels in a biethnic population. *Diabetes Care.* 18, pp. 992-1000.

van Hoek M, Dehghan A, Zillikens MC, Hofman A, Witteman JC & Sijbrands EJ. (2008). An RBP4 promoter polymorphism increases risk of type 2 diabetes. *Diabetologia.* 51(8), pp. 1423-8.

Vasseur F, Helbecque N, Dina C, Lobbens S, Delannoy V, Gaget S, Boutin P, Vaxillaire M, Leprêtre F, Dupont S, Hara K, Clément K, Bihain B, Kadowaki T & Froguel P. (2002). Single-nucleotide polymorphism haplotypes in the both proximal promoter and exon 3 of the APM1 gene modulate adipocyte-secreted adiponectin hormone levels and contribute to the genetic risk for type 2 diabetes in French Caucasians. *Hum Mol Genet.* 11(21), pp. 2607-14.

Vendrell J, Fernandez-Real JM, Gutierrez C, Zamora A, Simon I, Bardaji A, Ricart W & Richart C. (2003). A polymorphism in the promoter of the tumor necrosis factor-alpha gene (-308) is associated with coronary heart disease in type 2 diabetic patients. *Atherosclerosis.* 167(2), pp. 257-64.

Viitanen L, Pihlajamäki J, Miettinen R, Kärkkäinen P, Vauhkonen I, Halonen P, Kareinen A, Lehto S & Laakso M. (2001). Apolipoprotein E gene promoter (-219G/T) polymorphism is associated with premature coronary heart disease. *J Mol Med.* 79, pp. 732-7.

Wang H, Chu WS, Hemphill C & Elbein SC. (2002). Human resistin gene: molecular scanning and evaluation of association with insulin sensitivity and type 2 diabetes in Caucasians. *J Clin Endocrinol Metab.* 87(6), pp. 2520-4.

Wang H, Chu WS, Lu T, Hasstedt SJ, Kern PA &Elbein SC. (2004). Uncoupling protein-2 polymorphisms in type 2 diabetes, obesity, and insulin secretion. *Am J Physiol Endocrinol Metab* 286, pp. E1-E7.

Wannamethee SG, Lowe GD, Rumley A, Cherry L, Whincup PH & Sattar N. (2007). Adipokines and risk of type 2 diabetes in older men. *Diabetes Care.* 30, pp. 1200–1205.

Wauters M, Mertens I, Rankinen T, Chagnon M, Bouchard C & Van Gaal L. (2001). Leptin receptor gene polymorphisms are associated with insulin in obese women with impaired glucose tolerance. *J Clin Endocrinol Metab.* 86(7), pp. 3227-32.

Wauters M, Considine RV, Chagnon M, Mertens I, Rankinen T, Bouchard C & Van Gaal LF.(2002). Leptin levels, leptin receptor gene polymorphisms, and energy metabolism in women. *Obes Res.* 10(5), pp. 394-400.

Weinstein SP, O'Boyle E & Haber RS. (1994). Thyroid hormone increases basal and insulin-stimulated glucose transport in skeletal muscle. The role of GLUT4 glucose transporter expression. *Diabetes.* 43(10), pp. 1185-9.

Weiss EP, Brown MD, Shuldiner AR & Hagberg JM. (2002). Fatty acid binding protein 2 gene variants and insulin resistance: gene and gene-environmental interaction effects. *Physiol Genomics.* 10, pp. 145–57.

Xu K, Zhang M, Cui D, Fu Y, Qian L, Gu R, Wang M, Shen C, Yu R & Yang T. (2011). UCP2 -866G/A and Ala55Val, and UCP3 -55C/T polymorphisms in association with type 2 diabetes susceptibility: a meta-analysis study. *Diabetologia.* 54(9), pp. 2315-24.

Yamada K, Yuan X, Ishiyama S, Koyama K, Ichikawa F, Koyanagi A, Koyama W& Nonaka K. (1997). Association between Ala54Thr substitution of the fatty acid-binding protein 2 gene with insulin resistance and intra-abdominal fat thickness in Japanese men. *Diabetologia.* 40(6), pp. 706-10.

Yamamoto J, Kageyama S, Sakurai T, Ishibashi K, Mimura A, Yokota K, Aihara K, Taniguchi I, Yoshida H & Tajima N. (1999). Insulin resistance and angiotensin converting enzyme polymorphism in Japanese hypertensive subjects. *Hypertens Res.* 22(2), pp. 81-4.

Yang Q, Graham TE, Mody N, Preitner F, Peroni OD, Zabolotny JM, Kotani K, Quadro L & Kahn BB. (2005). Serum retinol binding protein 4 contributes to insulin resistance in obesity and type 2 diabetes. *Nature.* 436(7049), pp. 356-62.

Zee RY, Ridker PM & Chasman DI. (2011). Mitochondrial uncoupling protein gene cluster variation (UCP2-UCP3) and the risk of incident type 2 diabetes mellitus: the Women's Genome Health Study. *Atherosclerosis* 214, pp. 107- 109.

Zeggini E, Scott LJ, Saxena R, Voight BF, Marchini JL, Hu T, de Bakker PI, Abecasis GR, Almgren P, Andersen G, Ardlie K, Boström KB, Bergman RN, Bonnycastle LL, Borch-Johnsen K, Burtt NP, Chen H, Chines PS, Daly MJ, Deodhar P, Ding CJ, Doney AS, Duren WL, Elliott KS, Erdos MR, Frayling TM, Freathy RM, Gianniny L, Grallert H, Grarup N, Groves CJ, Guiducci C, Hansen T, Herder C, Hitman GA, Hughes TE, Isomaa B, Jackson AU, Jørgensen T, Kong A, Kubalanza K, Kuruvilla FG, Kuusisto J, Langenberg C, Lango H, Lauritzen T, Li Y, Lindgren CM, Lyssenko V, Marvelle AF, Meisinger C, Midthjell K, Mohlke KL, Morken MA, Morris AD, Narisu N, Nilsson P, Owen KR, Palmer CN, Payne F, Perry JR, Pettersen E, Platou C, Prokopenko I, Qi L, Qin L, Rayner NW, Rees M, Roix JJ, Sandbaek A, Shields B, Sjögren M, Steinthorsdottir V, Stringham HM, Swift AJ, Thorleifsson G, Thorsteinsdottir U, Timpson NJ, Tuomi T, Tuomilehto J, Walker M, Watanabe RM, Weedon MN, Willer CJ; Wellcome Trust Case Control Consortium, Illig T, Hveem K, Hu FB, Laakso M, Stefansson K, Pedersen O, Wareham NJ, Barroso I, Hattersley AT, Collins FS, Groop L, McCarthy MI, Boehnke M & Altshuler D. (2008). Meta-analysis of genome-wide association data and large-scale replication identifies additional susceptibility loci for type 2 diabetes. *Nat Genet.* 40(5), pp. 638-45.

Zimmerman AW & Veerkamp JH. (2002). New insights into the structure and function of fatty acid-binding proteins. *Cell Mol Life Sci.* 59(7), pp. 1096-116.

Zinman B, Hanley AJ, Harris SB, Kwan J& Fantus G. (1999). Circulating tumor necrosis factor α concentrations in a native Canadian population with high rates of type 2 diabetes mellitus. *J Clin Endocrinol Metab.* 84, pp. 272–8.

Section 2

Epidemiology of Insulin Resistance

Chapter 4

The Metabolic Syndrome in Hispanics – The Role of Insulin Resistance and Inflammation

Pablo I. Altieri, José M. Marcial, Nelson Escobales,
María Crespo and Héctor L. Banchs

Additional information is available at the end of the chapter

http://dx.doi.org/10.5772/50337

1. Introduction

The acknowledgment of the metabolic syndrome (MetS) as a pathological entity is one of the most important advancements in the management of cardiovascular disease in the last 2 decades. Increasing awareness and research of this syndrome has led to a deeper understanding of how different metabolic risk factors such as inflammation, insulin resistance and vascular pathologies such as coronary heart disease (CHD) interact and aggravate one another. The existence of MetS may imply uniformity in pathology across a range of populations. However, this is not the case: the mechanisms that underlie MetS and the cardiometabolic consequences they hold may very well vary between ethnicities. The following chapter aims to encompass MetS from its most fundamental principles with a focus on inflammation and insulin resistance to the novel research pertaining to its pathophysiology and management, with an emphatic eye on the Hispanic population.

2. Metabolic syndrome in Hispanics

The inner workings of MetS have yet to be fully elucidated; thus it remains difficult to evaluate how they differ between specific ethnic populations. Nevertheless, it remains a possibility that the processes involved in the syndrome, such as insulin resistance and inflammation, differ in degree and function with relation to Hispanic compared to non-Hispanic populations. It has been a recurring theme that the interactions between poor nutritional status, physical inactivity, and genetic predisposition might contribute to the disparities in the prevalence and characteristics of MetS and its components between ethnicities and the subgroups within; this subject has been studied to the extent that even the diagnostic criteria for MetS established by the AHA/NHLBI were challenged when adapted to a specific Andean population[1]. Moreover, researchers have found that a single DNA variation in the form of a guanine base pair on a gene already linked to a higher risk of Coronary Heart Disease (CHD) in other races confers a fivefold reduction in risk in African-Americans[2]. Lately, research has uncovered mutations in the Brain-derived neurotrophic factor (BDNF) gene, or *Bdnf* gene, which result in human obesity[58]. Mice having a truncated long *Bdnf* 3′ UTR genetic transcript developed severe hyperphagic obesity. In these mice, the ability of the adipocytokine leptin to activate hypothalamic neurons and inhibit food intake was compromised despite normal activation of leptin receptors. All these studies, whether they involve humans or mice, provide a window into a genetic basis for MetS.

Despite the obvious limits of studying a population that does not represent the entire Hispanic world, investigations exploring cardiovascular disease and MetS in Puerto Ricans provide invaluable information in understanding the interrelationship between genetics, environment and culture in the modification of cardiovascular health. Previous data support the fact that, given the same cardiovascular risk factors, Puerto Rico has a lower prevalence of CHD than other fully industrialized countries such as the United States[3]; however, the validity of these data may not be as strong today as when published nearly 3 decades ago: recent epidemiologic data show that, although mortality from CHD and stroke has been steadily decreasing in the United States in the past 4 decades, it has been increasing in Puerto Rico[4]. On the other hand, a recent investigation that examined the medical records of 173 patients with MetS who received treatment in the Cardiovascular Center of Puerto Rico and the Caribbean showed that these patients were devoid of aggressive CHD, meaning less ventricular tachycardia, less myocardial infarctions and less strokes, and had a relatively normal lipid profile (except for a mild elevation in serum triglycerides)[5], supporting the notion that island-based Puerto Ricans acquire a milder form of MetS than mainland populations (this notion extends to Hispanics and Caucasians living in the continental U.S.).[6] Furthermore, several investigators have reported that the incidence of ventricular tachycardia, a complication caused by remodeling and ischemia of the heart, is lower in Puerto Rico than in the United States[7], even when adjusting for a higher prevalence of MetS in Puerto Rico[8]. Interestingly, the number of cases recorded in this study showed an increased incidence of atrial fibrillation[9]; this may be thought to be a result of differential remodelling of the left ventricle and atrial function between ethnicities. In addition, the prevalence of CHD is lower in Puerto Rico than in the United States, despite a higher incidence of Diabetes Mellitus in the island than in the U.S. (16% vs. 8%)[10]. Nonetheless, the prevalence of CHD in Puerto Rico is increasing: In the 1980s, it was 50% lower than in the United States; it is only 20% lower today[10]. This is most likely due to external factors such as the increasingly unhealthy diet and sedentary lifestyle of many of the island's inhabitants.

3. Importance of the Renin-Angiotensin System (RAS)

The RAS is a complicated and essential system in the regulation of vascular homeostasis. Angiotensin II (AngII) is cleaved from angiotensin I (AngI) by angiotensin converting enzyme (ACE), which is localized on the surface of endothelial cells and in the media and adventia of the aorta[11]; a soluble form of ACE is also found in plasma. AngI is formed from angiotensinogen, which is secreted from the liver and cleaved by renin, which in turn is found in the juxta-glomerular cells in the kidney[12]. The traditional RAS inhibitors, angiotensin-converting enzyme inhibitors (ACE inhibitors) and angiotensin receptor blockers (ARBs), target the main RAS axis described above. However, there are additional enzymes associated with the production of AngII, such as by Cathepsin G[13], as well as other, more novel angiotensin molecules that serve as potential therapeutic targets: the ACE2/Ang-(1–9) axis is a new and important pathway to compensate for the vasoconstrictive and hyperproliferative RAS axis. A direct mechanism implicated in the production of these distinctive angiontensin molecules involves ACE2[14], a novel component of the RAS that converts AngI to Ang-(1-9) and AngII to Ang-(1-7), a peptide with vasodilator and anti-proliferative properties. The induction of ACE2 not only holds therapeutic promise by producing the anti-inflammatory Ang-(1-7), but also by reducing AngII levels, thereby conferring a twofold protection against cardiovascular remodeling from ongoing hypertension and inflammation.

Concomitant to the progression of the RAS, hyperglycemia promotes the deposition of advanced glycation end products (AGEs) that are formed from the non-enzymatic glycation of proteins and lipids after contact with reducing sugars[15]. The accumulation of AGEs is an important factor in the development and progression of vascular injury in diabetes-associated atherosclerosis. Both hyperglycemia and induction of the main RAS axis will increase oxidative stress and increase the rate of the atherosclerotic process that ultimately end in apoptosis and necrosis of myocytes[16, 17], hence propagating the deleterious effects of inflammation, insulin resistance and endothelial dysfunction.

The inhibition of the RAS by ACE inhibitors and ARBs has been mainstay therapy to reduce the onset and/or progression of hypertension, left ventricular dysfunction, diabetic renal disease and atherosclerosis. For example, inhibitors of the RAS seem to be more effective than other medications in halting the progression of dilated cardiomyopathy in hamsters that have an inherited mutation that predisposes to such a disease[18]. In rodents, pharmacological or genetic disruption of RAS action prevents weight-gain, promotes insulin sensitivity and relieves hypertension[19], suggesting that ACE inhibitors or ARBs may present an effective treatment for MetS in humans. In addition, when obese individuals lose weight, both adipose tissue mass and systemic RAS activity are reduced[20,21]. An increase in adipose tissue angiotensinogen has been reported in diet-induced obesity[22,23]: further evidence that lifestyle changes are integral to targeting the underlying mechanisms of MetS.

4. Inflammation and insulin resistance

Systemic inflammation[24-25] is a fundamental process in the development of cardiovascular disease in patients with MetS, and this process starts with the activation of the neuro-hormonal system; we have data that shows elevated intra-coronary levels of AngII and endothelin I (EI) in some patients with Diabetes Mellitus Type 2 (DMT2). We measured these peptides in 5 patients with DMT2 and concomitant MetS, normal coronary arteries and sub-normal ejection fraction (49 ± 5%), and discovered that the levels of AngII and EI were elevated in the coronary sinus (coronary efflux) and aorta of these patients when compared to the control group, which consisted of 5 patients with DMT2 but without MetS that were catheterized and found to have normal coronary arteries and a normal ejection fraction[26]. In the former, MetS group, AngII levels inside the coronary sinus and aorta were 46 ± 18 and 35 ± 15 pg/ml, respectively, while AngII levels were 10 ± 2 pg/ml inside both chambers of the control group ($P < 0.001$). Furthermore, in the group with MetS, the EI levels inside the coronary sinus and aorta were elevated at 14 ± 4 and 13 ± 6 pg/ml in both chambers, respectively, compared to 3 ± 1 pg/ml inside both chambers of the control group ($P < 0.001$).

This elevation of AngII and EI will activate angiotensin II receptor type 1 (AT1) and produce inflammatory cytokines, increase macrophage chemo-attractants and activate reactive oxygen species that produce oxidative stress in myocytes and smooth muscle cells[27]. This will not only induce the apoptosis and necrosis of myocytes, but also promote the proliferation and migration of smooth muscle cells, resulting in the atherosclerotic lesions that increase the incidence of myocardial infarcts[28]. Likewise, AngII, acting via angiotensin II receptor type 2 (AT2), has potent pro-inflammatory, pro-oxidant and pro-thrombotic effects[29]. Moreover, it has been shown that infusion of AngII in rats increases serum levels of AGEs. The oxidative and apoptotic effects of both hyperglycemia and AngII are most likely key in inducing diabetic cardiomyopathy[27,28], which explains why our patients with MetS have a subnormal ejection fraction, as opposed to the patients without MetS who have a normal ejection fraction, despite normal coronary arteries in both groups.

Omega-3, eicosapentaenoic acid (EPA) and docosahexaenoic acid (OHA) have also been shown to be anti-inflammatory; they are enzymatically converted to resolvins, which are very potent anti-inflammatory agents[30]. Resolvins diminish the activation and production of superoxide, increase nitric oxide and decrease inflammatory cytokines- this mechanism will counterbalance inflammation and, as a consequence, insulin resistance. It has been shown that Omega-3 in high doses will reduce the incidence of myocardial infarction and, in some patients, revert insulin resistance. We have reported the normalization of the 2-hour post-prandial levels of blood sugar with the use of Omega-3[6]. The mean 2-hour post-prandial glucose levels in 10 patients decreased from a mean value of 205±40mg/dl to 119±13mg/dl ($P<0.003$). This change occurred after using 6000mg per day of pure Omega-3 for about 6 months. The effect of Omega-3 is mediated through the insulin receptors of the cells. At present, we are studying these receptors in order to explain this increase in insulin sensibility.

Adipose tissue is a hormonally active endocrine tissue, producing cytokines, which influence other body tissues. Adiponectin is one such adipocytokine that protects cardiovascular tissue from ischemic injury and increases insulin sensitivity by stimulating fatty acid oxidation, decreasing plasma triglycerides and improving glucose metabolism[33,34]. Another adipocytokine, secreted-frizzled-related-protein-5 (Sfrp5), has been found to have significant metabolic consequences; incorporation of Wnt signaling pathways, which classically regulate developmental processes in many organisms, in adipocytes has led to evidence that obesity induces a reduction in the Sfrp5 production along with an increase in Wnt5a expression, leading to augmented inflammatory signalling and insulin resistance[36]. Conversely, Sfrp5 acts as an anti-inflammatory molecule, restraining the chronic inflammatory state and improving insulin sensitivity. On the other hand, tumor necrosis factor- α (TNF-α) and interleukin-6 (IL-6) are insulin antagonizing adipocytokines[37] that are associated to augmentation of inflammation and insulin resistance. As seen, inflammation is a complicated issue in obesity that has to be stopped due to deleterious effects produced in the cardiovascular system, such as the reduction in ejection fraction observed in our sample of patients with MetS and normal coronaries: a diabetic cardiomyopathy undoubtedly brought on by chronic inflammation and insulin resistance[40].

Insulin resistance is a fundamental mechanism underlying MetS and its components. Insulin is an anabolic hormone that exerts its effects primarily by promoting glycogen synthesis in the liver and muscle, increasing triglyceride synthesis in adipose tissue, and augmenting protein synthesis and inhibiting proteolysis. Therefore, the consequences of insulin resistance are multiple-fold. Truly, there are other processes involved in the development of insulin resistance other than inflammation. Abnormalities in fat storage and mobilization have been implicated in the pathogenesis of insulin resistance[38]. Abdominal obesity in particular has been shown to be most associated with insulin resistance and MetS. However, it has been observed that general obesity is not universal in MetS and insulin resistance. In addition, many obese subjects do not have metabolic abnormalities. Systemic chronic inflammation[39], on the other hand, paints the most complete picture of insulin resistance as it is the result of all altered cytokine production and signaling pathways in the body. A more accessible marker for this inflammation can be obtained by measuring C-reactive protein (CRP); 40% of our patients with MetS had an elevated CRP. Clinically, each of the diagnostic component criteria of the metabolic syndrome has been associated with increased levels of CRP[41], elevation of which bears a negative prognostic implication in the population involved - this biomarker has been associated to the development of heart disease, although this observation is not totally clear[31,32]. CRP production is located in the liver, a process induced by pro-inflammatory cytokines; this non-specific marker of inflammation has an important role in the host innate defense mechanism, but also regulates the amount of inflammatory response by activating the complement system. CRP can be used to monitor the status of the inflammatory system, and has been used to monitor the effect of statins in the inflammatory process of MetS[35]. In the Jupiter trial, rosuvastatin (20mg/day) reduced the systemic marker of CRP.

Finally, a novel and important piece in the development of insulin resistance consists of aldosterone-induced insulin resistance through the increase in insulin-like growth factor-1 (IGF-1) and hybrid receptors[42]. This research has demonstrated that aldosterone induces vascular remodeling through the IGF-1 and hybrid receptors and suggests that blocking the effects of aldosterone may attenuate and reduce angiopathy in hypertensive patients with hyperinsulinemia.

5. Circadian rhythm and the metabolic syndrome

Common disorders of circadian behavior and sleep, such as night-shift work and jetlag, are associated with increased hunger, decreased glucose and lipid metabolism and changes in hormonal processes involved in satiety[43]. Short-duration and poor-quality sleep have been shown to predict the development of DMT2 and obesity after age, BMI and various other confounding variables are considered and taken into account[44]. In addition, the induction of hunger may be associated to a reduction in circulating levels of leptin brought on by sleep deprivation[45]. Cardiovascular disease and hypertension are also related with sleep loss, as the risk of a fatal heart attack increases 45% in individuals who chronically sleep 5 hours per night or less[46]. Disruption of the circadian clock can lead to obesity, inflammation and insulin resistance[47].

6. Management

6.1. Diet and exercise

Lifestyle approaches to treating and preventing MetS greatly improve metabolic parameters by reducing body weight and increasing the level of physical activity. Multiple studies of obese patients with DMT2, hypertension or hypercholesterolemia have shown that weight improves the cardiovascular profile, including glycemic control, in both diabetic and non-diabetic individuals. Furthermore, lifestyle changes[48] comprising reduced total/saturated fat intake and increased polyunsaturated fat/fiber intake have been shown to significantly reduce multiple metabolic and inflammatory parameters such as CRP, central obesity and triglyceride levels. The ATTICA[49] epidemiological study showed that adherence to the Mediterranean diet was associated with 20% lower odds of having MetS, irrespective of age, sex, physical activity, lipids and blood pressure levels. On the other hand, consumption of a high fat diet induces changes in the fat microbia, producing inflammation that is associated with hyperphagia and an obese phenotype. In addition, data on the Hispanic and Asian diets with relation to diabetes have demonstrated that rice consumption is associated to an elevated risk of developing DMT2, presumably due to the higher glycemic index of rice when compared to whole grain[50]. Physical activity is a cornerstone in weight balance. However, only part of the beneficial effect of physical activity on the metabolic and cardiovascular profile is mediated through body weight changes. Physical activity improves insulin sensitivity, increases HDL levels, lowers blood pressure and maintains immune system health, which is very important in reducing inflammation and, as a consequence, insulin resistance[51].

6.2. Pharmacotherapy

Although intensified therapeutic lifestyle modifications may prevent the onset and progression of MetS, some patients may require drug therapy. While the individual components (e.g. glucose intolerance, hypertension, dyslipidemia) are all appropriate targets for treatment, newer therapies that manage the syndrome centrally may benefit from such a collective approach and thus prove more effective. Although traditional approaches to the separate risk factors have proven effective, increasing attention is now being directed at the management of insulin resistance, obesity and inflammation. Orlistat, sibutramine, and rimonabant are approved for long-term treatment of obesity; however, sibutramine is known to cause secondary hypertension and thus is not the ideal choice of therapy in obese patients with MetS. As was mentioned above, statins and RAS inhibitors have proven anti-inflammatory properties that may augment insulin sensitivity. Glitazones and metformin have been used increasingly over the recent years for the management of insulin resistance. The ongoing search for new strategies to combat the MetS has shed light on new molecules that may prove to be effective therapeutic targets in treating the syndrome; in vivo studies have established that atherosclerosis driven by the inhibition of stearoyl-coenzyme A desaturase 1 (SCD1), an enzyme involved in fatty acid metabolism, can be completely prevented by the omega-3 polyunsaturated fatty acids in dietary fish-oils[52]. Moreover, our data showing that in some patients, high doses of omega-3 polyunsaturated fatty acids will normalize the 2-hour post-prandial glucose levels in a sample from Puerto Rico is promising.

6.3. Bariatric surgery

Given that lifestyle changes and pharmacology may not be sufficient to achieve durable and effective weight loss, surgery to treat obesity and MetS has become an attractive alternative. In addition to weight loss, patients may enjoy improvement in other metabolic parameters such as insulin resistance and other obesity-related comorbidies. Bariatric surgery has been shown to reverse diabetes, hypertension, sleep apnea and hyperlipidemia[53], however, selection of candidates must be a strict process in view of peri- and postoperative complications and costs associated with different surgical procedures.

7. Social importance

The economic cost of combating obesity and associated comorbidies is estimated to exceed $100 billion annually in the United States[54]. With recent data showing the increasing burden of obesity throughout the world, it can be expected that the rates of MetS will be increasing. A study that aims to assess the independent contributions of MetS and its individual components to 10-year medical costs among a sample of elderly individuals showed that total costs to Medicare were 20% higher among participants with the MetS[55]. Another study found that risk factors for metabolic syndrome, such as obesity, high blood pressure, and elevated blood lipid levels, can increase a person's healthcare costs nearly 1.6-fold, or about $2,000 per year; for each additional risk factor those costs rise an average of 24%[56]. These figures are even more alarming in the context of the prevalence of the MetS in relation to socio-economic position: social class has been shown to have an inverse relation to MetS[57].

8. Conclusion

In an age when millions of people are estimated to be afflicted by the MetS, new perspectives into this cluster of risk factors are imperative if we are to evolve its management: the focus on inflammation and insulin resistance is crucial in order to halt or delay the disease as soon as it is detected. Moreover, the public health of Hispanic populations throughout the world has been evidenced to pose a significant public health problem that should be addressed specifically because of the distinct metabolic characteristics this ethnicity may hold. Likewise, this approach should prompt further investigation into parallel cardiometabolic particularities in other ethnicities.

Author details

Pablo I. Altieri, José M. Marcial, Nelson Escobales, María Crespo and Héctor L. Banchs
Department of Medicine and Physiology, University of Puerto Rico, Medical Sciences Campus, San Juan, Puerto Rico and The Cardiovascular Center of Puerto Rico and the Caribbean, Puerto Rico

9. References

[1] Medina-Lezama, J., *et al.* Optimal definitions for abdominal obesity and the metabolic syndrome in Andean Hispanics: the PREVENCION study. *Diabetes Care* 33, 1385-1388 (2010).

[2] Brian G. Kral, R.A.M., Bhoom Suktitipat, Ingo Ruczinski, Dhananjay Vaiya, Lisa R. Yanek, Arshed A. Quyyumi, Riyaz S. Patel, A Maziar Zafari, Viola Vaccarino, Elizabeth R. Hauser, William E. Kraus, Lewes C. Becker, Diane M. Becker. A common variant in the CD2KN2B gene on chromosome 9p21 protects against coronary artery disease in Americans of African ancestry. *Journal of Human Genetics* (2011).

[3] Garcia Palmieri MR, C.R., Cruz VW, Cortes AM, Colon A, Filiberty M, Ayala AM, PAttern D, Sobrino R, Torres R, Navarro M. Risk factors and prevalence of Coronary Heart Disease in Puerto Rico. *Circulation* 42, 541-542 (1970).

[4] Capewell, S., *et al.* Cardiovascular risk factor trends and potential for reducing coronary heart disease mortality in the United States of America. *Bull World Health Organ* 88, 120-130 (2010).

[5] Altieri P, B.H., Escobales N, Crespo M & Figueroa Y A Less Aggressive Metabolic Syndrome In Puerto Rico than in the United States. *J Investigative Med.* 2009: P2.

[6] Altieri P, B.H., Escobales N & Crespo M. . Metabolic Syndrome - Variability In Cultures and Interventional Management. 2nd World Congress On Interventional Therapies For Type 2 Diabetes. 2011: P4.

[7] Altieri, P., Garcia Palmieri MR. Sudden Death in Puerto Rico: A United States Caribbean Island. *Revista Latina de Cardiologia.* 1993: 14-17.

[8] Marcial J, Altieri PI, Banchs HL, Escobales N, Crespo M. Metabolic Syndrome among Puerto Ricans and others Hispanic populations. PRHSJ. 2011; 30 (3): 145-151.

[9] Altieri P, Figueroa Y, Banchs H, Henandez Gil de Lamadrid, Escobales N, Crespo M. Higher incidence of atrial fibrillation in the metabolic syndrome: A Hispanic population study. Boletín Asociación Médica de Puerto Rico, Año 103. 2011; 4: 24-27.

[10] U.S.Government Medical Statistics-2010

[11] Armal JF, Battle T, Rasetti C, Challah M, Costerousse O, Vincaut E, Michel JB, Alhene-Gelas F. ACE in three tunicae of rat aorta expression in smooth muscle and effect of renovascular hypertension. AMJ Physiol 1994; 267: H1777-H1784

[12] Woodman ZL, Oppong SY, Cooks Hooper NM, Schwager SL, Brand WF, Ehlers MR, Sturrock ED. Shedding of somatic angiotensin converting enzyme (ACE) is inefficient compared with testis ACE despite cleavage at identiacal stalk sites. Biochem J. 2000; 347:711-718.

[13] Rykl, J., *et al.* Renal cathepsin G and angiotensin II generation. *J Hypertens* 24, 1797-1807 (2006).

[14] Ocaranza, M.P. & Jalil, J.E. Protective Role of the ACE2/Ang-(1-9) Axis in Cardiovascular Remodeling. *Int J Hypertens* 2012, 594361 (2012).

[15] Yasunarik K, Kohono M, Kano H, Yakokawa K, Horio T, Yushikawa J. Aldose Hyperproliferation and hypertrophy of cultured rat vascular smooth muscle cell induced by high glucose. Arterioscler Thromb Vasc Biol. 1995; 15:2207-2212.

[16] Goldin, Beckman JA, Schmidt AM, Creager MA. Advanced glycation end products sparking the development of diabetic vascular injury. *Circulation*. 2006; 114:597-605.

[17] Guzik T, Mussa S, Gastald D, Sadowski J, Ratnatunga C, Pillai R, Channon KM. Machanism of increased vascular superoxide production in human diabetes mellitus. *Circulation*. 2002; 105:1656-1662.

[18] Crespo, M.J., Cruz, N., Altieri, P.I. & Escobales, N. Enalapril and losartan are more effective than carvedilol in preventing dilated cardiomyopathy in the Syrian cardiomyopathic hamster. *J Cardiovasc Pharmacol Ther* 13, 199-206 (2008).

[19] de Kloet, A.D., Krause, E.G. & Woods, S.C. The renin angiotensin system and the metabolic syndrome. *Physiol Behav* 100, 525-534 (2010).

[20] Strazzullo, P. & Galletti, F. Impact of the renin-angiotensin system on lipid and carbohydrate metabolism. *Curr Opin Nephrol Hypertens* 13, 325-332 (2004).

[21] Engeli, S., *et al.* Weight loss and the renin-angiotensin-aldosterone system. *Hypertension* 45, 356-362 (2005).

[22] Boustany, C.M., *et al.* Activation of the systemic and adipose renin-angiotensin system in rats with diet-induced obesity and hypertension. *Am J Physiol Regul Integr Comp Physiol* 287, R943-949 (2004).

[23] Rahmouni, K., Mark, A.L., Haynes, W.G. & Sigmund, C.D. Adipose depot-specific modulation of angiotensinogen gene expression in diet-induced obesity. *Am J Physiol Endocrinol Metab* 286, E891-895 (2004).

[24] Fuster V., Badimon JJ, Chesebro JH. The pathogenesis of Coronary Artery Disease and Acute Coronary Syndrome. *N Engl J Med*. Part 1 and 2, 1992; 326, 242-50, 310-8.

[25] Fuster V, Lewis A. Conner Memorial Lecture. Mechanism Leading to Myocardial Infarction: In Sights from Studies of Vascular Biology. *Circulation*. 1994; 90:2126-46.

[26] Altieri P., Alvarado S., Banchs H., Escobales N., Crespo M. The role of Angiotensin II and Endothelin I in the cardiomyopathy of diabetic patients. *J Investigative Med* 2012; 81

[27] Heeneman S, Sluimer J, Daemen Mat JAP. Angiotensin converting enzyme and vascular remodeling. *Circ Res*. 2007; 101:441-454.

[28] Goldberg IJ, Dansky HM, Diabetic vascular disease. *Arterioscler Thromb Vasc. Biol*. 2006; 26:1693-1701.

[29] Kaschina E, Grzesiak A, Li J, et al. Angiotensin II Type II receptor stimulation. A novel option of therapeutic interference with the renin-angiotensin system in myocardial infarction. *Circulation*. 2008; 118:2523-2532.

[30] Spite M, Serham CN. Novel lipid mediators promote resolution of acute inflammation-impact of aspirin and statins. *Cir Res*. 2010; 107:1170-1184.

[31] Kanes R, Rosuvastatin Inflammation, C-Reactive Protein, Jupiter and Primary Prevention of Cardiovascular Disease a Perspective. *Drug Des Devel Ther*. 2010 Dec 9; 4: 383-413.

[32] Elkind MS, Tai Coates K, Daik MC, Saccor L. High Sensitivity C-Reactive Protein, Lipoprotein-Associated Phospholipase A 2 and Outcome After Ischemic Stroke. Arch Intern Med 2006 Oct 23; 166 (19): 2073-80.

[33] Ouchi N, Kihara S, Funahashi T, Matsuzawa Y, Walsh K. Obesity, adiponectin and vascular inflammatory disease. Curr Opin Lipidol. 2003 Dec;14(6):561-6.

[34] R Shibata et al. Adiponectin protects against myocardial ischemia-reperfusion injury through AMPK- and COX-2–dependent mechanisms. Nat Med 11. 2005; 1096-1103.

[35] Davignon J, Jacob RF, Mason RP. The Antioxidant Effect of Statins. Coron Artery Dis. 2004 Aug; 15(5): 251-8.

[36] Ouchi, Noriyuki; Higuchi, Akiko; Ohashi, Koji; Oshima, Yuichi; Gokce, Noyan; Shibata, Rei; Akasaki, Yuichi; Shimono, Akihiko; Walsh, Kenneth. Sfrp5 Is an Anti-Inflammatory Adipokine That Modulates Metabolic Dysfunction in Obesity. Science 2010; 329: 454-457.

[37] Pittas, A.G., Joseph, N.A. & Greenberg, A.S. Adipocytokines and insulin resistance. *J Clin Endocrinol Metab* 89, 447-452 (2004)..

[38] Lewis GF, Carpentier A, Adeli K, Giacca A. Disordered fat storage and mobilizatin in the pathogenesis of insulin resistance and Type 2 diabetes. Endocr Rev. 2002; 23:201-29.

[39] Sjostrand M, Eriksson JVV. Neuroendocrine mechanisms in insulin resistance. Mol Cell Endocrinol. 2009; 297:104-111.

[40] Altieri P, Albarado S, Banchs H, Escobales N, Crespo M. The role of angiotensin II and Endothelin I in the cardiomyopathy of diabetic patients. J Investigative Med. 2012: 81.

[41] Ridker PM, Buring JE, Cook NR & Rifai N. C-reactive protein, the metabolic syndrome, and risk of incident cardiovascular events: an 8-year follow-up of 14,719 initially healthy American women. Circulation 2003; 107:391-397.

[42] Sherajee S, Fujita Y, Rafig K, et al. Aldosterone induces vascular insulin like growth factor I receptor and hybrid receptor. Arterioscler Thromb Vasc Biol. 2012; 32:257-263.

[43] Knutson, K.L. & Van Cauter, E. Associations between sleep loss and increased risk of obesity and diabetes. *Ann N Y Acad Sci* 1129, 287-304 (2008).

[44] Lumeng, J.C., *et al.* Shorter sleep duration is associated with increased risk for being overweight at ages 9 to 12 years. *Pediatrics* 120, 1020-1029 (2007).

[45] Taheri, S., Lin, L., Austin, D., Young, T. & Mignot, E. Short sleep duration is associated with reduced leptin, elevated ghrelin, and increased body mass index. *PLoS Med* 1, e62 (2004).

[46] Ayas, N.T., *et al.* A prospective study of sleep duration and coronary heart disease in women. *Arch Intern Med* 163, 205-209 (2003).

[47] Challet E, Delezie J. Interactions between metabolism and circadian clocks: reciprocal disturbances. An NY Acad Sci. 2011 Dec; 1243:30-46.

[48] Bo, S., *et al.* Effectiveness of a lifestyle intervention on metabolic syndrome. A randomized controlled trial. *J Gen Intern Med* 22, 1695-1703 (2007).

[49] Panagiotakos, D.B., *et al.* Impact of lifestyle habits on the prevalence of the metabolic syndrome among Greek adults from the ATTICA study. *Am Heart J* 147, 106-112 (2004).

[50] Sun A, Spegelman D, Van Dam R et. al. White rice, brown rice, and risk of diabetes type 2 in U.S. men and women. Arch Inter Med. 2010; 170:961-9.

[51] Walsh NP, Gleeson M, Pyne DB et. al. Position statement. Part two: Maintaining immune health. Exerc Immunol Rev. 2011; 17:64-103.

[52] Brown, J.M., *et al.* Combined therapy of dietary fish oil and stearoyl-CoA desaturase 1 inhibition prevents the metabolic syndrome and atherosclerosis. *Arterioscler Thromb Vasc Biol* 30, 24-30 (2010).

[53] Buchwald, H., *et al.* Bariatric surgery: a systematic review and meta-analysis. *JAMA* 292, 1724-1737 (2004).

[54] Wolf, A.M. & Colditz, G.A. Current estimates of the economic cost of obesity in the United States. *Obes Res* 6, 97-106 (1998).

[55] Curtis, L.H., *et al.* Costs of the metabolic syndrome in elderly individuals: findings from the Cardiovascular Health Study. *Diabetes Care* 30, 2553-2558 (2007).

[56] Boudreau, D.M., *et al.* Health care utilization and costs by metabolic syndrome risk factors. *Metab Syndr Relat Disord* 7, 305-314 (2009).

[57] Ramsay, S.E., Whincup, P.H., Morris, R., Lennon, L. & Wannamethee, S.G. Is socioeconomic position related to the prevalence of metabolic syndrome?: influence of social class across the life course in a population-based study of older men. *Diabetes Care* 31, 2380-2382 (2008).

[58] Liao, G.Y., *et al.* Dendritically targeted Bdnf mRNA is essential for energy balance and response to leptin. *Nat Med* 18, 564-571 (2012).

Section 3

Role of Obesity and Neuropeptides in Insulin Resistance

Chapter 5

Appetite Regulatory Peptides and Insulin Resistance

Maria Orbetzova

Additional information is available at the end of the chapter

http://dx.doi.org/10.5772/50977

1. Introduction

The discovery of leptin in 1994 provoked the interest in the adipose tissue which was no longer considered as an inert tissue storing energy in the form of triglycerides but as the greatest endocrine organ in human body [1, 2]. As a growing number of people suffer from obesity and metabolic syndrome, understanding the mechanisms by which various hormones and neurotransmitters have influence on energy balance, weight control and insulin resistance has been a subject of intensive research.

The regulation of appetite and feeding is a homeostatic mechanism. A powerful and complex physiological system exists to balance energy intake and expenditure, in order that sufficient energy is available and body weight remains stable [2, 3]. This system is composed of both afferent signals and efferent effectors. A large number of factors originating throughout the body send afferent signals to a smaller number of functional centers in the central nervous system (CNS), that then mediate interactions with efferent pathways to regulate energy expenditure and energy intake [4]. Thus, central circuits in the brain rely on peripheral signals indicating satiety levels and energy stores, as well as higher cortical factors such as emotional and reward pathways [5].

There are numerous peptides involved in the regulation of energy homeostasis, some of which are produced centrally and others peripherally in the gastrointestinal tract (GI), with some produced at both locations. These peptides are known as members of the 'gut-brain axis' [6]. Since the discovery of secretin, which was confirmed to stimulate pancreatic exocrine secretion, more than 40 other GI tract hormones have been discovered. Anticipation of a meal and the presence of food in the stomach and the small intestine stimulate secretion of many of these hormones from the gut through mechanical and chemical stimuli. These signals are involved in the initiation of food intake as well as termination of meals [7]. However, many of the same hormones are also expressed in the

CNS, acting to translate metabolic information between the GI tract and the brain [8]. In normal subjects, body weight is tightly regulated despite day-to-day variations in food intake and energy expenditure. Obesity is due to a state in which energy intake exceeds energy expenditure over a prolonged period of time. In humans it is also of note that psychological and emotional factors can drive food intake in excess of actual need [7].

In summary, signals relaying information such as the nutritional and energy status of the body converge within the CNS. Thus, CNS mediates energy balance in the body, the hypothalamus playing a main role in this process. The arcuate nucleus (ARC) is a key hypothalamic nucleus in the regulation of appetite and is involved in integrating peripheral satiety and adiposity signals via orexigenic and anorexigenic neuropeptide transmission to other hypothalamic and extrahypothalamic brain regions [9]. Proximity of ARC to the median eminence and the fact that it is not fully insulated from the circulation by the blood brain barrier makes it strategically positioned to integrate the great number of peripheral signals controlling food intake [5]. There are two major neuronal populations in the ARC implicated in the regulation of feeding. One population co-expresses Neuropeptide Y (NPY) and agouti-related protein (AgRP) and increases food intake. The second population of neurons co-expresses cocaine- and amphetamine-related transcript (CART) and pro-opiomelanocortin (POMC), the precursor to the melanocortin receptor agonist, α-melanocyte-stimulating hormone (α-MSH), and inhibits food intake. Neuronal projections from these two populations then communicate with other hypothalamic areas involved in appetite regulation such as the paraventricular nucleus (PVN), ventromedial nucleus (VMN), dorsomedial nucleus (DMN) and lateral hypothalamic area (LHA) [10].

Receptors for leptin and insulin are expressed on both of these types of neurons, suggesting that they are responsive to circulating levels of these hormonal signals, acting as effectors for altering food intake in response to variations in energy balance as indicated by body adiposity [11]. Leptin is secreted by adipocytes and circulates at concentrations proportional to fat mass. Restriction of food intake for a relatively longer period, results in a supression of leptin levels, which can be reversed by refeeding or administration of insulin. Insulin is a major metabolic hormone. Like leptin, levels of plasma insulin vary directly with changes in adiposity being influenced to a great extent by peripheral insulin sensitivity. The latter is related to total body fat stores and fat distribution, with visceral fat being the key determinant [12]. Plasma insulin increases at times of positive energy balance and decreases at times of negative energy balance. However, unlike leptin, insulin secretion increases rapidly after a meal, whereas leptin levels are relatively insensitive to meal ingestion. Both leptin and insulin cross the blood-brain barrier, stimulate anorexigenic α-MSH/CART neurons and inhibit orexigenic NPY/AgRP neurons, thus activating the catabolic pathways and inhibiting the anabolic pathways (Figure 1). When energy stores are low, production of leptin from adipose tissue, and thus circulating leptin concentrations fall, leading to increased production of hypothalamic neurotransmitters that strongly increase food intake, such as NPY, galanin, and AgRP and decreased levels of α-MSH, CART, and neurotensin that reduce food intake and increase energy expenditure [8, 13].

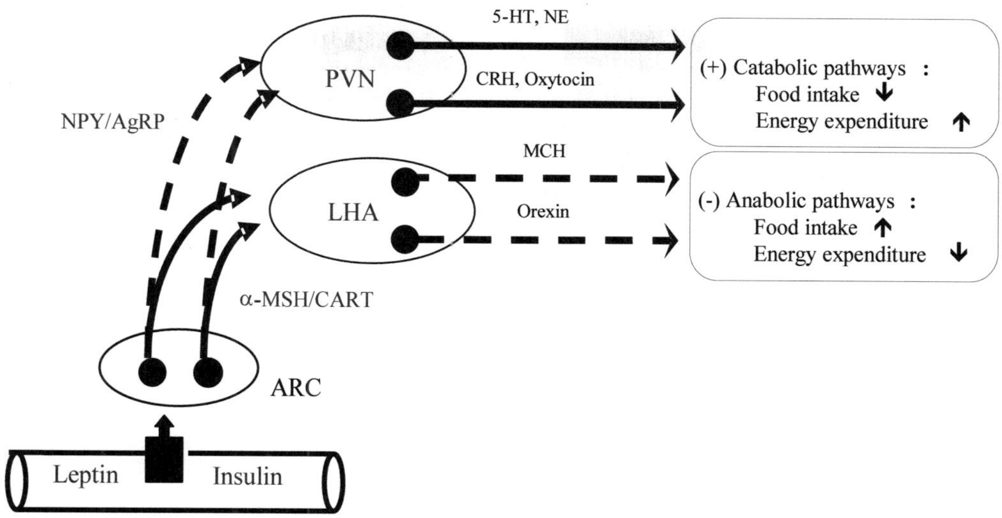

CRH, corticotrophin-releasing hormone; MCH, melanin-concentrating hormone, 5-HT, 5-hydroxytryptamine; NE, norepinephrine; (- - →) inhibition; (→) stimulation.

Figure 1. Schematic action of leptin and insulin on the hypothalamus.

In addition to leptin and insulin, receptors for ghrelin are also located on arcuate AgRP/NPY neurons, which are activated by central ghrelin administration. Furthermore, peripheral ghrelin administration activates neurons in the ARC and AgRP and NPY have been demonstrated to be requisite mediators of the hyperphagia induced by systemic ghrelin [11]. So, meal-generated satiety signals from the GI tract do interact with longer-term adiposity signals, such as insulin and leptin in energy balance [8].

NPY is one of the most abundant peptides of the hypothalamus and one of the most potent orexigenic factors. The majority of neurons expressing NPY in the hypothalamus are found within the ARC and most co-express AgRP [14]. Synthesis and release of NPY are both regulated by leptin binding to its hypothalamic receptor. NPY links afferents reflecting the nutritional status of the organism from endocrine, gastrointestinal, and central and peripheral nervous systems to effectors of energy intake and expenditure [15]. NPY stimulates appetite inducing hyperphagia, increase of fat depots, decrease of thermogenesis, and suppression of sympathetic activity. NPY is known to be involved in other physiological functions, such as cardiovascular regulation, affective disorder, memory retention, neuroendocrine control. When leptin levels increase after food intake, the latter binds to its receptors in the hypothalamus which leads to discontinuation of NPY secretion [5, 16]. The decrease of NPY concentration in obesity probably plays a role of a counter-regulatory factor intended to prevent further weight gain. Thus, NPY becomes one of the main regulators of food intake, body weight and energy expenditure.

Ghrelin is a fast-acting hormone, seemingly playing a role in meal initiation. Secreted predominantly from the stomach, ghrelin is the natural ligand for the growth hormone secretagogue-receptor (GHS-R) in the pituitary gland, thus fulfilling the criteria of a brain–

gut peptide [5, 6]. Although the majority of ghrelin is produced peripherally, there are ghrelin immunoreactive neurons within the hypothalamus that have terminals on hypothalamic NPY/AgRP, POMC and corticotropin releasing hormone (CRH) neurons [17], as well as orexin fibres in the LHA [18]. It was found that ghrelin acts to promote appetite in two ways—directly, by depolarizing the orexigenic NPY/AgRP neurons, and indirectly, by increasing the tonic inhibition exerted by the NPY/AgRP neurons over the anorexigenic POMC/CART neurons. Both of these ultimately enhance appetite [4, 17, 18]. The ability of ghrelin to increase food intake and body weight is mediated through the stimulation of NPY production in the hypothalamic ARC, where it antagonizes the inhibitory effect on NPY secretion displayed by leptin and insulin [19].

The purpose of this chapter is to provide background information on the relationship between the main appetite regulatory peptides NPY and ghrelin, and insulin resistance. The role of NPY and ghrelin in food intake and body weight control in humans, and their mechanism of action are discussed, focusing on association with glucose metabolism and insulin resistance.

2. Neuropeptide Y (NPY)

NPY is one of the most abundant peptides of the hypothalamus and one of the most potent orexigenic (appetite-increasing) factors [20]. It is a 36-amino acid peptide that was first isolated from porcine brain in 1982 [21] (Fugure 2). It is a member of the PP-fold family of peptides which consists of NPY, peptide YY (PYY), pancreatic polypeptide (PP) and peptide Y (PY) [22].

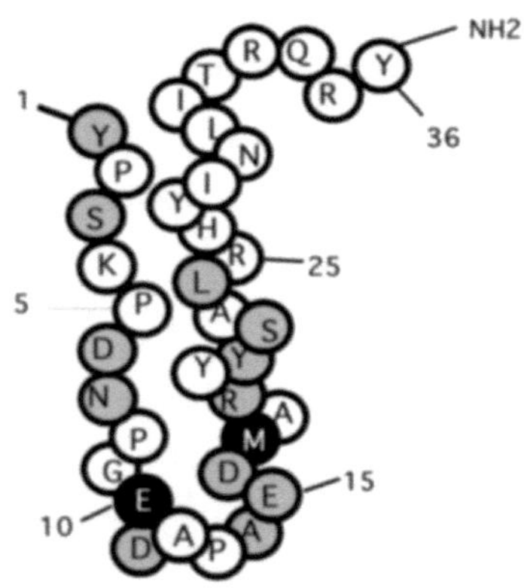

Figure 2. Structure of NPY.

NPY is synthesized by cell bodies in the ARC and transported axonally to the PVN where the highest concentrations are found [23]. NPY-expressing neurons are prominent also in the DMN and the VMN [24]. All these regions of the brain influence feeding behavior and energy balance.

NPY is also found in circulating blood, where it comes mainly from the adrenal medulla and sympathetic nerves, but this peripheral hormone does not cross the blood-brain barrier [25,

26]. NPY is present in the pancreas, in both the islet cells and in sympathetic nerve terminals [27, 28].

Regulation of NPY synthesis and release

The levels of hypothalamic NPY mRNA and NPY release increase with fasting and decrease after refeeding [29-31]. When fed with a high-carbohydrate diet; diabetic rats exhibit increased gene expression of the NPY in the hypothalamic ARC, and high-fat diet suppressed NPY expression [32]. Thus, NPY synthesis as well as its receptorial expression are sensitive to changes in the metabolic status and food availability. While starvation and food deprivation increase NPY release [30], in obese subjects the activity of NPY neurones is down-regulated in the attempt to restrain overeating of palatable food [33]. These facts support the existence of a long loop control system in energy metabolism between the brain and adipose tissue. Several peripheral factors are involved in the modulation of this system. Among them insulin and leptin display an inhibitory effect; glucocorticoids and ghrelin act as stimulatory afferent signals [34].

It has been reported that *leptin* is a major inhibitory regulator of the activation by ghrelin of the orexigenic network of NPY [35]. Circulating leptin crosses the blood brain barrier and binds to the long form of the leptin receptor, Ob-Rb, in the hypothalamus [36]. The Ob-Rb is expressed widely within the hypothalamus but particularly in the ARC, VMN, DMN and LHA. Several experimental studies demonstrate that systemic administration of leptin inhibits NPY gene overexpression through a specific action in the ARC. Cells within the ARC express both NPY and leptin receptors, and leptin directly activates anorectic POMC neurons and inhibits orexigenic AgRP/NPY neurons [37]. All available data can be summarized as follows: when leptin levels increase after food intake, the latter binds to its receptors in the hypothalamus which leads to discontinuation of NPY secretion. When production of leptin from adipose tissue is reduced, the circulating leptin concentrations fall, and this lead to enhanced production of NPY that strongly increase food intake.

Receptors for *ghrelin* are also located on arcuate AgRP/NPY neurons, which are activated by central ghrelin administration. Ghrelin acts by depolarizing the orexigenic NPY/AgRP neurons, and by increasing the tonic inhibition exerted by the NPY/AgRP neurons over the anorexigenic POMC/CART neurons [11]. c-Fos expression increases within NPY-synthesizing neurons in the ARC after peripheral administration of ghrelin [38], and ghrelin fails to increase food intake following ablation of the ARC [39]. Studies of knockout mice demonstrate that both NPY and AgRP signalling mediate the effect of ghrelin, although neither neuropeptide is obligatory [40].

Insulin is a major metabolic hormone produced by the pancreas and the first adiposity signal to be described. Little or no insulin is produced in the brain itself [41, 42]. Insulin levels are dependent on peripheral insulin sensitivity that is related to total body fat stores and fat distribution, with visceral fat being a key determinant of insulin sensitivity [12]. Once insulin enters the brain, it acts as an anorexigenic signal, decreasing food intake and subsequently body weight. It was found that both the NPY and melanocortin systems are important downstream targets for the effects of insulin on food intake and body weight. Insulin penetrates the blood–brain barrier via a saturable, receptor-mediated process, at levels which are proportional to the circulating insulin [43]. Insulin receptors are widely distributed in the brain, with highest concentrations found in the olfactory bulbs and the hypothalamus [44]. Within the hypothalamus, there is particularly high expression of insulin receptors in the ARC; they are also present in the DMH, PVN, and suprachiasmatic and periventricular regions [45]. Hypothalamic NPY is a potential mediator of the regulatory effects of insulin. The increase of NPY levels in the PVN and prepro-NPY mRNA in the ARC during fasting are inhibited by intracerebroventricular (icv) administration of insulin. Fasting, therefore, increases NPY biosynthesis along an ARC-PVN pathway in the hypothalamus via a mechanism dependent on low insulin levels [46]. NPY expression is increased in insulin-deficient, streptozocin-induced diabetic rats and this effect is reversed with insulin therapy [47, 48]. Insulin receptors have been found also on POMC neurons in the ARC [49]. Administration of insulin into the third ventricle of fasted rats increases POMC mRNA expression and the reduction of food intake caused by icv injection of insulin is blocked by a POMC antagonist [49]. Furthermore, POMC mRNA is reduced by 80% in rats with untreated diabetes, and this can be attenuated by peripheral insulin treatment which partially reduces the hyperglycaemia [50].

Glucocorticoid hormones play a critical role in energy balance and also appear to mediate at least some of their actions through the central NPY axis. They may regulate NPY-induced insulin release and NPY signaling within the VMH of the hypothalamus. Glucocorticoid-receptor immunoreactivity is found within the rat CNS, including the ARC, VMH, and PVN [51]. Many of these receptors are expressed at the nucleus of NPY-containing, endocrine-related neurons and coexist in regions containing high NPY receptor density [52]. In rats, excessive corticosterone promotes body fat gain and hyperinsulinemia [53] and also increases NPY synthesis and Y1-receptor mRNA expression, at least within the ARC ([54, 55]. Conversely, removal of glucocorticoids by adrenalectomy reduces hyperphagia and body weight of obese (*fa/fa*) rats [56], abolishes obesity induced by VMH lesions [57], and prevents obesity induced by chronic central NPY infusion in normal rats [58]. However, it has been reported that adrenalectomy does not alter NPY-1 (Y1)-receptor mRNA expression in the ARC [54]. Chronic icv infusion of NPY induces hyperphagia, hyperinsulinemia, and insulin resistance in rats, and these effects are blocked by previous adrenalectomy [59]. Wisialowski et al. [60] have demonstrated that adrenalectomy also abolishes the insulin release caused by an acute icv injection of NPY and this is associated with significant reduction in Y1- and Y5-receptor mRNA expression specifically within the VMH. These experiments imply that glucocorticoids are necessary for icv NPY to stimulate insulin release and suggest that the latter manifest this regulatory role through alterations in Y1- and Y5-receptor expression in the VMH [60]. Taken together, all these observations indicate that glucocorticoids have a regulatory role in long-term central NPY signaling.

As concerns plasma NPY, its concentrations rise in response to muscular exercise [61] and in disorders such as pheochromocytoma and renal failure [62].

Mechanisms of action of NPY – NPY receptors

PP-fold family of peptides bind to seven transmembrane-domain G-protein-coupled receptors [63]. Heterogeneity among NPY (and PYY) receptors was first proposed on the basis of studies on sympathetic neuroeffector junctions, where NPY (and PYY) can exert three types of action: 1) a direct (e.g., vasoconstrictor) response; 2) a postjunctional potentiating effect on norepinephrine (NE)-evoked vasoconstriction; and 3) a prejunctional suppression of stimulated NE release. The two latter phenomena are probably reciprocal, since NE affect NPY mechanisms similarly [**64**]. Six different NPY receptors have been identified ([65], of which five have been cloned and characterized. Y1–Y5 receptors have been demonstrated in rat brain, but Y6, identified in mice, is absent in rats and inactive in primates [66]. The Y1, Y2, Y4 and Y5 receptors, cloned in the hypothalamus, have all been postulated to mediate the orexigenic effects of NPY. Biological redundancies are likely to exist between Y1 and Y5 receptor signaling [67].

NPY initiates appetite drive directly through its receptors, particularly the Y1-5 (NPY5-R), and by the simultaneous inhibition of anorexigenic melanocortin signalling in the ARC [68]. NPY5-R is thought to be the main receptor involved in NPY-induced food intake since a reduction in food intake after an icv injection of antisense oligonucleotides directed against NPY5-R is demonstrated in rats [69].

Although the large number of Y receptors has made it difficult to delineate their individual contributions, recent studies analyzing NPY and Y receptor-overexpressing, knockout, and conditional-knockout mouse models have started to unravel some of the complexity. To elucidate the role of NPY1-R in food intake, energy expenditure, and other possible functions, Kushi et al. [70] have generated NPY1-R-deficient mice (Y1-R-/-) by gene targeting. Contrary to their hypothesis that the lack of NPY signaling via Y1-R would result in impaired feeding and weight loss, Y1-R-/- mice showed a moderate obesity and mild hyperinsulinemia without hyperphagia. The authors suggest either that the Y1-R in the hypothalamus is not a key molecule in the leptin/NPY pathway, which controls feeding behavior, or that its deficiency is compensated by other receptors, such as NPY5-R. Probably the mild obesity found in Y1-R-/- mice was caused by the impaired control of insulin secretion and/or low energy expenditure [70]. This model could be useful for studying the mechanism of mild obesity and abnormal insulin metabolism in noninsulin-dependent diabetes mellitus.

In order to investigate the role of different Y receptors in the NPY-induced obesity syndrome, Lin et al. [71] used recombinant adeno-associated viral vector to overexpress NPY in mice deficient of selective single or multiple Y receptors (including Y1, Y2, and Y4). Results from this study demonstrated that long-term hypothalamic overexpression of NPY lead to marked hyperphagia, hypogonadism, body weight gain, enhanced adipose tissue accumulation, hyperinsulinemia, and other hormonal changes characteristic of an obesity syndrome. NPY-induced hyperphagia, hypogonadism, and obesity syndrome persisted in all genotypes studied ($Y1^{-/-}$, $Y2^{-/-}$, $Y2Y4^{-/-}$, and $Y1Y2Y4^{-/-}$ mice). However, triple deletion of Y1, Y2, and Y4 receptors prevented NPY-induced hyperinsulinemia. These findings suggest that Y1, Y2, and Y4 receptors under this condition are not crucially involved in NPY's hyperphagic, hypogonadal, and obesogenic effects, but they are responsible for the central regulation of circulating insulin levels by NPY [71].

A lot of investigators' data point that NPY5-R mediates the feeding response to exogenous and endogenous NPY. It may be involved in energy balance and is, therefore, a susceptibility candidate gene for obesity and related disorders such as the metabolic syndrome and type 2 diabetes mellitus. It is hypothesized that the feeding effect of NPY may indeed be mediated by a combination of receptors rather than a single one. Also, increasing evidence points to the existence of other as yet unidentified Y receptors, which may mediate NPY's orexigenic actions, and it remains possible that, under certain physiological conditions, NPY may bind and activate receptors for which it normally has no or only low affinities.

Analogs of NPY with high selectivity for the Y1 and Y5 receptor subtypes strongly stimulate food intake in rodents, and icv administration of specific Y5 receptor agonists increases food intake and body weight in mice [72]. A clinical study examining a therapeutic intervention based on the NPY system has been performed by Erundu et al. [73]. The authors tested the hypothesis that blockade of the NPY5-R will lead to weight loss in humans using MK-0557, a potent, highly selective, orally active NPY5-R antagonist. MK-0557 has no significant binding to the human NPY1-R, NPY2-R, NPY4-R, or mouse NPY6-R at concentrations of 10 μM. These data indicate a >7500-fold selectivity for the NPY5-R relative to the other NPY receptor subtypes. MK-0557 was administered to 547 obese subjects, who showed statistically significant weight loss at 12 weeks compared to subjects treated with placebo [73]. These observations clearly indicate that antagonizing the NPY5-R induces weight loss in humans. After that a long-term trial over 52 weeks was performed in 1661 subjects (832 completed). There was a a mean weight loss of 3.4 kg in those who completed the trial, which was significantly greater than the weight loss seen in the placebo-treated group. Significantly more subjects lost ≥5% and ≥10% of initial body weight with the NPY5-R antagonist than did so on placebo. The authors conclude, however, that the magnitude of the weight loss observed was not clinically significant, and this conclusion is supported by the observation that there were no significant improvements in secondary endpoints such as glucose and lipid levels and blood pressure measurements [73]. While several potential new obesity therapies that act through the CNS pathways or peripheral adiposity signals are in early-phase clinical trials, the above study serves to point out that manipulation of the homeostatic mechanisms involving hypothalamic/brainstem pathways for a clinically significant outcome in obese patients remains a major challenge [74].

Link between NPY, obesity and insulin resistance

NPY is a powerful stimulant of food intake. Numerous studies in rodent models have demonstrated that administration of NPY into the PVN stimulates feeding [75, 76] and that repeated injections of NPY result in persistent feeding and the development of obesity by promoting fat accumulation [77, 78]. Central administration of NPY was found to reduce energy expenditure, resulting in reduced brown fat thermogenesis [79], suppression of sympathetic nerve activity [80] and inhibition of the thyroid axis [81]. There are some data that NPY activates hypothalamic-pituitary-adrenal axis (HPA) [82], that is implicated in the regulation of metabolism and energy balance. An acute injection of NPY into the PVN produces increases in circulating ACTH and corticosterone in both conscious and anesthetized rats [83]. ARC NPY neurons project to the ipsilateral PVN [84], and repeated icv injection of NPY into the PVN in normal rats causes hyperphagia, an increase in basal plasma insulin level and morning cortisol level, independent of increased food intake, increased metabolic activity of white adipose tissue and muscle insulin resistance, and results in obesity [85, 86]. Several of these metabolic effects are still present when increased food intake is prevented by food restriction [85]. It was shown that Y5 receptor subtype is involved in the activation of HPA axis mediated by NPY [82].

Interestingly, injection of NPY directly into the VMH significantly increases food intake [75], and NPY-induced feeding is enhanced in VMH-lesioned rats [87]. Lesions of the VMH in rodents also cause multiple changes in metabolic status, including hyperphagia, hyperglycemia, and hyperinsulinaemia [88]. Enhanced NPY expression in the VMH is associated with obesity [89]. Furthermore, NPY has been shown to directly inhibit over one fifth of spontaneously active rat VMH neurons, and this inhibition is potentiated by overfeeding [90]. Therefore, the mechanism by which acute icv NPY stimulates insulin release in the absence of feeding may be by inhibiting the spontaneous activity of the VMH through Y1 and Y5 receptors. A reduction of these receptors with adrenalectomy would then reduce the ability of NPY to inhibit VMH neurons. These data suggest the VMH may also be a site of action for NPY in the development of obesity; however, the mechanisms by which NPY is involved in each aspect of central energy regulation remain to be defined.

Some investigators found that acute icv NPY administration had no affect on plasma glucose levels, indicating that NPY-induced insulin release is not simply a secondary response to changes in peripheral glucose [60, 91]. The decreased basal insulin levels and lack of insulin release in response to NPY injection in adrenalectomized rats with downregulation of Y1-and Y5-receptor mRNA in the VMH, demonstrated in the study of Wisialowski et al. [60], highlights the role for Y1-and Y5-receptors in the etiology of NPY-induced hyperinsulinemia, insulin resistance, and obesity.

Van den Hoek et al. [92] found that icv administration of NPY in the third ventricule in rats acutely hampers the capacity of insulin to suppress endogenous glucose production via activation of sympathetic nerves innervating the liver The authors discusssed a possible explanation for the role of NPY in sympathetic overdrive and hepatic insulin resistance that are typical for obese subjects with the metabolic syndrome [92]. In a study of Singhal et al. [93] the ability of resistin to increase hepatic insulin resistance and modulate the levels of various mediators in the liver was abolished in mice lacking NPY as well as in mice pretreated with icv NPY Y1 receptor antagonist. The authors established a crucial link between NPY and resistin's ability to regulate hepatic insulin resistance possibly via induction of SOCS3 (suppressor of cytokine signaling-3), tumor necrosis factor (TNF)-α and interleukin 6 (IL6). Additionally, NPY is critical to mediating the decrease in STAT3 (signal transducer-activated transcript-3) phosphorylation by central resistin [93].

It was found that the obesity syndrome, induced by injection of NPY into the CNS of rats, closely resembles the phenotype of either leptin deficient *ob/ob* mice, or leptin resistant *db/db* mice [58, 85]. In these animals, genetic alterations of the satiety effect of leptin within the hypothalamus result in an overexpression of NPY leading to a complex syndrome including hyperphagia, increased fat storage and obesity. The experimental studies in *ob/ob* mice demonstrate that systemic administration of leptin inhibits NPY gene overexpression through a specific action in the ARC and exerts a hypoglycemic action that is partly independent of its weight-reducing effects. It must be pointed that both effects occur before reversal of the obesity syndrome. Defective leptin signaling due to either leptin deficiency (in *ob/ob* mice) or leptin resistance (in *db/db* mice) therefore leads directly to hyperglycemia and the overexpression of hypothalamic NPY, that is implicated in the pathogenesis of the obesity syndrome [94]. Moreover, the obesity syndrome produced by icv administration of NPY is characterised by increased expression of the *ob* gene in adipose tissue [58]. On the other hand leptin, the *ob* gene product, has been shown to inhibit NPY synthesis and release from hypothalamic nuclei in *ob/ob* mice. Correction of the obese state induced by genetic leptin deficiency reduces elevated levels of both blood glucose and hypothalamic NPY mRNA [95].

Although NPY seems to be an important orexigenic signal, NPY-null mice have normal body weight and adiposity [96, 97]. This absence of an obese phenotype may be due to the presence of compensatory mechanisms or alternative orexigenic pathways, such as those which signal via AgRP [98]. It is possible that there is evolutionary redundancy in orexigenic signalling in order to avert starvation. This redundancy may also contribute to the difficulty elucidating the receptor subtype that mediates NPY-induced feeding [99].

In searching the role of NPY in human obesity and metabolic disorders, polymorphisms in the NPY5-R gene have been studied by other authors in several populations. Thus, NPY5-R gene was sequenced by Jenkinson et al. [100], and several single nucleotide polymorphisms (SNPs) were genotyped in the Pima Indians with three novel SNPs being identified, which were described as polymorphism 1, 2, and 3 (P1, P2, and P3). All three SNPs are in non-coding regions. There were genotype differences in lean and obese Pima Indians for P2 and for a 3 SNP haplotype [100]. A silent single nucleotide polymorphism within the NPY5-R coding sequence showed no evidence of association with BMI in children and adolescents [101]. In contrast, a novel polymorphism in the intervening segment between exons of the genes encoding NPY1-R and NPY5-R was associated with reduced serum triglyceride (TG) levels and HDL-cholesterol in a severely obese cohort [102] that should be considered as a protective lipid profile. Roche et al. [103] investigated the potential implication of NPY, NPY-Y1 and -Y5 subtype receptors [rNPY-Y1/-Y5] in the development of human obesity. Two complementary genetic approaches were used: 1) linkage analyses between obesity and polymorphic markers located nearby NPY and rNPY-Y1/-Y5 genes in 93 French Caucasian morbidly obese families; 2) single strand conformation polymorphism (SSCP) scanning of the coding region of the NPY and rNPYY1 genes performed in 50 unrelated obese patients ascertained. No evidence of linkage between morbid obesity or obesityrelated quantitative traits and NPY and rNPY-Y1/Y5 regions was found in this population. Moreover, SSCP scanning revealed no mutation in the coding region of NPY and rNPY-Y1 genes among obese subjects. The authors suggest that NPY and NPY-Y1/ Y5 receptors are unlikely to be implicated in the development of human morbid obesity, at least in the French Caucasian population [103].

In addition to the above data, genetic association of NPY receptor Y5 (NPY5R) SNPs with metabolic syndrome was studied in 439 Mexican American individuals by Coletta et al. [104]. Minor alleles for five of nine genetic variants (rs11100493, rs12501691, P1, rs11100494, rs12512687) of the NPY5-R SNPs were found to be significantly associated with both increased plasma TG levels and decreased high-density lipoprotein (HDL) concentrations [104]. In addition, the minor allele for SNP P2 was significantly associated with a decreased homeostasis model assessment of β-cell function (HOMA-%β). Linkage disequilibrium between SNPs pairs indicated one haplotype block of five SNPs (rs11100493), and low HDL-cholesterol are highly associated with insulin resistance states, such as type 2 diabetes mellitus, obesity, and the metabolic syndrome. So, these results provide evidence for association of SNPs in the NPY5R gene with atherogenic dyslipidemia in insulin resistance. In the course of identification of genes implicated in the development of human obesity, further genome-wide searches could be successful for identifying multiple predisposing loci.

It has become apparent, that upon vigorous electrical stimulation or intense stressors motor neurons on the sympathetic nerve system (SNS) may secrete NPY as well as NE [105]. Acting through NPY receptors on vascular and adipose tissue, secreted NPY may play an important role in the pathophysiology of obesity and metabolic syndrome. Thus, Kuo et al. [105] demonstrated that stress exaggerated diet-induced obesity through a peripheral mechanism in the abdominal white adipose tissue that is mediated by NPY. The authors found that stressors such as exposure to cold or aggression lead to NPY release from SNS, which in turn upregulates NPY and its Y2 receptors (NPY2-R) in a glucocorticoid-dependent manner in the abdominal fat. This positive feedback response by NPY lead to abdominal fat enhancement. Release of NPY and activation of NPY2-R stimulated fat angiogenesis, macrophage infiltration, and the proliferation and differentiation of new adipocytes, resulting in abdominal obesity and a metabolic syndrome-like condition. NPY, like stress, stimulated fat growth, whereas pharmacological inhibition or fat-targeted knockdown of NPY2R is anti-angiogenic and anti-adipogenic. Thus, manipulations of NPY2-R activity within fat tissue offer new ways to remodel fat and treat obesity and metabolic syndrome [105].

NPY may be an important intra-islet paracrine hormone [38]. When produced by pancreatic islets, its expression is dependent on the prevailing endocrine environment. Islet NPY appears to constrain insulin release under a variety of conditions. Whether peripheral NPY has a hormone-like action and directly influences glucose metabolism and/or insulin secretion *in vivo* is under investigation. It this context NPY, at high concentrations, may contribute to the modulation of insulin secretion *in vitro*. NPY nerve fibers occur in the mouse pancreas and that most of these NPY nerve fibers are nonadrenergic. Furthermore, in the mouse, NPY enhances basal plasma insulin levels at high dose levels under *in vivo* conditions. At lower dose levels it inhibits glucose-induced, but not cholinergically induced insulin secretion [106]. It has also been reported that NPY may reduce plasma glucose concentrations during exercise by inhibiting glycogen breakdown in the splanchnic compartment [107, 108]. Moreover, the potential relation between circulating NPY and the pathophysiological consequences of obesity need further investigation.

Vettor et al. [109] found that peripheral NPY infusion in normal rats increased the overall rate of glucose disposal by increasing insulin responsiveness in skeletal muscle. Plasma leptin was significantly increased by hyperinsulinaemia, but was not affected by NPY infusion. Both the early and late phase of the insulin response to hyperglycaemia were significantly reduced by NPY. Based on their data for an increased glycolytic flux combined with a blunted increase in lactate, the authors suggested that NPY may raise insulin mediated glucose disposal by increasing its utilisation through the oxidative pathways. Intravenous NPY did not influence glucose metabolism in adipose tissue and leptin release [109].

The above data indicate that NPY has different effects on insulin secretion when administered acutely via intracerebroventricular or intravenous routes. Thus, peripheral NPY plays a clear inhibitory role in glucose-induced insulin secretion. It is also possible that the duration of treatment, and not just the route of administration, may be a relevant factor.

Several appetite-regulating genes (MCH, CRH, NPY, cholecystokinin, etc.) as well as their corresponding receptors, are expressed in the adipose tissue. The coexistance of locally produced NPY and NPYR-2 suggests a NPY autocrine/paracrine system of regulation of adipocyte function. Kos et al. reported that NPY is not only expressed but also secreted by human adipose tissue and insulin increases NPY secretion [110]. Direct effects of NPY on adipocyte function are also described. Thus, NPY was as potent as insulin in increasing both leptin and resistin secretion from pre-adipocytes from visceral fat in vitro [105]. Treatment of human subcutaneous adipocytes with recombinant human NPY downregulates leptin receptor [110], exerts an anti-lipopytic effect probably mediated by adenylate cyclase inhibition [111], and promotes the proliferation of pre-adipocytes [105, 112]. Probably, the enhanced local expression of NPY within visceral adipose tissue may contribute to the molecular mechanisms underlying increased visceral adiposity. The anti-lipolytic action on NPY can promote an increase in adipocyte size in hyperinsulinaemic conditions, such as abdominal obesity and metabolic syndrome.

As compared to the numerous experimental and genetic studies, the clinical studies on circulatory NPY in obesity are not so many. It is interesting that significant alteration of NPY circulatory levels is not found in adults after weight reduction [113] as well as in adolescents [114] besides the progressive decrease of leptin levels. Probably, the leptin control on hypothalamic production of NPY cannot be estimated by the levels of the latter in peripheral circulation.

In one of our recent studies on different morphological types of obesity [115], NPY levels in obese women were lower than those of the normal weight controls, the differences being significant when comparing the obese group as a whole and the subgroup with android obesity only (Table 1). There was a reverse correlation between NPY and body weight, and percentage body fat. In analogy with the comparisons regarding NPY, leptin levels did not differ significantly between the two groups of obese women. Our data are in accordance with the data of Zahorska-Markiewicz et al. in obese women and in women with normal weight [113]. Notwithstanding the absence of statistically significant differences in leptin and NPY levels between our obese patients, we observed that at relatively highest leptin levels NPY had relatively lowest levels, and vice versa. This was supported by the ascertained negative correlation between the two hormones. In the control group, significantly lower leptin levels were associated with significantly higher NPY levels as compared to the obese group. We can suggest that the decrease of NPY concentration in obesity may play a role of a counter-regulatory factor intended to prevent further weight gain. In this and previous study of ours [116] we did not find significant differences in circulatory levels of resistin and TNFα between lean women and women with both gynoid and android obesity. The latter were insulin-resistant with significantly higher basal insulinaemia and HOMA-index, respectively (Table 1).

Hormones	Leptin (ng/ml)	Resistin (ng/ml)	TNFα (pg/ml)	NPY (ng/ml)	Insulin (μIU/ml)	HOMA index
Android obesity (n=32)	21.28±11.14*	2.35±0.59	15.75±6.79	4.59±1.13*	20.13±8.17*#	4.34±1.68*#
Gynoid obesity (n=27)	17.14±9.05	2.24±0.76	18.18±6.07	5.21±1.19	10.47±5.24	2.18±1.34
Controls (n=24)	10.02±5.98	2.09±1.19	19.17±9.08	5.99±1.18	8.03±3.22	1.69±0.98

(All data are expressed as mean±SD.* - significant difference as compared to the control group; # - significant difference as compared to the group with gynoid obesity)

Table 1. Hormonal parameters and HOMA-index in the women with obesity and normal weight women [115].

The NPY levels were found similar in a group of patients with gestational diabetes mellitus and in pregnant women with normal glucose tolerance in a study of Ilhan et al [117]. Notably, the NPY concentration correlated positively with insulin levels in patients with type 2 diabetes mellitus [117]. These data suggest a potential involvement of circulating NPY in diabetes pathology that needs further purposeful studies.

NPY and reproductive function

Having in mind the fact, that NPY secretion is increased in response to metabolic challenges that inhibit luteinizing hormone releasing hormone (LHRH) secretion (e.g., fasting) and decreased by treatments that restore the metabolic deficit and reinstate reproductive function (e.g., re-feeding) [20], several studies have focused on the role of NPY in reproductive processes.

A modulating action of NPY on the gonadotropic and somatotropic systems in experimental animals has been reported. NPY affects luteinizing hormone (LH) and follicle-stimulating hormone (FSH) release from anterior pituitary cells *in vitro* and enhances LHRH-induced LH secretion [118]. In female rats NPY decreased LH release in pituitary cell culture *in vitro* [119]. Barb et al. [120] conducted 2 experiments in ovariectomized prepubertal gilts to test the hypothesis that NPY stimulates appetite and modulates LH and growth hormone (GH) secretion, and that leptin modifies such acute effects of NPY on feeding behavior and LH and GH secretion. In the first one, gilts received icv injections of NPY. In the second one gilts received icv injections of leptin, NPY or NPY + leptin, and feed intake was measured. The authors found that NPY suppressed LH secretion and the 100 μg dose stimulated GH secretion. NPY reversed the inhibitory effect of leptin on feed intake and suppressed LH secretion, but serum GH concentrations were unaffected [120]. In another experiment in prepubertal gilts, Barb et al. [121] demonstrated that NPY did not alter basal LH secretion nor 10(-8) M LHRH-induced increase in LH secretion but 10(-9) M LHRH-stimulated LH secretion was reduced by NPY and was not different from control or LHRH alone. At the same time NPY increased basal GH secretion and enhanced the GH response to growth hormone releasing factor (GRF) at the level of the pituitary gland [121]. These data support the modulating role of NPY on GH and LH secretion. Experimental evidence in rodents and monkeys suggests that NPY preferentially exerts inhibitory effects on LHRH-LH secretion when estrogen levels are low [122, 123]. In primates, the role of NPY as a regulator of gonadotropin secretion is complicated by the observation that age may influence the effects of NPY (inhibitory or stimulatory), as does the site of exogenous NPY administration [124, 125]. An important physiological role for NPY as a modulator of neuroendocrine activity which culminates in the preovulatory surge of LH is discussed [118]

All above mentioned and many similar results support the hypothesis that NPY modulates feed intake, and LH and GH secretion and may serve as a neural link between metabolic state and the reproductive, as well as the growth axis.

Clinical evidence suggests that NPY exerts primarily an inhibitory effect on the hypothalamic-pituitary-ovarian (HPO) axis in humans. Thus, a role for NPY in hypothalamic amenorrhea is inferred from the observation that NPY levels in the cerebrospinal fluid and serum are elevated in underweight amenorrheic women, and are returned to normal after long-term weight restoration in women who resumed normal menstrual cycling [126-128]. Starvation-induced alterations of neuropeptide activity probably contribute to neuroendocrine dysfunctions in anorexia nervosa. Kaye et al. [126] made the conclusion, that in girls with anorexia nervosa a disturbance of CNS corticotropin releasing hormone (CRH) activity is likely to be responsible for hypercortisolemia, while a disturbance of CNS NPY may contribute to amenorrhea [126]. In addition, disturbances of these neuropeptides could contribute to other symptoms such as increased physical activity, hypotension, reduced sexual interest, depression, and pathological feeding behavior [129].

Similarly, a role for NPY in the initiation of puberty is suggested by the observation that concentrations of NPY in girls with delayed puberty are higher than in girls matched for weight and body composition who exhibited normal pubertal development [130]. Higher concentrations of NPY in girls with constitutional delay of puberty (CDP) may be responsible for the disorder and reduced levels of IGF-I. Correlation of NPY with % body fat suggests an involvement of this neuropeptide in the process of fat accumulation associated with CDP [130].

Of great interest is to focus on the role of NPY in one of the most common endocrine-metabolic diseases, affecting up to 10% of women of reproductive age, the polycystic ovary syndrome (PCOS) [131, 132]. It is widely accepted that PCOS is a prototype of a sex specific metabolic syndrome [132-134]. Obesity is present in 30–70% of affected women depending on the setting of the study and the ethnical background of the subjects, and it is characterized by central distribution of fat [133, 135, 136]. In women with PCOS, hyperinsulinemia, dyslipidemia, and/or hypertension are highly dependent on obesity, which worsens all of the clinical manifestations of PCOS [133, 136-138]. At present there is an increasing body of evidence of high levels of atherogenic adipocytokines and low levels of adiponectin in women with PCOS that change according to variations of fat mass [139]. Endocrine function of the adipocytes is regulated mainly by nutritional status, and both these factors are complexly interweaved in the energy storing mechanism in the adipose tissue [140]. It is still not fully elucidated if there are consistent differences in the levels or in the effects of appetite-regulating hormones as is NPY in PCOS.

Manneras et al. [141] demonstrated an enhanced mesenteric (visceral) adipose tissue expression of NPY in a rat model of PCOS in comparison with normal rats. Exercise reduced adiposity and adipose NPY expression and additionally normalized ovarian cyclicity [141].

Women with PCOS may exhibit altered leptin sensitivity of the hypothalamic NPY neurons to leptin inhibition, and higher plasma NPY levels have been observed in women with PCOS compared to nonPCOS controls; this may perturb LHRH secretion [142]. Thus, Baranowska et al. [143] found elevated NPY levels in both lean and overweight women with anovulatory PCOS. The increase in NPY in their study was independent of the increase in BMI. In obese women with PCOS, plasma leptin was increased compared to lean women [143]. Bidzińńska-Speichert et al. [144] also found higher leptin and NPY levels and lower galanin levels in PCOS women as compared to healthy controls [144]. These data are in conformity with observations from our recent on-going study where we found significantly higher NPY and leptin levels in obese insulin-resistant PCOS women as compared to nonPCOS weight matched women [Orbetzova, unpublished data]. It can be suggested that the feedback system in the interaction between leptin and NPY is disturbed in PCOS.

In contrast, Romualdi et al. [145] demonstrated that in basal conditions, obese PCOS women exhibited lower NPY levels than obese controls. Ghrelin injection markedly increased NPY in controls, whereas PCOS women showed a deeply blunted NPY response to the stimulus. Metformin treatment induced a significant decrease in insulin levels and the concomitant recovery of NPY secretory capacity in response to ghrelin in PCOS women. Leptin levels, which were similar in the two groups, were not modified by ghrelin injection; metformin did not affect this pattern. The authors conclude that hyperinsulinaemia seems to play a pivotal role in the alteration of NPY response to ghrelin in obese PCOS women. This derangement could be implicated in the pathophysiology of obesity in these patients [145]. The limitations of this very interesting study on the ghrelin–NPY relationship in PCOS is the small number of patients (seven obese, hyperinsulinaemic subjects with PCOS and seven obese control women) and the data need further purposeful investigation.

Interventions that influence reproductive and metabolic function in PCOS may also affect levels of the adipose tissue hormones and regulators of appetite, such as NPY. It has been postulated that some of the effects of insulin-sensitizing agents in PCOS may be mediated through changes in adipocytokines levels. Some authors demonstrated that treatment of women with PCOS with insulin-sensitising agents induces a reduction in serum leptin levels [146-149]. In this context our recent data from a study comprising of 2 groups of overweight insulin-resistant PCOS women [150] showed that a 3-month treatment with metformin (Group 1) and rosiglitazone (Group 2), added to an oral hormone contraceptive (OHC) (a standard combination of ethynil oestradiol 35 μg plus cyproterone acetate 2 mg) resulted in decrease of atherogenic adipocytokines (leptin, resistin, and TNFα) (Table 2) that may have beneficial effects in the future prevention of atherosclerosis and cardiovascular diseases in this risk cohort of young women. But the serum concentrations of NPY also decreased that is in support of some our previous [151] and other authors [143, 144] data for impaired NPY-leptin link in PCOS. The change of NPY and adipocytokines was associated with weight loss only in the metformin group that is an expected effect of the drug and in conformity with other studies [150].

Groups / Parameters	Group 1 (n=32) Metformin + OHC		Group 2 (n= 34) Rosiglitazone +OHC	
	0 months	3 months	0 months	3 months
Leptin (ng/ml)	13.17±3.42	6.40±1.40**	15.54±4.49	7.17±1.59**
Resistin (ng/ml)	2.19±0.67	1.63±0.45**	2.61±0.79	1.68±0.41**
TNFα (pg/ml)	12.52±5.78	8.47±3.09***	13.45±4.30	9.60±4.16****
NPY (ng/ml)	4.51±1.18	3.64±0.46*	4.54±1.47	3.21±1.25****
Weight (kg)	78.24±20.14	75.50±18.66**	82.41±16.17	82.23±15.80
BMI (kg/m²)	28.45±4.38	27.45±3.73**	29.27±4.24	29.22±4.27
Waist (cm)	88.69±7.72	86.63±5.92*	88.97±8.05	88.24±7.63
Fats (%)	35.56±10.10	33.98±8.77	35.55±12.40	34.72±13.09
Fats (kg)	29.77±15.20	27.23±13.39*	32.30±17.86	31.33±17.94

*- p<0.05 – vs basal; **- p<0.01 – vs basal; ***- p=0.001 – vs basal; ****- p<0.001 – vs basal

Table 2. NPY, adipose tissue hormones, and some clinical characteristics of the groups before and after treatment [150]

Having in mind that the decrease in NPY and adipocytokines was not in parallel with changes in body weight and composition in the rosiglitazone group and was associated with only slignt and non significant influence on hyperinsulinaemia, resp. insulin resistance, additional direct adipose tissue and/or disease specific effects of the treatment may come into consideration that needs further elucidation.

3. Ghrelin

Ghrelin was discovered by Kojima et al. [152] in rat stomach extracts in 1999. This peptide has been identified in many species, including mammals, avians, amphibians, reptiles, and fish [153-159] and the sequence of first seven amino acids of the N-terminal region of ghrelin are highly conserved between species [160].

Ghrelin is an orexigenic factor released primarily from the oxyntic cells of the stomach, but also from duodenum, ileum, caecum and colon [161, 162]. Gastric ghrelin cells had been classified as X/A-like cells by their round, compact, electron-dense secretory granules that distinguish them electron-microscopically from other previously characterized gastric endocrine cell types before the discovery of ghrelin [161, 163]. Ghrelin has also been detected in many other organs, such as the bowel, pancreas, kidney, placenta, lymphatic tissue, gonads, thyroid, adrenal, lung, pituitary and hypothalamus, and in different human neoplastic tissues and related cancer cell lines, such as gastric and intestinal carcinoids, lymphomas and thyroid, breast, liver, lung and prostate carcinomas. Levels of ghrelin expression in these normal and tumoral tissues or cell lines are lower than in the stomach, and although the potential physiological role of ghrelin as an autocrine/paracrine factor in these tissues is still under investigation [164].

In mice, rats and humans, ghrelin is an acyl-peptide consisting of 28 amino acids, sharing a 36% structural resemblance to motilin [165]. A hydroxyl group of serine at position 3 of the ghrelin molecule is esterified with an octanoic acid. The esterification increases the hydrophobicity of the ghrelin molecule, and is essential for most of its biological activities [152,166-168]. An enzyme that catalyses the acyl-modification of ghrelin was discovered in 2008 by Yang et al. [169], was renamed ghrelin O-acyltransferase (GOAT). In vivo studies showed that GOAT gene disruption in mouse models completely abolished ghrelin acylation [170, 171]. GOAT inhibition leading to weight reduction and beneficial metabolic effects [172] is therefore a useful target for future development of therapeutic compounds for obesity and metabolic syndrome.

Ghrelin receptor

Ghrelin was discovered via its growth hormone releasing effect as an endogenous agonist of the GHS-R, that is still the only receptor so far described [152, 173, 174]. The GHS-R was first identified in 1996 as a seven transmembrane domain peptide totaling 366 amino acids. It is a G protein-coupled receptor (GPCR) that is linked to both Gq and Gs signaling pathways. It generates intracellular signaling through its $G\alpha 11$ subunit, although the specific intracellular pathways elicited by this receptor are dependent on the tissue type in which it is expressed [175].

There are two splice variants - GHS-R type 1a that is the receptor to which ghrelin binds and through which it exerts its stimulatory effects on growth hormone release [152, 161, 176, 177], and GHS-R type 1b, which is a COOH-terminal truncated form of the type 1a receptor, and is physiologically inactive [178]. Ghrelin administration does not increase food intake in mice lacking GHS-R type 1a, suggesting that the orexigenic effects may be mediated by the above receptor; however, these mice have normal appetite and body composition [173, 179].

Ghrelin exists as two different molecular forms in both gastric ghrelin-producing cells and circulation: 1) acylated ghrelin (with the n-octanoic acid at the serine-3 position), which is essential for activation of GHS-R1a and modulation of neuroendocrine and orexigenic effects; and 2) nonacylated ghrelin (des-acyl ghrelin), which is the most abundant form in the stomach and circulation but is unable to activate GHS-R1a, and to exhibit further GH-releasing activity [180] (Figure 3). Nonetheless, food intake is induced by des-acyl ghrelin, administered by icv injection, to the same extent as ghrelin [181]. Nonacylated ghrelin exerts some cardiovascular and antiproliferative actions. Because the genome database does not contain another GPCR that resembles GHS-R, probably des-acyl ghrelin acts by binding different GHS-R subtypes or as yet unidentified receptor families [178, 182].

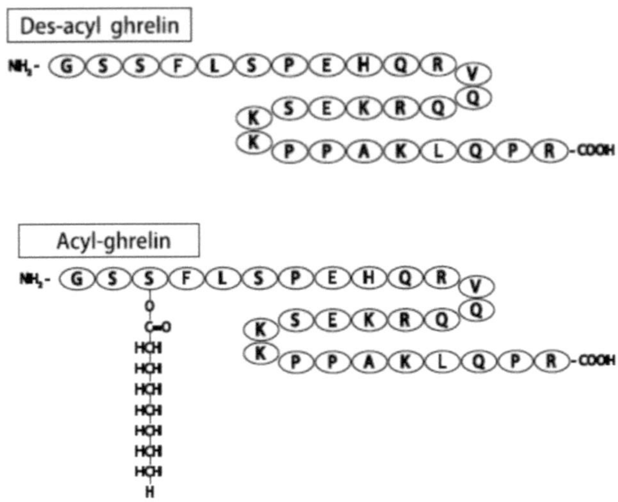

Figure 3. Structure of nonacylated and acylated ghrelin

GHS-R1a is widely distributed in the body with high expression levels in the hypothalamus and in all three components of the dorsal vagal complex, including the area postrema, the nucleus of the solitary tract (NTS), the dorsal motor nucleus of the vagus and parasympathetic preganglionic neurons [183]. Low expression is detected in other brain areas and in numerous other tissues including the myocardium, stomach, small intestine, pancreas, colon, adipose tissue, liver, kidney, lung, placenta and peripheral T-cells [152, 161, 182, 184-187].

The ghrelin receptor is well conserved across all vertebrate species examined, including a number of mammals, bird and fish. This strict conservation suggests that ghrelin and its receptor serve essential physiological functions [188]. Some studies have also described ghrelin analogues which show dissociation between the feeding effects and stimulation of GH, suggesting that GHS-R type 1a may not be the only receptor mediating the effects of ghrelin on food intake [189].

The gene encoding ghrelin also encodes another peptide, called *obestatin*. The administration of obestatin reduces food intake and weight gain in rats via activation of GPR3, an orphan G-protein coupled receptor [190, 191]. Therefore, one gene produces two products with opposing metabolic effects, which are exercised through different receptors [192].

Ghrelin as a member of the 'gut-brain axis'

The human body is endowed with a complex physiological system that maintains relatively constant body weight and fat stores despite the wide variations in daily energy intake and energy expenditure. With weight loss, compensatory physiological adaptations result in increased hunger and decreased energy expenditure, while opposite responses are triggered when body weight increases. This regulatory system is formed by multiple interactions between the gastrointestinal tract (GIT), adipose tissue, and the CNS and is influenced by behavioural, sensorial, autonomic, nutritional, and endocrine mechanisms [2, 3].

The hypothalamus (particularly the ARC) and the brain (particularly the NTS) are the main sites of convergence and integration of the central and peripheral signals that regulate food intake and energy expenditure [193, 194]. There are mechanisms of short-term regulation (satiety signals) which determine the beginning and the end of a meal (hunger and satiation) and the interval between meals (satiety) [195], and long-term regulatory factors (signals of adiposity) which help the body to regulate energy depots. Thus, meal-generated satiety signals from the GIT do interact with longer-term adiposity signals, such as insulin and leptin in maintaining energy balance. Satiety signals from the GIT are transmitted primarily through vagal and spinal nerves to the NTS. There is, however, a large integration and convergence of these signals by neural connections between the ARC nucleus, NTS, and vagal afferent fibres. The nervous system, in turn, influences gastric and pancreatic exocrine secretion, gastrointestinal motility, blood supply, and secretion of gut hormones [191].

The GIT contributes with several peptides that have incretin-, hunger-, and satiety-stimulating actions, such as ghrelin, glucagon-like peptide 1 (GLP-1), peptide YY (PYY), oxyntomodulin (OXM), and cholecystokinin (CCK) and that are considered as members of the 'gut-brain axis'. Many of the GIT hormones that affect food intake are also synthesized in the brain, such as CCK, GLP-1, apolipoprotein A-IV, gastrin-releasing peptide, PYY, and ghrelin. Generally, peptides that reduce (or increase) food intake when administered systemically usually have the same action when administered centrally. This has been demonstrated for CCK, GLP-1, apolipoprotein A-IV, gastrin-releasing peptide, neuromedin B, and ghrelin [5, 6, 191].

Ghrelin is expressed in a group of neurons adjacent to the third ventricle, between the DMN, VMN, PVN and ARC. These neurons terminate on NPY/AgRP, POMC and corticotrophin-releasing hormone neurons, and are able to stimulate the activity of ARC NPY neurons, forming a central circuit which could mediate energy homeostasis [17]. The central ghrelin neurons also terminate on orexin-containing neurons within the LHA [18], and icv administration of ghrelin stimulates orexin-expressing neurons [18, 196]. The feeding response to centrally administered ghrelin is attenuated after administration of anti-orexin antibody and in orexin-null mice [18].

Ghrelin reaches the hypothalamus through the circulation, and the brain stem through vagal innervation. The integrity of the vagus nerve is crucial for ghrelin effects since vagotomy prevents its orexigenic effect in animal models and humans. Ghrelin is thought to exert its orexigenic action via the ARC in a pattern representing a functional antagonism to leptin. c-

Fos expression increases within ARC NPY-synthesizing neurons after peripheral administration of ghrelin [197], and ghrelin fails to increase food intake following ablation of the ARC [198]. Studies of knockout mice demonstrate that both NPY and AgRP signalling mediate the effect of ghrelin, although neither neuropeptide is obligatory [179]. GHS-R are also found on the vagus nerve [185], and administration of ghrelin leads to c-Fos expression in the area postrema and NTS [196, 199], suggesting that the brainstem may also participate in ghrelin signalling. The orexigenic action of ghrelin occurs independently of its stimulatory effects on GH secretion [176, 198, 200]. It is more likely that the physiological role of ghrelin is to prepare the body for an influx of metabolic energy [201-203].

Administration of ghrelin, either centrally or peripherally, increases food intake and body weight and decreases fat utilization in rodents [176, 204]. Furthermore, central infusion of anti-ghrelin antibodies in rodents inhibits the normal feeding response after a period of fasting, suggesting that ghrelin is an endogenous regulator of food intake [199]. Human subjects who receive ghrelin intravenously demonstrate a potent increase in food intake of 28% [205], and rising pre-prandial levels correlate with hunger scores in humans initiating meals spontaneously [202]. Chronic administration increases body weight, not only by stimulating food intake, but also by decreasing energy expenditure and fat catabolism [165, 176, 199].

In summary, the orexigenic effect of hypothalamic ghrelin is regulated through a neuronal network involving food intake. Fasting results in increased release of ghrelin from the stomach (the exact mechanism of this remains obscure) leading to increased plasma ghrelin levels, which reach the hypothalamus either via the blood stream directly in areas with no blood–brain barrier, or by crossing the blood–brain barrier via a saturable transport system or via the vagus nerve and the NTS [206]. Ghrelin's effect on appetite is mediated by an effect both on the hypothalamus and the NTS.To stimulate the release of the orexigenic peptides, ghrelin-containing neurons send efferent fibers onto NPY/AgRP-expressing neurons. On the other hand, to suppress the release of the anorexigenic peptide, ghrelin-containing neurons send efferent fibers onto POMC neurons [17]. Leptin directly inhibits appetite-stimulating effects of NPY and AgRP, whereas hypothalamic ghrelin augments NPY gene expression and blocked leptin-induced feeding reduction. Thus, ghrelin and leptin have a competitive interaction in feeding regulation [188].

Regulation of ghrelin secretion

Serum ghrelin concentrations vary widely throughout the day. The most known factor for the regulation of ghrelin secretion is feeding [201] - ghrelin decreases after food intake, and increases when fasting with higher values during the night sleep [180, 201, 207]. In people on a fixed feeding schedule, circulating ghrelin levels are thought to be regulated by both calorie intake and circulating nutritional signals [162, 176]. Thus, blood glucose levels may play an important role in the regulation of ghrelin secretion: oral or intravenous administration of glucose decreases plasma ghrelin concentration [208]. Ghrelin levels fall in response to the ingestion of food, but not following gastric distension by water intake suggesting that mechanical distension of the stomach alone clearly does not induce ghrelin release [176, 209, 210]. In healthy subjects, a longer fasting period during the day (i.e. irregular meal pattern typical for several eating disorders) increases ghrelin concentration, but does not affect postprandial ghrelin response to a mixed meal [211]. The described pattern of secretion raised the concept of ghrelin as a hunger hormone, responsible for meal initiation. However, one study has failed to show a correlation between the ghrelin level and the spontaneous initiation of a meal in humans [212], and an alteration of feeding schedule in sheep has been shown to modify the timing of ghrelin peaks [213]. Recently Schüssler et al. showed that ghrelin levels increased significantly during a 30-min. interval following a presentation of pictures with food in healthy volunteers and suggested that in addition the sight of food can elevate ghrelin levels [214].

The most remarkable inhibitory input on ghrelin secretion is represented by the activation of somatostatin (SS) receptors as indicated by evidence that native SS, its natural analog cortistatin, and a synthetic analog such as octreotide lower circulating ghrelin levels in humans [215]. Ghrelin secretion in humans is under the stimulatory control of the cholinergic, namely muscarinic receptors, and acetylcholine is the first stimulatory neurotransmitter shown to play a stimulatory role on ghrelin secretion in humans [216].

In rats, ghrelin shows a bimodal peak, which occurs at the end of the light and dark periods [217]. In humans, ghrelin levels vary diurnally in phase with leptin, which is high in the morning and low at night [201].

It should be considered that ghrelin secretion may be a conditioned response which occurs to prepare the metabolism for an influx of calories. But, whatever the precise physiological role of ghrelin, it appears not to be an essential regulator of food intake, as ghrelin-null animals do not have significantly altered body weight or food intake on a normal diet [218].

Relationship between ghrelin and glucose-insulin homeostasis

Current extensive study data of ghrelin's role in metabolic processes indicate its unambiguous relation with control on glucose homeostasis and β-cell function. Both GHS-R1a and GHS-R1b are present in animal and human endocrine pancreas [219, 220]. Ghrelin is also present in pancreas, and epsilon pancreatic cells have been suggested to be a putative ghrelin-expressing cell type [221]. Moreover, a specific receptor able to bind both acylated and nonacylated ghrelin has also been demonstrated within the human pancreas; this is therefore a non-GHS-R1a [168, 222]. Ongoing studies support the hypothesis that ghrelin, independently of its acylation, modulates glucose metabolism at the hepatic level [223].

Exogenic ghrelin *short-tem effects* induce hyperglycaemia in experimental rodents via an GH-independent mechanism of action [224]. In contrast, ghrelin-receptor antagonists may improve glucose tolerance in rats, with no weight gain due to increased insulin secretion [225]. Acute administration of ghrelin to humans increases plasma glucose levels and amplifies the hyperglycaemic effect of arginine [226]. This hyperglycaemic effect might result from the endocrine effects of ghrelin as well as from direct effects on hepatocytes in which it modulates glycogen synthesis and gluconeogenesis [227]. Although data of ghrelin *long-term effects* are insufficiently clarified, a tendency of an increase in plasma glucose levels appears to be presented [224]. Many of the studies in patients with type 1 diabetes show low ghrelin levels, probably as a manifestation of a compensatory mechanism against hyperglycaemia [225].

Numerous studies indicate a negative association between systemic ghrelin and insulin levels [184, 228]. Thus, ghrelin is found to inhibit insulin secretion both *in vitro* and *in vivo* in most human and animal studies [226, 229]. In humans the acute administration of ghrelin inhibits spontaneous and arginine-stimulated insulin secretion but does not affect the insulin response to the oral glucose tolerance test (OGTT) [226, 230, 231]. In addition, the regulation of insulin secretion by ghrelin is closely related to the blood glucose level. Date et al. [232] reported that ghrelin stimulates insulin release in the presence of high levels of glucose (8.3mM) that could independently cause insulin release from cultured islet cells. In contrast, ghrelin had no effect on insulin release in the context of a basal level of glucose (2.8 mM) [232]. Antagonism of the pancreatic ghrelin can enhance insulin release to meet increased demand for insulin in high-fat diet-induced obesity of mice [233].

Ghrelin might influence some of the peripheral effects of insulin. Thus, it is found to stimulate hepatic glucose production [227], reinforce the action of insulin on glucose disposal in mice [234], inhibit adinopectin secretion [235] and stimulate secretion of the counter-regulatory hormones, including GH, cortisol, adrenaline [236] and possibly glucagon [237]. In healthy subjects, in the absence of GH and cortisol secretion, ghrelin acutely decreased peripheral, but not hepatic, insulin sensitivity together with stimulation of lipolysis. These effects occurred without detectable suppression of AMP-activated protein kinase phosphorylation (an alleged second messenger for ghrelin) in skeletal muscle [238]. So, ghrelin also exerts direct metabolic effects towards induction of insulin resistance independent of the regulation by counter-regulatory hormones.

Insulin in turn decreases ghrelin levels, regardless of changes in glucose concentrations [239]. Broglio et al. [240] have found that both oral and intravenous insulin suppress ghrelin, although they exhibit opposite effects on glucose levels. The same authors have shown that protein-induced inhibition of ghrelin is enabled by oral administration, while intravenous arginine does not lead to ghrelin reduction regardless of insulin elevations, which is a fact of interest and of relation to protein diets [240].

Given all the above data, it is proposed that ghrelin could have an important function in glucose homeostasis and insulin release, independent of GH secretion [241]. Data of administration of GHSR1a antagonists suggest that these compounds improve long-term glucose tolerance and insulin resistance. Since there are some differences about the role of ghrelin on insulin secretion [188], further research on ghrelin-insulin interrelationship is expected. At least theoretically, ghrelin and/or its signalling manipulation could be used for the treatment or prevention of diseases of glucose homeostasis.

Ghrelin in obesity, diabetes mellitus and metabolic syndrome

In addition to a probable role in meal initiation, ghrelin seems to be an adiposity-related hormone that is involved in the long-term regulation of body weight Plasma ghrelin levels are inversely correlated with body mass index and current evidence strongly suggests that ghrelin could contribute to obesity and the metabolic syndrome [225]. Variations within the ghrelin gene may contribute to early-onset obesity [242, 243] or be protective against fat accumulation [225], but the role of ghrelin polymorphisms in the control of body weight continues to be controversial [244, 245].

It has been shown that ghrelin secretion differs between lean and obese subjects. Thus, plasma ghrelin concentration is found to be low in obese people and high in lean people in some studies [207, 208, 246]. The expression of ghrelin receptors in the hypothalamus increases markedly with either fasting or chronic food restriction [247], as does the hypothalamic response to a ghrelin-receptor agonist [248], which is consistent with a feed-forward loop that enhances ghrelin-mediated stimulation of appetite during energy deficit. Anorexic individuals have high circulating ghrelin which falls to normal levels after weight gain [249]. The suppressed plasma ghrelin levels in obese subjects normalize after diet-induced weight loss [250]. The postprandial falls of serum ghrelin concentrations are proportional to energy intake in lean subjects, but not in obese subjects. Unlike lean individuals, obese subjects do not demonstrate the same rapid post-prandial drop in ghrelin levels [251]. Moreover, obesity is associated with much lower overall reduction of postprandial ghrelin levels and an absence of nocturnal elevations as seen in subjects of normal weight [194, 195, 210]. This may result in increased food intake and contribute to obesity. The fall in plasma ghrelin concentration after bariatric surgery, despite weight loss, is thought to be partly responsible for the suppression of appetite and weight loss seen after these operations [252].

The severe hyperphagia seen in Prader–Willi syndrome is associated with elevated ghrelin levels [253] that is in contrast to other forms of obesity, and it has been hypothesized that ghrelin might contribute to the nature of this syndrome. Moreover, there are similarities between the clinical features of Prader–Willi syndrome and those predicted from overstimulation of NPY by ghrelin (e.g. hyperphagic obesity, hypogonadotropic hypogonadism and dysregulation of GH) and the correlation between ghrelin levels and hyperphagia and excessive obesity, in these patients [254]. Indeed, the high ghrelin levels in obese people with Prader–Willi syndrome make the carriers of the syndrome logical first-line candidates for testing the weight reducing effects of ghrelin-blocking agents

Recently, the role of ghrelin in diabetes mellitus has been investigated: polymorphisms of the ghrelin gene are associated with the risk of diabetes [255], ghrelin promotes regeneration of b-cells in streptozocin-treated newborn rats, preventing the development of diabetes in disease-prone animals after b-cell destruction [256], and ghrelin antagonists partially reverse hyperphagia in uncontrolled, streptozocin-diabetic rats [257]. It has been found that fasting ghrelin concentrations are lower in people with type 2 diabetes mellitus than in non-diabetic people, even after adjusting for BMI. It has also been shown that the decrease in circulating ghrelin is proportionate to the degree of insulin insensitivity. We also found significant negative correlation between ghrelin and fasting insulin, and HOMA-index, respectively, in insulin resistant women with type 2 diabetes mellitus [258]. These observations suggest that ghrelin and insulin sensitivity are linked. All the data indicate that ghrelin might have a role in the pathogenesis and therapy of diabetes, contributing to either the impairment of insulin sensitivity or to the restraint of body-mass gain. Nonetheless, because of the controversy about the cause-and-effect relationship between ghrelin levels and diabetes mellitus, further investigations are needed to elucidate the precise role of ghrelin (and its variants) in the development and treatment of this disease.

Low plasma ghrelin levels are associated with metabolic cluster per se, which indicates that ghrelin might be a useful biomarker for the metabolic syndrome [228, 259]. Thus, conditions of severe metabolic syndrome due to insulin resistance, such as in obese Pima Indians, are related with reduced fasting ghrelin plasma levels [207]. In a study on the relation between metabolic parameters, ghrelin, leptin and IGF-1 in a cohort of 1,045 individuals, Ukkola et al. [260] have found that low ghrelin levels are associated with metabolic syndrome and type 2 diabetes mellitus only in presence of insulin and leptin resistance. At high leptin levels, ghrelin concentrations decrease linearly with increasing the number of metabolic syndrome components [260]. In patients on haemodialysis, fasting ghrelin levels negatively correlate with metabolic syndrome manifestation, ghrelin shows a tendency to decrease with increasing the number of the metabolic syndrome components, and the waist circumference appears to be an independent predictor of its levels [261].

In patients with the metabolic syndrome and low ghrelin levels, intraarterial administration of ghrelin rapidly improves endothelial function [262]. Similar to insulin, ghrelin stimulates an increased nitrogen oxide (NO) production in cultured bovine aortic endothelial cells in a dose- and time-dependent manner. It has been found that ghrelin-induced NO production in human aortic endothelial cells is arrested by their pre-treatment with a NO-synthase inhibitor, phosphatidylinositol synthase (PI 3)-kinase inhibitor, selective GHSR-1a antagonist or "exclusion" of these receptors. On the other hand, ghrelin has been found to stimulate enhanced phosphorylation of Akt (Ser^{473}) and endothelial NO-synthase in human aortic endothelial cells, as well as phosphorylation of mitogen-activated protein (MAP) kinase, but not of MAP-kinase-dependent production of the vasoconstrictor endothelin-1 in bovine aortic endothelial cells. With regard to these data it may be concluded that ghrelin exhibits characteristic, rapid vascular effects, presented as stimulated NO production in the endothelium via signal pathways including the GHSR-1a, PI 3-kinase, Akt and endothelial NO-synthase, which may be taken into consideration for the development of innovative therapeutic strategies for endothelial dysfunction in diabetes and insulin resistance [262].

Vlasova et al. have found that peripheral injection of a ghrelin antagonist in experimental animals (rats) increases arterial pressure and pulse rate via at least partial activation of the sympathetic nervous system [263]. These findings direct our attention to eventual cardiovascular adverse effects, when administering ghrelin antagonists as a therapeutic strategy for reducing food intake, particularly in patients at a high cardiovascular (CV) risk (e.g., patients with metabolic syndrome).

Ghrelin's role in processes of reproduction and PCOS

Presently not so much is known of ghrelin effects on processes of reproduction. Experimental models in rats have shown that ghrelin plays a role at different levels of the hypothalamic-pituitary-ovary axis regulation. Its central route of administration in female rats results in suppression of the LH secretion at various stages of estrus [264]. In *in vitro* settings, ghrelin also inhibits gonadotropin-releasing hormone (GnRH) secretion from the hypothalamus [264]. At a pituitary level, ghrelin exhibits either stimulating or inhibiting action on basal LH secretion, depending on the menstrual cycle stage. However, the *in vitro* GnRH-stimulated LH release is inhibited by ghrelin, regardless of the steroid medium [265]. In rhesus monkeys, the confirmed inhibitory effect of ghrelin on the GnRH-LH system suggests that in primates, ghrelin exhibits a central regulatory effect on processes of reproduction [266].

It was shown by Kluge et al. that ghrelin suppresses the secretion of LH and FSH in healthy women [267]. Ghrelin levels have been found to be higher in anovulatory women with excessive physical loading-induced anorexia nervosa and amenorrhea, as well as in normal weight-women with hypothalamic amenorrhea [268-270]. In normal-weight women with amenorrhea, the increased ghrelin levels have been associated with disturbed dietary habits and regimen [271]. It is not clear whether disturbances in ghrelin secretion play a direct role in neuroendocrine regulation of the hypothalamic-pituitary-ovary axis or present a marker of the metabolic status itself.

In males, ghrelin has an additional inhibitory role, decreasing human chorionic gonadotropin (hCG)- and cAMP-stimulated testosterone secretion [272] and the expression of the gene encoding stem cell factor that is a key mediator of spermatogenesis and a putative regulator of Leydig-cell development [273]. In hypogonadal males, a positive correlation between ghrelin and androgens persists after testosterone replacement therapy [274].

There is no consensus on whether alterations in levels of appetite-regulating hormones, such as ghrelin, are associated with PCOS. Fasting ghrelin levels were found decreased in most [275-279], but not in all studies [280, 281] in women with PCOS. Thus in 2002, Pagotto et al. [275] first demonstrated that ghrelin levels were lower in obese women with PCOS, compared with these in weight-matched healthy controls. Ghrelin has been inversely correlated with insulin resistance markers. These correlations have persisted even after therapy (hypocaloric diet plus metformin or placebo) for improving insulin sensitivity. In both groups, weight reduction has resulted in minimal changes of plasma ghrelin levels. The observed negative correlation between ghrelin and androstenedione, but not between ghrelin and testosterone or other androgens, is interesting [275]. In PCOS, Schofl et al. have confirmed lower ghrelin levels that are in a close correlation with insulin resistance rates [276]. After therapy with metformin in insulin-resistant women, ghrelin levels have increased, but in insulin-sensitive women with PCOS, ghrelin levels have been comparable to these in controls. Furthermore, the authors have found no correlation between ghrelin and the body mass index (BMI) [276], which suggests a ghrelin-insulin resistance interrelation apart from ghrelin activity in controlling appetite, body weight, respectively. Panidis et al. [282] have reported that women with PCOS and hyperandrogenaemia have significantly lower ghrelin levels compared to healthy controls and PCOS carriers with clinical hyperandrogenism but normal androgen levels. Ghrelin levels in the latter are lower than these found in the control group, but the differences are not statistically significant. The authors have concluded that PCOS-associated hyperandrogenaemia results in reduced ghrelin concentrations [282]. Although PCOS-associated hyperandrogenaemia and 17-OH-progesterone levels are inversely related to ghrelin levels, anovulation and polycystic ovary morphology are associated with higher ghrelin concentrations [283]. Thus, it has been hypothesized that different clinical and biochemical manifestations of the syndrome might be associated with different concentrations of ghrelin.

In support of the relation between PCOS and ghrelin, there are data of increased ghrelin levels after a 3-month treatment with an oral contraceptive containing both ethinyl oestradiol and drospirenone in women with PCOS [284]. Similar to other studies, ghrelin is negatively correlated with the BMI, waist/hip ratio, insulin, homeostatic model assessment (HOMA) index and free testosterone [284]. According to a study conducted by Fusco et al., ghrelin administration in normal weight-women and obese PCOS patients has exerted glucose-enhancing and insulin-lowering effects, the latter absent in the normal weight-controls [285], which supports the relation between ghrelin and hormonal/metabolic disorders in PCOS.

One of studies that have not confirmed changes in ghrelin levels in women with PCOS is this conducted by Orio et al. [280]. The authors have found no correlation between ghrelin and either of the hormonal or biochemical parameters (including insulin and insulin resistance markers), but only a correlation between ghrelin and the BMI [280]. These data support the relation determined between ghrelin and the body weight only and exclude the effects of the disease itself. These findings are in a sense similar to those observed by Bik et al., who have not found significant differences in ghrelin levels between a group of normal weight PCOS women and a group of normal weight healthy women; however, ghrelin was significantly lower in healthy obese women compared to lean women with PCOS [286].

Impaired ghrelin suppression after a test meal and increased feeling of hunger and decreased feeling of satiety (according to visual analogue scales) have been described in a small group of obese women with PCOS, even after weight reduction [287], which has been also confirmed by another study, comparing lean and obese women with PCOS and relevant, weight-matched controls [288]. Romualdi et al. [289] gave more detailed evaluation of ghrelin and polypeptide YY responses following oral load with a test meal (527 kcal, distributed by contents in 24.1% fats, 54.4% carbohydrates and 21.5% proteins) in women with PCOS. Low baseline ghrelin levels and reduced suppression after meals, more pronounced in the obese than in the lean patients was shown. The authors have found no correlation between ghrelin and the androgens; however, a negative correlation has been established between ghrelin and the HOMA-index. Compared to controls, PCOS women had a significantly suppressed neuropeptide Y response to injected ghrelin, as the response has restored after treatment with metformin and significant insulin reduction. In this experimental setting, leptin has undergone no significant changes [289]. Obviously, hyperinsulinaemia is the factor which exerts effect on the ghrelin-neuropeptide Y relation.

We found significantly lower ghrelin levels in women with PCOS compared to healthy controls (21.78 ± 2.12 ng/ml versus 34.67 ± 3.57 ng/ml; $p = 0.04$), as ghrelin was inversely correlated with insulin levels at a degree similar to these of insulin resistance markers.

Negative correlations were also found with the BMI, waist measurement and waist-to-hip ratio, in conformity with most of the studies at present. Furthermore, the observed negative correlation between ghrelin and testosterone ($r = -0.315$; $p < 0.05$), and this between ghrelin and leptin ($r = -0.306$; $p<0.05$) disappear after the exclusion of BMI, waist-to-hip ratio and HOMA-index [290]. In a comparative study on ghrelin levels in insulin-resistant women with PCOS and women with type 2 diabetes and higher insulin resistance, ghrelin levels have been significantly lower in syndrome carriers versus diabetics [291]. Based on our data we consider that ghrelin levels in women with PCOS reflect both the metabolic and hormonal disturbances, typical for the syndrome.

A recent study conducted by Panidis et al. [292] has confirmed that alterations in ghrelin secretion are intrinsic for the disease itself and has demonstrated that active (acetylated) ghrelin/total ghrelin ratio is decreased in normal weight-women with PCOS, as the anomalies are most pronounced in the severe forms of the syndrome, including all diagnostic criteria: hyperandrogenia, chronic anovulation and morphologically polycystic ovaries [292]. Based on the proven changes in women with PCOS and various phenotype manifestations, some authors have even suggested ghrelin to be used as a predictive marker of PCOS and have found through a plot-analysis of the receiver operating characteristic curve (ROC) a sensitivity of 70% and specificity of 86% with a cut-off value of 34.1 ng/ml, below which the diagnosis of PCOS is likely, while a cut-off ghrelin value below 9 ng/ml is highly specific for PCOS [293].

In conclusion, there is, probably, an anomaly in ghrelin regulation in PCOS, related not only to overweight and insulin resistance. The mechanisms associating abnormal ghrelin regulation with the disease are still to be elucidated. However, the pathological and therapeutic importance of this association is unclear. Independent effects of ghrelin on the hypothalamic-pituitary-gonadal axis with an inhibitory effect on the LH secretion and a decreased LH response to GnRH, typical for the syndrome, may also be taken into consideration.

4. Conclusion

Given the growing epidemic of obesity, it has become increasingly important to understand the physiological processes that regulate body weight. Regulation of food intake and metabolism is maintained by complex pathways and neuronal circuits which themselves receive peripheral signals such as gut hormones. Metabolically important abdominal obesity with an excess of visceral fat accumulation results in altered release of adipokines, leading to CNS mediated skeletal muscle and hepatic insulin resistance. The central regulation of energy balance has become even more fascinating and complex with the characterization of mechanisms of action of NPY, the most abundant hypothalamic orexigenic factor. Much attention has recently centered on ghrelin, the only known circulating orexigen. Insulin resistance and compensatory hyperinsulinemia are independently associated with suppression of ghrelin that furthers our understanding of the variable expression of ghrelin in humans.

With continued research, it should be possible to elucidate exactly how the associations among insulin resistance, hyperinsulinemia, and orexigens (NPY and ghrelin) participate in the more intricate web of factors that regulate body weight. Better understanding of the mechanisms involved in the regulation of energy metabolism will become a background for development of new therapeutic approaches against obesity, insulin resistance, metabolic syndrome, and other nutritional disorders.

Author details

Maria Orbetzova
Clinic of Endocrinology and Metabolic Diseases, "Sv.Georgy" University Hospital, Medical University, Plovdiv, Bulgaria

5. References

[1] Ahima RS, Filer J (2000) Adipose tissue as an endocrine organ. Trends. Endocrinol. Metab. 11; 327-329.
[2] Milcheva B, Orbetzova M (2004) Adipose tissue – an endocrine organ. Endokrinologiya 9(2): 64-72 (in Bulgarian).
[3] Wilding JP (2002) Neuropeptides and appetite control. Diabet. Med. 19: 619-627.
[4] Lopaschuk GD, Ussher JR, Jaswal JS (2010) Targeting intermediary metabolism in the hypothalamus as a mechanism to regulate appetite. Pharmacol. Rev. 62: 237–264.
[5] Simpson KA, Martin NM, Bloom SR (2009) Hypothalamic regulation of food intake and clinical therapeutic applications. Arq. bras. Endocrinol. Metab. 53(2): 120-128.
[6] Higgins S, Gueurguiev M, Korbonits M (2007) Ghrelin, the peripheral hunger hormone. Annals med. 39: 116–136.
[7] Suzuki K, Simpson KA, Minnion JS, Shillito JC, Bloom SR (2010) The role of gut hormones and the hypothalamus in appetite regulation. Endocrine J. 57 (5), 359-372.
[8] Zhang Y, Ning G, Handelsman Y, Bloomgarden ZT (2010) Gut hormones and the brain. J. Diab. 2: 138–145.
[9] Schwartz MW, Woods SC, Porte DJr, Seeley RJ, Baskin DG (2000) Central nervous system control of food intake. Nature 404: 661–671.
[10] Bouret SG, Draper SJ, Simerly RB (2004) Formation of projection pathways from the arcuate nucleus of the hypothalamus to hypothalamic regions implicated in the neural control of feeding behavior in mice. J. Neurosci. 24(11): 2797-2805.
[11] Benoit SC, Tracy AL, Davis JF, Choi D (2008) Novel functions of orexigenic hypothalamic peptides: From genes to behavior. Nutrition 24(9): 843–847.
[12] Porte D Jr, Baskin DG , Schwartz MW (2002) Leptin and insulin action in the central nervous system. Nutrition Rev. 60: S20–S29.
[13] Cowley MA, Smart JL, Rubinstein M, Cerdan MG, Diano S, Horvath TL, Cone RD, Low MJ (2001) Leptin activates anorexigenic POMC neurons through a neural network in the arcuate nucleus. Nature 411(6836): 480-484.
[14] Bagnol D, Lu XY, Kaelin CB, Day HE, Ollmann M, Gantz I, Akil H, Barsh GS, Watson SJ (1999) Anatomy of an endogenous antagonist: relationship between Agouti-related protein and proopiomelanocortin in brain. J. Neurosci. 19(18): RC26.

[15] Rosenbaum M, Leibel RL, Hirsch J (1997) Obesity. NEJM 337(6): 396-407.

[16] Wynne K, Stanley S, McGowan B, Bloom S (2005) Appetite control. J. Endocrinol. 184: 291–318.

[17] Cowley MA, Smith RG, Diano S, Tschop M, Pronchuk N, Grove KL, Strasburger CJ, Bidlingmaier M, Esterman M, Heiman ML, Garcia-Segura LM, Nillni EA, Mendez P, Low MJ, Sotonyi P, Friedman JM, Liu H, Pinto S, Colmers WF, Cone RD, Horvath TL (2003) The distribution and mechanism of action of ghrelin in the CNS demonstrates a novel hypothalamic circuit regulating energy homeostasis. Neuron 37(4): 649-661.

[18] Toshinai K, Date Y, Murakami N, Shimada M, Mondal MS, Shimbara T, Guan JL, Wang QP, Funahashi H, Sakurai T, Shioda S, Matsukura S, Kangawa K, Nakazato M (2003) Ghrelin-induced food intake is mediated via the orexin pathway. Endocrinology 144(4): 1506-1512.

[19] Greenman Y, Golani N, Gilad S, Yaron M, Limor R, Stern N (2004) Ghrelin secretion is modulated in a nutrient- and gender-specific manner. Clin. Endocrinol. 60, 382–388.

[20] Van Vugt DA, Lujan ME, Froats M, Krzemien A, Couceyro PR, Reid RL (2006) Effect of fasting on cocaine-amphetamine-regulated transcript, neuropeptide Y, and leptin receptor expression in the non-human primate hypothalamus. Neuroendocrinology 84(2): 83–93.

[21] Tatemoto K (1982) Neuropeptide Y: complete amino acid sequence of the brain peptide. Proc Natl. Acad. Sci. USA 79: 5485–5489.

[22] Cerda-Reverter JM, Larhammar D (2000). Neuropeptide Y family of peptides: structure, anatomical expression, function, and molecular evolution. Biochem. Cell Biol. 78: 371-392.

[23] Frankish HM, Dryden S, Hopkins D, Wang Q, Williams G (1995) Neuropeptide Y, the hypothalamus, and diabetes: insights into the central control of metabolism. Peptides 16: 757-771.

[24] Dryden S, Frankish H, Wang Q, Williams G (1994) Neuropeptide Y and energy balance: one way ahead for the treatment of obesity? Eur. J. Clin. Invest. 24: 293–308.

[25] Zukowska-Grojec Z (1995) Neuropeptide Y: a novel sympathetic stress hormone and more. Ann. N Y Acad. Sci. 771: 219-233

[26] Taborsky GJ, Beltramini LM, Brown M, Veith RC, Kowalyk S (1994) Canine liver releases neuropeptide Y during sympatheticnerve stimulation. Am.j. physiol. 266: E804-E812.

[27] Sundler F, Ekblad E, Hakanson R (1991) The neuroendocrine system of the gut - an update. Acta oncol. 30: 419-427.

[28] Pettersson M, Ahren B, Lundquist I, Bottcher G, Sundler F (1987) Neuropeptide Y: intrapancreatic neuronal localization and effects on insulin secretion in the mouse. Cell tissue res. 248: 43-48.

[29] Sanacora G, Kershaw M, Finkelstein JA, White JD (1990) Increased hypothalamic content of preproneuropeptide Y messenger ribonucleic acid in genetically obese Zucker rats and its regulation by food deprivation. Endocrinology 127: 730-737.

[30] Kalra SP, Dube MG, Fournier A, Kalra PS (1991) Structurefunction analysis of stimulation of food intake by neuropeptide Y: effects of receptor agonists. Physiol. Behav. 50: 5–9.
[31] Swart I, Jahng JW, Overton JM, Houpt TA (2002) Hypothalamic NPY, AGRP, and POMC mRNA responses to leptin and refeeding in mice. Am. J. Physiol. 283: R1020-R1026.
[32] Chavez M, Seeley RJ, Havel PJ, Friedman M, Woods SC, Schwartz MW (1998). Effect of a high-fat diet on food intake and hypothalamic neuropeptide gene expression in streptozotocin diabetes. J. Clin. Invest. 102: 340-346.
[33] Widdowson PS, Upton R, Henderson L, Buckingham R, WilsonS, Williams G (1997) Reciprocal regional changes in brain NPY receptor density during dietary restriction and dietary-induced obesity in the rat. Brain Res. 774: 1–10.
[34] Arora S, Anubhuti. (2006) Role of neuropeptides in appetite regulation and obesity–a review. Neuropeptides 40: 375–401.
[35] Kalra SP, Ueno N, Kalra PS (2005) Stimulation of appetite by ghrelin is regulated by leptin restraint: peripheral and central sites of action. J. Nutrition 135: 1331–1335.
[36] Faouzi M, Leshan R, Bjornholm M, Hennessey T, Jones J, Munzberg H (2007) Differential accessibility of circulating leptin to individual hypothalamic sites. Endocrinology 148(11): 5414-5423.
[37] Mercer JG, Hoggard N, Williams LM, Lawrence CB, Hannah LT, Morgan PJ, Trayhurn P (1996) Coexpression of leptin receptor and preproneuropeptide Y mRNA in arcuate nucleus of mouse hypothalamus. J. Neuroendocrinol. 8(10):733–735.
[38] Wang ZL, Bennet WM,Wang RM, Ghatei MA (1994) Evidence of a paracrine role of neuropeptide Y in the regulation of insulin
[39] Tamura H, Kamegai J, Shimizu T, Ishii S, Sigihara H, Oikawa S (2002) Ghrelin stimulates GH but not food intake in arcuate nucleus ablated rats. Endocrinology 143(9): 3268-3275.
[40] Chen HY, Trumbauer ME, Chen AS, Weingarth DT, Adams JR, Frazier EG, Shen Z, Marsh DJ, Feighner SD, Guan XM, Ye Z, Nargund RP, Smith RG, van der Ploeg LH, Howard, AD, MacNeil DJ, Quian S (2004) Orexigenic action of peripheral ghrelin is mediated by neuropeptide Y (NPY) and Agouti-related protein (AgRP). Endocrinology 145 (10): 1210.
[41] Woods SC, Seeley RJ, Baskin DG, Schwartz MW (2003) Insulin and the blood-brain barrier. Curr. pharm. des. 9: 795–800.
[42] Banks WA (2004) The source of cerebral insulin. Eur. J. Pharmacol. 490: 5–12.
[43] Baura GD, Foster DM, Porte D Jr, Kahn SE, Bergman RN, Cobelli C, Schwartz MW (1993) Saturable transport of insulin from plasma into the central nervous system of dogs in vivo. A mechanism for regulated insulin delivery to the brain. J. Clin. Invest. 92: 1824–1830.
[44] Marks JL, Porte DJr, Stahl WL, Baskin DG (1990) Localization of insulin receptor mRNA in rat brain by in situ hybridization. Endocrinology 127: 3234–3236.
[45] Corp ES, Woods SC, Porte DJr, Dorsa DM, Figlewicz DP, Baskin DG (1986) Localization of 125I-insulin binding sites in the rat hypothalamus by quantitative autoradiography. Neurosci. Lett. 70: 17–22.

[46] Schwartz MW, Sipols AJ, Marks JL, Sanacora G, White JD, Scheurink A, Kahn SE, Baskin DG, Woods SC, Figlewicz DP (1992) Inhibition of hypothalamic neuropeptide Y gene expression by insulin. Endocrinology 130: 3608–3616.

[47] Williams G, Gill JS, Lee YC, Cardoso HM, Okpere BE, Bloom SR (1989) Increased neuropeptide Y concentrations in specific hypothalamic regions of streptozocin-induced diabetic rats. Diabetes 38: 321–327.

[48] White JD, Olchovsky D, Kershaw M, Berelowitz M (1990) Increased hypothalamic content of preproneuropeptide-Y messenger ribonucleic acid in streptozotocin-diabetic rats. Endocrinology 126: 765–772.

[49] Benoit SC, Air EL, Coolen LM, Strauss R, Jackman A, Clegg DJ, Seeley RJ, Woods SC (2002) The catabolic action of insulin in the brain is mediated by melanocortins. J. Neurosci. 22: 9048–9052.

[50] Sipols AJ, Baskin DG, Schwartz MW (1995) Effect of intracerebroventricular insulin infusion on diabetic hyperphagia and hypothalamic neuropeptide gene expression. Diabetes 44: 147–151.

[51] Fuxe K, Wikström AC, Okret S, Agnati LF, Härfstrand A, Yu ZY, Granholm L, Zoli M, Vale W, Gustafsson JA (1985) Mapping of glucocorticoid receptor immunoreactive neurons in the rat tel- and diencephalon using a monoclonal antibody against rat liver glucocorticoid receptor. Endocrinology 117: 1803–1812.

[52] Harfstrand A, Cintra A, Fuxe K, Aronsson M, Wikström AC, Okret S, Gustafsson JA, Agnati LF (1989) Regional differences in glucocorticoid receptor immunoreactivity among neuropeptide Y immunoreactive neurons of the rat brain. Acta Physiol. Scand. 135: 3–9.

[53] Rebuffe-Scrive M, Walsh UA, McEwen B, Rodin J (1992) Effects of chronic stress and exogenous glucocorticoids on regional fat distribution and metabolism. Physiol. Behav. 52: 583–590.

[54] Larsen PJ, Jessop DS, Chowdrey HS, Lightman SL, Mikkelsen JD (1994) Chronic administration of glucocorticoids directly upregulates prepro-neuropeptide Y and Y1-receptor mRNA levels in the arcuatenucleus of the rat. J. Neurendocrinol. 6: 153–159.

[55] Akabayashi A, WatanabeY, Wahlestedt C, McEwen BC, Paez X, Leibowitz SF (1994) Hypothalamic neuropeptide Y, its gene expression and receptor activity: relation to circulating corticosterone in adrenalectomized rats. Brain Res. 665: 201–212.

[56] Freedman MR, Horwitz BA, Stern JS (1986) Effect of adrenalectomy and glucocorticoid replacement on development of obesity. Am. J. Physiol. 250: R595–R607.

[57] King BM, Banta AR, Tharel GN, Bruce BK, Frohman LA (1983) Hypothalamic hyperinsulinaemia and obesity: role of adrenal glucocorticoids. Am. J. Physiol. 245: E194–E199.

[58] Sainsbury A, Cusin I, Doyle P, Rohner-Jeanrenaud F, Jeanrenaud B (1996) Intracerebroventricular administration of neuropeptide Y to normal rats increases obese gene expression in white adipose tissue. Diabetologia 39: 353–356.

[59] Sainsbury A, Cusin I, Rohner-Jeanrenaud F, Jeanrenaud B (1997). Adrenalectomy prevents the obesity syndrome produced by chronic central neuropeptide Y infusion in normal rats. Diabetes 46: 209–214.

[60] Wisialowski T, Parker Rl, Preston E, Sainsbury A, Kraegen E, Herzog H, Cooney G (2000) Adrenalectomy reduces neuropeptide Y–induced insulin release and NPY receptor expression in the rat ventromedial hypothalamus. J. Clin. Invest. 105:1253–1259
[61] Sundkvist G, Bramnert M, Bergstrom B, Manhem P, Lilja B, Ahren B (1992) Plasma neuropeptide Y (NPY) and galanin before and during exercise in type 1 diabetic patients with autonomic disfunction. Diabetes Res. Clin. Pract. 15: 219-226.
[62] Takahashi K, Mouri T, Itoi K, Sone M, Ohneda M, Murakami O, Nozuki M, Tachibana Y, Yoshinaga K (1987) Increased plasmaimmunoreactive neuropeptide Y concentrations in phaeochromocytoma and chronic renal failure. J. Hypertens. 5: 749-753
[63] Larhammar D (1996) Structural diversity of receptors for neuropeptide Y, peptide YY and pancreatic polypeptide. Regulatory Peptides 65: 165–174.
[64] Wahlestedt C, Grundemar L, Håkanson R, Heilig M, Shen GH, Zukowska-Grojec Z, Reis DJ (1990) Neuropeptide Y receptor subtypes, Y1 and Y2. Ann. N Y Acad. Sci. 611: 7-26.
[65] Blomqvist AG, Herzog H (1997) Y-receptor subtypes: how many more? Trends Neurosci. 20: 294–298.
[66] Inui A (1999) Neuropeptide Y feeding receptors: are multiple subtypes involved? Trends Pharmacol. Sci. 20: 43–46.
[67] Parker E, Van Heek M, Stamford A (2002) Neuropeptide Y receptors as targets for anti-obesity drug development: perspective and current status Eur. J. Pharmacol. 440: 173–187.
[68] Kalra SP, Kalra PS (2004) NPY and cohorts in regulating appetite, obesity and metabolic syndrome: beneficial effects of gene therapy. Neuropeptides 38: 201–211.
[69] Schaffhauser AO, Stricker-Krongrad A, Brunner L, Cumin F, Gerald C, Whitebread S, Criscione L, Hofbauer KG. (1997) Inhibition of food intake by neuropeptide Y Y5 receptor antisense oligodeoxynucleotides. Diabetes 46: 1792–1798.
[70] Kushi A, Sasai H, Koizumi H, Takeda N, Yokoyama M, Nakamura M (1998) Obesity and mild hyperinsulinemia found in neuropeptide Y-Y1 receptor-deficient mice. Proc. Natl. Acad. Sci. U S A. 95(26): 15659-15664.
[71] Lin E-JD, Sainsbury A, Lee NJ, Boey D, Couzens M, Enriquez R, Slack K, Bland R, During MJ, Herzog H (2006) Combined Deletion of Y1, Y2, and Y4 Receptors Prevents Hypothalamic Neuropeptide Y Overexpression-Induced Hyperinsulinemia despite Persistence of Hyperphagia and Obesity. Endocrinology 147: 5094-5101.
[72] Parker EM, Balasubramaniam A, Guzzi M, Mullins DE, Salisbury BG, Sheriff S, Witten MB, Hwa JJ (2000) [D-Trp^{34}] neuropeptide Y is a potent and selective neuropeptide Y Y_5 receptor agonist with dramatic effects on food intake. Peptides 21: 393–399.
[73] Erundu N, Gantz I, Musser B, Suryawanshi S, Mallick M, Addy C, Cote J, Bray G, Fujioka K, Bays H, Hollander P, Sanabria-Bohórquez SM, Eng WS, Långström B, Hargreaves RJ, Burns HD, Kanatani A, Fukami T, MacNeil DJ, Gottesdiener KM, Amatruda JM, Kaufman KD, Heymsfield SB (2006) Neuropeptide Y5 receptor antagonism does not induce clinically meaningful weight loss in overweight and obese adults. Cell Metab. 4(4): 275-282.
[74] Farooq S (2006) Treating obesity: Does antagonism of NPY fit the bill? Cell Metab. 4(4): 260-262.

[75] Stanley BG, Leibowitz SF (1985) Neuropeptide Y injected into the paraventricular hypothalamus: a powerful stimulant of feeding behavior. Proc. Natl. Acad. Sci. USA 82: 3940 –3943.

[76] Morley JE, Levine AS, Gosnell BA, Kneip J, Grace M (1987) Effect of neuropeptide Y on ingestive behaviors in the rat. Am. J. Physiol. 252: 599–609.

[77] Stanley BG, Anderson KC, Grayson MH, Leibowitz SF (1989) Repeated hypothalamic stimulation with neuropeptide Y increases daily carbohydrate and fat intake and body weight gain in female rats. Physiol. Behav. 46: 173–177.

[78] Beck B, Stricker-Krongrad A, Nicols JP, Burlet C (1992) Chronic and continuous intracerebroventricular infusion of neuropeptide Y in Long-Evans rats mimics the feeding of obese Zucker rats. Int. J. Obesity 16: 295–302.

[79] Billington CJ, Briggs JE, Grace M, Levine AS (1991) Effects of intracerebroventricular injection of neuropeptide Y on energy metabolism. Am. J. Physiol. – Regulatory, Integrative and Comparative Physiology 260: R321–R327.

[80] Egawa M, Yoshimatsu H, Bray GA (1991) Neuropeptide Y suppresses sympathetic activity to interscapular brown adipose tissue in rats. Am. j. physiol. – Regulatory, Integrative and Comparative Physiology 260: R328–R334.

[81] Fekete C, Sarkar S, Rand WM, Harney JW, Emerson CH, Bianco AC, Lechan RM (2002) Agouti-related protein (AGRP) has a central inhibitory action on the hypothalamic-pituitary-thyroid (HPT) axis; comparisons between the effect of AGRP and neuropeptide Y on energy homeostasis and the HPT axis. Endocrinology 143: 3846–3853.

[82] Kakui N, Kitamura K (2007) Direct Evidence that Stimulation of Neuropeptide Y Y_5 Receptor Activates Hypothalamo-Pituitary-Adrenal Axis in Conscious Rats via both Corticotropin-Releasing Factor- and Arginine Vasopressin-Dependent Pathway. Neuroendocrinology 148 (6): 2854

[83] Wahlestedt C, Skagerberg G, Ekman R, Heilig M, Sundler F, Hakanson R (1987) Neuropeptide Y (NPY) in the area of the hypothalamic paraventricular nucleus activates the pituitary-adrenocortical axis in the rat. Brain Res. 417: 33–38

[84] Bai FL, Yamano M, Shiotani Y, Emson PC, Smith AD, Powell JF, Tohyama M (1985) An arcuato-paraventricular and –dorsomedial hypothalamic neuropeptide Y-containing system which lacks noradrenaline in the rat. Brain Res. 331: 172–175.

[85] Zarjevski N, Cusin I, Vettor R, Rohner-Jeanrenaud F, Jeanrenaud B (1993) Chronic intracerebroventricular neuropeptide-Y administration to normal rats mimics hormonal and metabolic changes of obesity. Endocrinology 133: 1753–1758

[86] Vettor R, Zarjevski N, Cusin I, Rohner-Jeanrenaud F, Jeanrenaud B (1994) Induction and reversibility of an obesity syndrome by intracerebroventricular neuropeptide Y administration to normal rats. Diabetologia 37: 1202–1208

[87] Kalra PS, Dube MG, Xu B, Kalra SP (1997) Increased receptor sensitivity to neuropeptide Y in the hypothalamus may underlie transient hyperphagia and body weight gain. Regul. Pept. 72: 121–130

[88] Penicaud L, Kinebanyan MF, Ferré P, Morin J, Kandé J, Smadja C, Marfaing-Jallat P, Picon L (1989) Development of VMH obesity: in vivo insulin secretion and tissue insulin sensitivity. Am. J. Physiol. 257: E255–E260

[89] Guan XM, Yu H, Trumbauer M, Frazier E, Van der Ploeg LH, Chen H (1998) Induction of neuropeptide Y expression in dorsomedial hypothalamus of diet-induced obese mice. Neuroreport. 9: 3415–3419

[90] Heidel E, Plagemann A, Davidowa H (1999) Increased response to NPY of hypothalamic VMH neurons in postnatally overfed juvenile rats. Neuroreport. 10: 1827–1831.

[91] Leibowitz SF, Sladek C, Spencer L, Tempel D (1988) NeuropeptideY, epinephrine and norepinephrine in the paraventricular nucleus: stimulation of feeding and the release of corticosterone, vasopressin and glucose. Brain Res. Bull. 21: 905–912.

[92] van den Hoek AM, van Heijningen C, Schro¨der-van der Elst JP, Ouwens DM, Havekes LM, Romijn JA, Kalsbeek A, Pijl H (2008) Intracerebroventricular Administration of Neuropeptide Y Induces Hepatic Insulin Resistance via Sympathetic Innervation. Diabetes 57: 2304–2310.

[93] Singhal NS, Lazar MA, Ahima RS (2007) Central Resistin Induces Hepatic Insulin Resistance via Neuropeptide Y. J. Neurosci. 27(47): 12924 –12932.

[94] Schwartz MW, Baskin DG, Bukowski TR, Kuijper JL, Foster D, Lasser G, Prunkard DE, Porte D Jr, Woods SC, Seeley RJ, Weigle DS (1996) Specificity of leptin action on elevated blood glucose levels and hypothalamic neuropeptide Y gene expression in ob/ob mice. Diabetes 45(4): 531–535

[95] Stephens TW, Basinski M, Bristow PK, Bue-Valleskey JM, Burgett SG, Craft L, et al. (1995) The role of neuropeptide Y in the antiobesity action of the obese gene product. Nature 377: 530-532

[96] Thorsell A, Heilig M (2002) Diverse functions of neuropeptide Y revealed using genetically modified animals. Neuropeptides 36: 182–193.

[97] Bannon AW, Seda J, Carmouche M, Francis JM, Norman MH, Karbon B, McCaleb ML (2000) Behavioral characterization of neuropeptide Y knockout mice. Brain Res. 868: 79–87.

[98] Marsh DJ, Miura GI, Yagaloff KA, Schwartz MW, Barsh GS, Palmiter RD (1999) Effects of neuropeptide Y deficiency on hypothalamic agouti-related protein expression and responsiveness to melanocortin analogues. Brain Res. 848: 66–77

[99] Raposinho PD, Pedrazzini T, White RB, Palmiter RD, Aubert ML (2004) Chronic neuropeptide Y infusion into the lateral ventricle induces sustained feeding and obesity in mice lacking either Npy1r or Npy5r expression. Endocrinology 145: 304–310

[100] Jenkinson CP, Cray K, Walder K, Herzog H, Hanson R, Ravussin E (2000) Novel polymorphisms in the neuropeptide-Y Y5 receptor associated with obesity in Pima Indians. Int. J. Obes. 24: 580–584

[101] Rosenkranz K, Hinney A, Ziegler A, Vonprittwitz S, Barth N, Roth H (1998) Screening for mutations in the neuropeptide Y Y5 receptor gene in cohorts belonging to different weight extremes. Int .J. Obes. 22: 157–163

[102] Blumenthal JB, Andersen RE, Mitchell BD, Seibert MJ, Yang H, Herzog H, Beamer BA, Franckowiak SC, Walston JD (2002) Novel neuropeptide Y1 and Y5 receptor gene variants: associations with serum triglyceride and high-density lipoprotein cholesterol levels. Clin. Genet. 2002; 62:196 –202.

[103] Roche C, Boutin P, Dinal C, Gyapay G, Basdevant A, Hager J, Guy-Grand B, Cle´ment K, Froguel P (1997) Genetic studies of neuropeptide Y and neuropeptide Y receptors Y1 and Y5 regions in morbid obesity. Diabetologia 40: 671–675

[104] Colletta, DK, J Schneider J, Stern MP, Blangero J, Defronzo RA, Duggirala R, Jenkinson CP (2007) Association of neuropeptide Y receptor Y5 polymorphisms with dyslipidemia in Mexican Americans. Obesity 15: 809–815.

[105] Kuo LE, Kitlinska JB, Tilan JU, Li L, Baker SB, Johnson MD, Lee EW, Burnett MS, Fricke ST, Kvetnansky R, Herzog H, Zukowska Z (2007) Neuropeptide Y acts directly in the periphery on fat tissue and mediates stress-induced obesity and metabolic syndrome Nat. Med. 13(7): 803-811

[106] Petterson M, Ahren B (1990) Insulin secretion in rats: effects of neuropeptide Y and noradrenaline. Diabetes Res. 13: 35-42

[107] Ahlborg G, Weitzberg E, Sollevi A, Lundberg JM (1992) Splanchnic and renal vasoconstrictor and metabolic responses to neuropeptide Y in resting and exercising man. Acta Physiol. Scand. 145: 139-149.

[108] Ahlborg G, Lundberg JM (1994) Inhibitory effects of neuropeptide on splanchnic glycogenolysis and renin release in humans. Clin. Physiol. 14: 187-196.

[109] Vettor R, Pagano C, Granzotto M, Englaro P, Angeli P, BlumWF, Federspil G, Rohner-Jeanrenaud F, Jeanrenaud B (1998) Effects of intravenous neuropeptide Y on insulin secretion and insulin sensitivity in skeletal muscle in normal rats Diabetologia 41: 1361-1367.

[110] Kos K, Harte AL, James S, Snead DR, O'Hare JP, McTernan PG, Kumar S (2007) Secretion of neuropeptide Y in human adipose tissue and its role in maintenance of adipose tissue mass. Am. J. Physiol. Endocrinol. Metab. 293: E1335-E1340.

[111] Valet P, Berlan M, Beauville M, Crampes F, Montastruc JL, Lafoutan MJ (1990) Neuropeptide Y and Peptide YY Inhibit Lipolysis in Human and Dog Fat Cells through a Pertussis Toxin-sensitive G Protein. J. Clin. Invest. 85 : 291-295

[112] Yang K, Guan H, Arany E, Hill DJ, Cao X (2008) Neuropeptide Y is produced in visceral adipose tissue and promotes proliferation of adipocyte precursor cells via the Y1 receptor. FASEB J. 22: 2452-2464

[113] Zahorska-Markiewicz B, Obuchowicz E, Waluga M, Tkacz E, Herman ZS (2001) Neuropeptide Y in obese women during treatment with adrenergic modulation drugs. Med. Sci. Monit. 7(3): 403-408

[114] Moro D, Mazzilli G, Grugni G, Guzzaloni G, Tedeschi S, Morabito F (1998) Leptin and neuropeptide Y serum levels in young obese during weight loss. Minerva Endocrinol; 23(4): 105-110.

[115] Orbetzova M, Koleva D, Mitkov M, Atanassova I, Nikolova J, Atanassova P, Genchev G (2012) Adipocytokines, neuropeptide Y and insulin resistance in overweight women with gynoid and android type of adipose tissue distribution. Folia Medica (in press)

[116] Orbetzova M, Atanassova I, Milcheva B, Shigarminova R, Genchev G, Zacharieva S (2004) Adipose tissue hormones in women with different morphological types of overweight. Endokrinologyia 9(4): 214-223 (in Bulgarian).

[117] Ilhan A, Rasul S, Dimitrov A, Handisurya A, Gartner W, Baumgartner-Parzer S, Wagner L, Kautzky-Willer A, Base W (2010) Plasma neuropeptide Y levels differ in distinct diabetic conditions Neuropeptides 44 (6): 485–489.

[118] McDonald JK (1990) Role of neuropeptide Y in reproductive function. Ann. N Y Acad. Sci. 611: 258-272.

[119] Borowiec M, Wasilewska-Dziubiñska E, Chmielowska M, Woliñska-Witort E, Baranowska B (2002) Effects of leptin and neuropeptide Y (NPY) on hormones release in female rats. Neuro. Endocrinol. Lett. 23(2): 149-154.

[120] Barb CR, Kraeling RR, Rampacek GB, Hausman GJ (2006) The role of neuropeptide Y and interaction with leptin in regulating feed intake and luteinizing hormone and growth hormone secretion in the pig. Reproduction 131(6): 1127-1135.

[121] Barb CR, Barrettt GB (2005) Neuropeptide Y modulates growth hormone but not luteinizing hormone secretion from prepuberal gilt anterior pituitary cells in culture. Domest Anim Endocrinol. 29(3):548-555.

[122] Kaynard AH, Pau KY, Hess DL, Spies HG (1990) Third-ventricular infusion of neuropeptide Y suppresses luteinizing hormone secretion in ovariectomized rhesus macaques. Endocrinology 127(5): 2437–2444.

[123] Kalra SP, Horvath T, Naftolin F, Xu B, Pu S, Kalra PS (1997) The interactive language of the hypothalamus for the gonadotropin releasing hormone (GNRH) system. J. Neuroendocrinol. 9(8): 569–576.

[124] Plant TM, Shahab M (2002) Neuroendocrine mechanisms that delay and initiate puberty in higher primates. Physiol. Behav. 77(4–5): 717–722.

[125] Shahab M, Balasubramaniam A, Sahu A, Plant TM (2003) Central nervous system receptors involved in mediating the inhibitory action of neuropeptide Y on luteinizing hormone secretion in the male rhesus monkey (Macaca mulatta). J Neuroendocrinol. 15(10): 965–970.

[126] Kaye WH, Berrettini WH, Gwirtsman HE, Gold PW, George DT, Jimerson DC, Ebert MH (1989) Contribution of CNS neuropeptide (NPY, CRH, and beta-endorphin) alterations to psychophysiological abnormalities in anorexia nervosa. Psychopharmacol. Bull. 25(3): 433–438.

[127] Kaye WH (1996) Neuropeptide abnormalities in anorexia nervosa. Psychiatry Res. 62(1): 65–74.

[128] Ooewiecimska J, Ziora K, Geisler G, Broll-Waoeka K (2005) Prospective evaluation of leptin and neuropeptide Y (NPY) serum levels in girls with anorexia nervosa. Neuro Endocrinol. Lett. 26(4): 301–304.

[129] Mircea CN, Lujan ME, Pierson RA (2007) Metabolic Fuel and Clinical Implications for Female Reproduction. J. Obstet . Gynaecol. Can. 29(11): 887–902.

[130] Błogowska A, Krzyzanowska-Swiniarska B, Zieliñska D, Rzepka-Górska I (2006) Body composition and concentrations of leptin, neuropeptide Y, beta-endorphin, growth hormone, insulin-like growth factor-I and insulin at menarche in girls with constitutional delay of puberty. Gynecol. Endocrinol. 22(5): 274–278.

[131] Azziz R, Woods KS, Reyna R, Key TJ, Knochenhauer ES, Yildiz BO (2004) The prevalence and features of the polycystic ovary syndrome in an unselected population. J. Clin. Endocrinol. Metab. 89: 2745–2749.

[132] Orbetzova M (2009) Adipose tissue hormones in women with polycystic ovary syndrome. Nauka Endocrinologia, 6: 258-261 (in Bulgarian).

[133] Orbetzova M, Kamenov Z, Kolarov G, Orbetzova V, Andreeva M, Genchev G, Genov G, Zacharieva S (2003) Metabolic disturbances in women with polycystic ovary syndrome. Folia Medica 3: 12-20

[134] Hahn S, Tan S, Sack S, Kimmig R, Quadbeck B, Mann K, Janssen OE (2007) Prevalence of the metabolic syndrome in German women with polycystic ovary syndrome. Exp. Clin. Endocrinol. Diabetes 115: 130–135

[135] Martinez-Bermejo E, Luque-Ramirez M, Escobar- Morreale HF (2007) Obesity and the polycystic ovary syndrome. Minerva Endocrinol; 32: 129–140.

[136] Orbetzova M, Orbetzova V, Kamenov Z, Kolarov G, Andreeva M, Genchev G, Zacharieva S, Borissov I. Comparison of the diagnostic indexes for establishing disturbances in of carbohydrate metabolism in women with polycystic ovary syndrome (PCOS). Akusherstvo i Ginekologiya 2003; 42 (4): 10-15 (in Bulgarian)

[137] Vrbikova J, Hainer V (2009) Obesity and polycystic ovary syndrome. Obesity Facts 2: 26–35.

[138] Gambineri A, Pelusi C, Vicennati V, Pagotto U, Pasquali R (2002) Obesity and the polycystic ovary syndrome. Int. J. Obes. Relat. Metab. Disord. 26: 883–896

[139] Escobar-Morreale HF, Villuendas G, Botella-Carretero JI, Alvarez-Blasco F, Sanchon R, Luque-Ramirez M, San Millan JL (2006) Adiponectin and resistin in PCOS: a clinical, biochemical and molecular genetic study. Hum. Reprod. 21: 2257–2265

[140]Garruti G, Depalo R, Vita MG, Lorusso F, Giampetruzzi F, DamatoAB, Giorgino F (2009) Adipose tissue, metabolic syndrome and polycystic ovary syndrome: from pathophysiology to treatment. Reproduct. Biomed. Online 19 (4): 552–563

[141] Manneras L, Cajander S, Holmang A, Seleskovic Z, Lystig T, Lonn M, Stener-Victorin, E (2007) A new rat model exhibiting both ovarian and metabolic characteristics of polycystic ovary syndrome. Endocrinology 148: 3781-3791.

[142] Brannian JD, Hansen KA (2002) Leptin and ovarian folliculogenesis:implications for ovulation induction and ART outcomes. Seminars Reprod. Med. 20 103–112.

[143] Baranowska B, Radzikowska M, Wasilewska-Dziubińska E, Kapliński A,Roguski K, Płonowski A (1999) Neuropeptide Y, leptin, galanin and insulin in women with polycystic ovary syndrome. Gynecol. Endocrinol. 13(5): 344–351

[144] Bidzińńska-Speichert B, Lenarcik A, Tworowska-Bardzińńska U, Ślęęzak R, Bednarek-Tupikowska G, Milewicz A (2012) Pro12Ala PPAR γ2 gene polymorphism in PCOS women: the role of compounds regulating satiety Gynecol. Endocrinol. 28(3): 195-198.

[145] Romualdi D, De Marinis L, Campagna G, Proto C, Lanzone A, Guido M (2008) Alteration of ghrelin–neuropeptide Y network in obese patients with polycystic ovary syndrome: role of hyperinsulinism. Clin. Endocrinol. 69:562–567

[146] Krassas GE, Kaltsas TT, Pontikides N, Jacobs H, Blum W, Messinis I (1998) Leptin levels in women with polycystic ovary syndrome before and after treatment with diazoxide. Euro. J. Endocrinol. 139: 184–189.

[147] Morin-Papunen LC, Koivunen RM, Tomas C, Ruokonen A, Martikainen HK (1998) Decreased serum leptin concentrations during metformin therapy in obese women with polycystic ovary syndrome. J. Clin. Endocrinol. Metab. 83(7): 2566-2568.

[148] Pasquali R, Gambineri A, Biscotti D, Vicennati V, Gagliardi L, Colitta D, Fiorini S, Cognigni GE, Filicori M & Morselli-Labate AM (2000) Effect of long-term treatment with metformin added to hypocaloric diet on body composition, fat distribution, and androgen and insulin levels in abdominally obese women with and without the polycystic ovary syndrome. J. Clin. Endocrinol. Metab. 85(8): 2767 2774.

[149] Kowalska I, Kinalski M, Straczkowski M, Wolczyski S, Kinalska I (2001) Insulin, leptin, IGF-1 and insulin dependent protein concentrations after insulin sensitizing therapy in obese women with polycystic ovary syndrome. Eur. J. Endocrinol. 144: 509-515.

[150] Orbetzova M, Pehlivanov B, Mitkov M, Atanassova I, Kamenov Z, Kolarov G, Genchev G (2011). Effect of short-term standard therapeutic regimens on Neuropeptide Y and adipose tissue hormones in overweight insulinresistant women with polycystic ovary syndrome (PCOS). Folia Medica 3: 15-24.

[151] Orbetzova M, Kamenov Z, Zacharieva S, Hristov V, Kolarov G, Atanassova I, Shigarminova R, Milcheva B, Genchev G (2007) Adipose tissue hormones, anthropometric and metabolic parameters in women with polycystic ovarian syndrome (PCOS) before and after standard therapeutic regimens. Endokrinni Zaboliavaniya, 36(1): 3-27 (in Bulgarian).

[152] Kojima K, Hosoda H, Date Y, Nakazato M, Matsue H, Kangawa K (1999) Ghrelin is a novel growth-hormone releasing acylated peptide from stomach. Nature 402: 656-660.

[153] Kaiya H, Van Der Geyten S, Kojima M, Hosoda H, Kitajima Y, Matsumoto M, Geelissen S, Darras VM, Kangawa K (2002) Chicken ghrelin: purification, cDNA cloning and biological activity. Endocrinology 143: 3454–3463.

[154] Kaiya H, Kojima M, Hosoda H, Koda A, Yamamoto K, Kitajima Y, Matsumoto M, Minamitake Y, Kikuyama S, Kangawa K (2001) Bullfrog ghrelin is modified by n-octanoic acid at its third threonine residue. J. Biol. Chem. 276: 40441–40448.

[155] Kaiya H, Kojima M, Hosoda H, Riley LG, Hirano T, Grau EG, Kangawa K (2003) Identification of tilapia ghrelin and its effects on growth hormone and prolactin release in the tilapia, Oreochromis mossambicus. Comp. Biochem. Physiol. B 135: 421–429.

[156] Kaiya H, Kojima M, Hosoda H, Moriyama S, Takahashi A, Kawauchi H, Kangawa K (2003) Peptide purification, complementary deoxyribonucleic acid (DNA) and genomic DNA cloning, and functional characterization of ghrelin in rainbow trout. Endocrinology 144: 5215-5226.

[157] Kaiya H, Darras VM, Kangawa K (2007) Ghrelin in birds: its structure, distribution and function. J Poult. Sci. 44: 1–18.

[158] Kaiya H, Furuse M, Miyazato M, Kangawa K (2009) Current knowledge of the roles of ghrelin in regulating food intake and energy balance in birds. Gen. Compar. Endocrinol. 163 (1-2): 33–38.

[159] Miura T, Maruyama K, Kaiya H, Miyazato M, Kangawa K, Uchiyama M, Shioda S, Matsuda K (2009) Purification and properties of ghrelin from the intestin e of the goldfish, Carassius auratus. Peptides 30:758–765.

[160] Kojima M, Kangawa K (2010) Ghrelin: more than endogenous growth hormone secretagogue Ann. NY Acad. Sci. 1200: 140-148.

[161] Date Y, Kojima M, Hosoda H, Sawaguchi A, Mondal MS, Suganuma T, Matsukura S, Kangawa K, Nakazato M (2000) Ghrelin, a novel growth hormone-releasing acylated

peptide, is synthesized in a distinct endocrine cell type in the gastrointestinal tracts of rats and humans. Endocrinology 141: 4255-4261.

[162] Sakata I, K Nakamura, M Yamazaki, M Matsubara, Y Hayashi, K Kangawa, T Sakai (2002) Ghrelin-producing cells exist as two types of cells – closed- and opened-type cells, in rat gastrointestinal tract. Peptides 23: 531-536.

[163] Dornonville De La Cour C, Bjorkqvist M, Sandvik AK, Bakke I, Zhao CM, Chen D, Hakanson R (2001) A-like cells in the rat stomach contain ghrelin and do not operate under gastrin control. Regulat. Pept. 99: 141-150.

[164] Ghigo E, Broglio F, Arvat E, Maccario M, Papotti M, Muccioli G (2005) Ghrelin: More Than a Natural GH Secretagogue and/or an Orexigenic Factor. Clin. Endocrinol. 62 (1): 1-17.

[165] Asakawa A, Inui A, Kaga T, Yuzuriha H, Nagata T, Ueno N, Makino S, Fujimiya M, Niijima A, Fujino MA, Kasuga M (2001) Ghrelin is an appetite-stimulatory signal from stomach with structural resemblance to motilin. Gastroenterology 120: 337-345.

[166] Hosoda H, Kojima M, Matsuo H, Kangawa K (2000) Ghrelin and des-acyl ghrelin: two major forms of rat ghrelin peptide in gastrointestinal tissue. Biochem. Biophys. Res. Commun. 279: 909-913.

[167] Banks WA, Tschop M, Robinson SM, Heiman ML (2002) Extent and direction of ghrelin transport across the bloodbrain barrier is determined by its unique primary structure. J. Pharmacol. Exp. Ther. 302: 822-827.

[168] Broglio F, Benso A, Gottero C, Prodam F, Gauna C, Filtri L, Arvat E, van der Lely AJ, Deghenghi R, Ghigo E (2003) Non-acylated ghrelin does not possess the pituitaric and pancreatic endocrine activity of acylated ghrelin in humans. J. Endocrinol. Invest. 26: 192-196.

[169] Yang J, Brown MS, Liang G, Grishin NV, Goldstein JL (2008) Identification of the acyltransferase that octanoylates ghrelin, an appetite-stimulating peptide hormone. Cell 132: 387–396.

[170] Gutierrez JA, Solenberg PJ, Perkins DR, Willency JA, Knierman MD, Jin Z, Witcher DR, Luo S, Onyia JE, Hale JE (2008) Ghrelin octanoylation mediated by an orphan lipid transferase. PNAS 105: 6320–6325.

[171] Kirchner H, Gutierrez JA, Solenberg PJ, Pfluger PT, Czyzyk TA, Willency JA, Schurmann A, Joost HG, Jandacek RJ, Hale JE, Heiman ML, Tschop MH (2009) GOAT links dietary lipids with the endocrine control of energy balance. Nature Med. 15: 741–745.

[172] Barnett BP, Hwang Y, Taylor MS, Kirchner H, Pfluger PT, Bernard V, Lin YY, Bowers EM, Mukherjee C, Song WJ, Longo PA, Leahy DJ, Hussain MA, Tschop MH, Boeke JD, Cole PA (2010) Glucose and weight control in mice with a designed ghrelin O-acyltransferase inhibitor. Science 330, 1689-1692.

[173] Sun Y, Wang P, Zheng H, Smith RG (2004) Ghrelin stimulation of growth hormone release and appetite is mediated through the growth hormone secretagogue receptor. Proc. Natl. Acad. Sci. USA 101: 4679–4684.

[174] Zigman JM, Nakano Y, Coppari R, Balthasar N, Marcus JN, Lee CE, Jones JE, Deysher AE, Waxman AR, White RD, Williams TD, Lachey JL, Seeley RJ,Lowell BB, Elmquist JK

(2005) Mice lacking ghrelin receptors resist the development of diet-induced obesity. J. Clin. Invest. 115: 3564–3572.

[175] Soares JB, Roncon-Albuquerque R, Leite-Moreira A (2008) Ghrelin and ghrelin receptor inhibitors: agents in the treatment of obesity. Expert. Opin. Ther. Targets 12(9): 1177–1189.

[176] Tschop M, Smiley DL, Heiman ML (2000) Ghrelin induces adiposity in rodents. Nature 407: 908-913.

[177] Wren AM, Small CJ, Ward HL, Murphy KG, Dakin CL, Taheri S, Kennedy AR, Roberts GH, Morgan DG, Ghatei, MA, Bloom SR (2000) The novel hypothalamic peptide ghrelin stimulates food intake and growth hormone secretion. Endocrinology 141: 4325-4328.

[178] Kojima M, Kangawa K (2005) Ghrelin: structure and function. Physiol. Rev. 85: 495–522.

[179] Chen HY, Trumbauer ME, Chen AS, Weingarth DT, Adams JR, Frazier EG, Shen Z, Marsh DJ, Feighner SD, Guan XMYeZ, Nargund RP, Smith RG, Van der Ploeg LH, Howard AD, MacNeil DJ, Qian S (2004) Orexigenic action of peripheral ghrelin is mediated by neuropeptide Y and agouti-related protein. Endocrinology 145: 2607-2612.

[180] Ariyasu H, Takaya K, Tagami T, Ogawa Y, Hosoda K, Akamizu T, Suda M, Koh T, Natsiu K, Toyooka S, Shirakami G, Usui T, Shimatsu A, Doi K, Hosoda H, Kojima M, Kangawa K, Nakao K (2001) Stomach is a major source of circulating ghrelin and feeding state determines plasma ghrelin-like immunoreactivity levels in humans. J. Clin. Endocrinol. Metab. 86: 4753-4758.

[181] Toshinai K, Yamaguchi H, Sun Y, Smith RG, Yamanaka A, Sakurai T, Date Y, Mondal MS, Shimbara T, Kawagoe T, Murakami N, Miyazato M, Kangawa K, Nakazato M (2006) Des-acyl ghrelin induces food intake by a mechanism independent of the growth hormone secretagogue receptor. Endocrinology 147: 2306-2314.

[182] van der Lely AJ, Tschop M, Heiman ML, Ghigo E (2004) Biological, physiological, pathophysiological, and pharmacological aspects of ghrelin. Endocr. Rev. 25: 426–457.

[183] Zigman JM, Jones JE, Lee CE, Saper CB, Elmquist JK (2006) Expression of ghrelin receptor mRNA in the rat and the mouse brain. J. Comp. Neurol. 494: 528–548.

[184] Kojima S, Nakahara T, Nagai N, Muranaga T, Tanaka M, Yasuhara D, Masuda A, Date Y, Ueno H, Nakazato M, Naruo T (2005) Altered ghrelin and peptide YY responses to meals in bulimia nervosa. Clin. Endocrinol. (Oxf.) 62: 74–78.

[185] Date Y, Nakazato M, Hashiguchi S, Dezaki K, Mondal MS, Hosoda H, Kojima M, Kangawa K, Arima T, Matsuo H, Yada T, Matsukura S (2002) Ghrelin is present in pancreatic alpha-cells of humans and rats and stimulates insulin secretion. Diabetes 51: 124-129.

[186] Gualillo O, Caminos J, Blanco M, Garcia-Caballero T, Kojima M,Kangawa K, Dieguez C & Casanueva F 2001 Ghrelin, a novel placental-derived hormone. Endocrinology 142: 788–794.

[187] Hattori N, Saito T, Yagyu T, Jiang BH, Kitagawa K, Inagaki C (2001) GH, GH receptor, GH secretagogue receptor, and ghrelin expression in human T cells, B cells, and neutrophils. J. Clin. Endocrinol. Metab. 86: 4284–4291.

[188] Sato T, Nakamura Y, Shiimura Y, Ohgusu H, Kangawa K, Kojima M (2012) Structure, regulation and function of ghrelin. J. Biochem. 151(2): 119–128.

[189] Torsello A, Locatelli V, Melis MR, Succu S, Spano MS, DeghenghiR, Muller EE, Argiolas A (2000) Differential orexigenic effects of hexarelin and its analogs in the rat hypothalamus: indication for multiple growth hormone secretagogue receptor subtypes. Neuroendocrinology 72: 327–332.

[190] Zhang JV, Ren PG, Avsian-Kretchmer O, Luo CW, Rauch R, Klein C, Hsueh AJ (2005) Obestatin, a peptide encoded by the ghrelin gene, opposes ghrelin's effects on food intake. Science 310: 996–999.

[191] Zhang JV, Ning G, Handelsman Y, Bloomgarden ZT (2010) Gut hormones and the brain. J. Diab. 2: 138–145.

[192] Boguszewski CL, Paz-Filho G, Velloso LA (2010) Neuroendocrine body weight regulation: integration between fat tissue, gastrointestinal tract, and the brain. Pol. J. Endocrinol. 61 (2): 194–206.

[193] Horvath TL (2005) The hardship of obesity: a soft-wired hypothalamus. Nat. Neurosci. 8: 561–565.

[194] Murphy KG, Dhillo WS, Bloom SR (2006) Gut peptides in the regulation of food intake and energy homeostasis. Endocr. Rev. 27: 719–727.

[195] Cummings DE, Overduin J. Gastrointestinal regulation of food intake (2007) J. Clin. Invest. 117: 13–23.

[196] Lawrence CB, Snape AC, Baudoin FM, Luckman SM (2002) Acute central ghrelin and GH secretagogues induce feeding and activate brain appetite centers. Endocrinology 143: 155-162.

[197] Wang L, Saint-Pierre DH, Tache Y (2002) Peripheral ghrelin selectively increases Fos expression in neuropeptide Y-synthesizing neurons in mouse hypothalamic arcuate nucleus. Neurosci. Lett. 325: 4751.

[198] Tamura H, Kamegai J, Shimizu T, Ishii S, Sugihara H, Oikawa S (2002) Ghrelin stimulates GH but not food intake in arcuate nucleus ablated rats. Endocrinology 143: 3268–3275.

[199] Nakazato M, Murakami N, Date Y, Kojima M, Matsuo H, Kangawa K, Matsukura S (2001) A role for ghrelin in the central regulation of feeding. Nature 409: 194-198.

[200] Shintani M, Ogawa Y, Ebihara K, Izawa-Abe M, Miyanaga F, Takaya K, Hayashi T, Inoue G, Hosoda K, Kojima M, Kangawa K, Nakao K (2001) Ghrelin, an endogenous growth hormone secretagogue, is a novel orexigenic peptide that antagonizes leptin action through the activation of hypothalamic neuropeptide Y/Y1 receptor pathway. Diabetes 50: 227-232.

[201] Cummings DE, Purnell JQ, Frayo RS, Schmidova K, Wisse BE, Weigle DS (2001) A preprandial rise in plasma ghrelin levels suggests a role in meal initiation in humans. Diabetes 50: 1714-1719.

[202] Cummings DE, Frayo RS, Marmonier C, Aubert R, Chapelot D (2004) Plasma ghrelin levels and hunger scores in humans initiating meals voluntarily without time- and food-related cues. Am. J. Physiol. Endocrinol. Metab. 287: E297–E304.

[203] Drazen DL, Vahl TP, D'Alessio DA, Seeley RJ, Woods SC (2006) Effects of a fixed meal pattern on ghrelin secretion: evidence for a learned response independent of nutrient status. Endocrinology: 147: 23–30.

[204] Wren AM, Seal LJ, Cohen MA, Brynes AE, Frost GS, Murphy KG, Dhillo WS, Ghatei MA, Bloom SR (2001a) Ghrelin enhances appetite and increases food intake in humans. J. Clin. Endocrinol. Metab. 86: 5992.

[205] Wren AM, Small CJ, Abbott CR, Dhillo WS, Seal LJ, Cohen MA, Batterham RL, Taheri S, Stanley SA, Ghatei MA, Bloom SR (2001b) Ghrelin causes hyperphagia and obesity in rats. Diabetes 50: 2540-2547.

[206] Kola B, Korbonits M (2009) Shedding light on the intricate puzzle of ghrelin's effects on appetite regulation. J. Endocrinol. 202 (2): 191-198.

[207] Tschop M, Weyer C, Tataranni PA, Devanarayan V, Ravussin E, Heiman ML (2001) Circulating ghrelin levels are decreased in human obesity. Diabetes 50: 707-709.

[208] Shiiya T, Nakazato M, Mizuta M, Date Y, Mondal MS, Tanaka M, Nozoe S, Hosoda H, Kangawa K, Matsukura S (2002) Plasma ghrelin levels in lean and obese humans and the effect of glucose on ghrelin secretion. J. Clin. Endocrinol. Metab. 87: 240-244.

[209] Dzaja A, Dalal MA, Himmerich H, Uhr M, Pollmacher T, Schuld A (2004) Sleep enhances nocturnal plasma ghrelin levels in healthy subjects. Am. J. Physiol. Endocrinol. Metab. 286: E963-E967.

[210] Yildiz BO, Suchard MA, Wong ML, McCann SM, Licinio J (2004). Alterations in the dynamics of circulating ghrelin, adiponectin, and leptin in human obesity. Proc. Natl. Acad. Sci. USA 101: 10434-10439.

[211] Briatore L, Andraghetti G, Cordera R (2006) Effect of two fasting periods of different duration on ghrelin response to a mixed meal. Nutr. Metab. Cardiovasc. Dis. 16: 471-476.

[212] Callahan HS, Cummings DE, Pepe MS, Breen PA, Matthys CC, Weigle DS (2004) Postprandial suppression of plasma ghrelin level is proportional to ingested caloric load but does not predict intermeal interval in humans. J. Clin. Endocrinol. Metab. 89: 1319-1324.

[213] Sugino T, Yamaura J, Yamagishi M, Kurose Y, Kojima M, Kangawa K, Hasegawa Y, Terashima Y (2003) Involvement of cholinergic neurons in the regulation of the ghrelin secretory response to feeding in sheep. Biochem. Biophys. Res. Commun. 304: 308-312.

[214] Schüssler P, Kluge M, Yassouridis A, Dresler M, Uhr M, Steiger A (2012) Ghrelin Levels Increase After Pictures Showing Food. Obesity | doi:10.1038/oby.2011.385

[215] Norrelund H, Hansen TK, Ørskov H, Hosoda H, Kojima M, Kangawa K, Weeke J, Møller N, Christiansen JS, Jørgensen JO (2002) Ghrelin immunoreactivity in human plasma is suppressed by somatostatin. Clin. Endocrinol. (Oxf).57(4): 539-546.

[216] Broglio F, Gottero C, Van Koetsveld P, Prodam F, Destefanis S, Benso A, Gauna C, Hofland L, Arvat E, van der Lely AJ, Ghigo EJ (2004) Acetylcholine regulates ghrelin secretion in humans.Clin. Endocrinol. Metab. 89(5): 2429-2433.

[217] Murakami N, Hayashida T, Kuroiwa T, Nakahara K, Ida T, Mondal MS, Nakazato M, Kojima M, Kangawa K (2002) Role for central ghrelin in food intake and secretion profile of stomach ghrelin in rats. J. Endocrinol. 174: 283–288.

[218] Sun Y, Ahmed S, Smith RG (2003) Deletion of ghrelin impairs neither growth nor appetite. Mol. Cell. Biol. 23: 7973–7981.

[219] Gnanapavan S, Kola B, Bustin SA, Morris DG, McGee P, Fairclough P, Bhattacharya S, Carpenter R, Grossman AB, Korbonits M (2002) The tissue distribution of the mRNA of

ghrelin and subtypes of its receptor, GHS-R, in humans. J. Clin. Endocrinol. Metab. 87: 2988–2991.

[220] Anderson LL, Jeftinija S, Scanes CG, Stromer MH, Lee J-S, Jeftinija K, Glavaski-Joksimovic A (2005) Physiology of ghrelin and related peptides. Domest. Anim. Endocrinol. 29: 111–144.

[221] Wierup N, Yang S, McEvilly RJ, Mulder H, Sundler F (2004) Ghrelin is expressed in a novel endocrine cell type in developing rat islets and inhibits insulin secretion from INS-1 (832/13) cells. J. Histochem. Cytochem. 52: 301–310.

[222] Muccioli G, Papotti M, Locatelli V, Ghigo E, Deghenghi R (2001) Binding of 125I-labeled ghrelin to membranes from human hypothalamus and pituitary gland. J. Endocrinol. Invest. 24: RC7-RC9.

[223] Gauna C, Delhanty P, Hofland L, Broglio F, Janssen J, Ross R, Ghigo E, van der Lely AJ (2004) Ghrelin and des-octanoyl ghrelin modulate glucose output by primary hepatocytes. In: The Endocrine Society's 86th Annual Meeting, June 1619 2004, New Orleans, USA

[224] Soriano-Guillen L, Barrios V, Campos-Barros A, Argente J (2004) Ghrelin levels in obesity and anorexia nervosa: effect of weight reduction or recuperation. J. Pediatr. 144: 30–35.

[225] Ukkola O (2009) Ghrelin and metabolic disorders. Curr. Protein Pept. Sci. 10 (1): 2–7.

[226] Broglio F, Gottero C, Benso A, Prodam F, Destefanis S, Gauna C, Maccario M, Deghenghi R, van der Lely AJ, Ghigo E (2003) Effects of ghrelin on the insulin and glycemic responses to glucose, arginine, or free fatty acids load in humans. J. Clin. Endocrinol. Metab. 88: 4268-4272.

[227] Murata M, Okimura Y, Iida K, Matsumoto M, Sowa H, Kaji H, Kojima M, Kangawa K, Chihara K (2002) Ghrelin modulates the downstream molecules of insulin signaling in hepatoma cells. J. Biol. Chem. 277: 5667–5674.

[228] Pöykkö SM, Kellokoski E, Hörkköe S, Kauma H, Kesäniemi YA, Ukkola O (2003) Low plasma ghrelin is associated with insulin resistance, hypertension, and the prevalence of type 2 diabetes. Diabetes 52(10): 2546–2553.

[229] Egido EM, Rodriguez-Gallardo J, Silvestre RA, Marco J (2002) Inhibitory effect of ghrelin on insulin and pancreatic somatostatin secretion. Europ. J. Endocrinol. 146: 241-244.

[230] Broglio F, Arvat E, Benso A, Gottero C, Muccioli G, Papotti M, van der Lely AJ, Deghenghi R, Ghigo E (2001) Ghrelin, a natural GH secretagogue produced by the stomach, induces hyperglycemia and reduces insulin secretion in humans. J. Clin. Endocrinol. Metab. 86: 5083-5086.

[231] Arosio M, Ronchi CL, Gebbia C, Cappiello V, Beck-Peccoz P, Peracchi M (2003) Stimulatory effects of ghrelin on circulating somatostatin and pancreatic polypeptide levels. J. Clin. Endocrinol. Metab. 88: 701-704.

[232] Date Y, Nakazato M, Murakami N, Kojima M, Kangawa K, Matsukura S (2001) Ghrelin acts in the central nervous system to stimulate gastric acid secretion. Biochem. Biophys. Res. Commun. 280 (3): 904-907.

[233] Dezaki K, Sone H, Koizumi M, Nakata M, Kakei M, Nagai H, Hosoda H, Kangawa K, Yada T (2006) Blockade of pancreatic islet-derived ghrelin enhances insulin secretion to prevent high-fat dietinduced glucose intolerance. Diabetes 55: 3486-3493.

[234] Heijboer AC, van den Hoek AM, Parlevliet ET, Havekes LM, Romijn JA, Pijl H, Corssmit EP M (2006) Ghrelin differentially affects hepatic and peripheral insulin sensitivity in mice. Diabetologia 49: 732–738.

[235] Ott V, Fasshauer M, Dalski A, Meier B, Perwitz N, Klein HH, Tschöp M, Klein J (2002) Direct peripheral effects of ghrelin include suppression ofadiponectin expression. Horm. Metab. Res. 34: 640–645.

[236] Malagón MM, Luque RM, Ruiz-Guerrero E, Rodríguez-Pacheco F, García-Navarro S, Casanueva FF, Gracia-Navarro F, Castaño JP (2003) Intracellular signalling mechanisms mediating ghrelin-stimulated growth hormone release in somatotropes. Endocrinology 144, 5372–5380

[237] Salehi A, Dornonville de la Cour C, Håkanson R, Lundquist I (2004) Effects of ghrelin on insulin and glucagons secretion: a study of isolated pancreatic islets and intact mice. Regul. Pept. 118: 143–150.

[238] Vestergaard ET, Gormsen LC, Jessen N, Lund S, Hansen TK, Moller N, Jorgensen JO (2008) Ghrelin Infusion in Humans Induces Acute Insulin Resistance and Lipolysis Independent of Growth Hormone Signaling. Diabetes 57: 3205–3210.

[239] Flanagan DE, Evans M L, Monsod TP, Rife F, Heptulla RA, Tamborlane WV, Sherwin RS (2003) The influence of insulin on circulating ghrelin. Am. J. Physiol. Endocrinol. Metab. 284: E313–E316.

[240] Broglio F, C Gottero, F Prodam, Destefanis S, Gauna C, Me E, Riganti F, Vivenza D, Rapa A, Martina V, Arvat E, Bona G, van der Lely AJ, Ghigo E (2004) Ghrelin secretion is inhibited by glucose load and insulin-induced hypoglycaemia but unaffected by glucagon and arginine in humans. Clin. Endocrinol. (Oxf); 61:503–509.

[241] Leite-Moreira AF, Soares J-B (2007) Physiological, pathological and potential therapeutic roles of ghrelin. Drug Discov. Today 12, 7/8: 276-288.

[242] Korbonits M, Gueorguiev M, O'Grady E, Lecoeur C, Swan DC, Mein CA, Weill J, Grossman AB, Froguel P (2002) A variation in the ghrelin gene increases weight and decreases insulin secretion in tall, obese children. J. Clin. Endocrinol. Metab. 87: 4005–4008.

[243] Miraglia dG, Santoro N, Cirillo G, Raimondo P, Grandone A, D'Aniello A, Di Nardo M, Perrone L (2004) Molecular screening of the ghrelin gene in Italian obese children: the Leu72 Met variant is associated with an earlier onset of obesity. Int. J. Obes. Relat. Metab. Dis. 28: 447–450.

[244] Hinney A, Hoch A, Geller F, Schafer H, Siegfried W, Goldschmidt H, Remschmidt H, Hebebrand J (2002) Ghrelin gene: identification of missense variants and a frameshift mutation in extremely obese children and adolescents and healthy normal weight students. J. Clin. Endocrinol. Metab. 87: 2716–2719.

[245] Wang HJ, Geller F, Dempfle A, Schauble N, Friedel S, Lichtner P, Fontenla-Horro F, Wudy S, Hagemann S, Gortner L et al. (2004) Ghrelin receptor gene: identification of several sequence variants in extremely obese children and adolescents, healthy normal-

weight and underweight students, and children with short normal stature. J. Clin. Endocrinol. Metab. 89 157–162.

[246] Bellone S, Rapa A, Vivenza D, Castellino N, Petri A, Bellone J, Me E, Broglio F, Prodam F, Ghigo E, Bona G (2002) Circulating ghrelin levels as function of gender, pubertal status and adiposity in childhood. J. Endocrinol. Invest. 25: RC13-RC15

[247] Kurose Y, Iqbal J, Rao A, Murata Y, Hasegawa Y, Terashima Y, Kojima M, Kangawa K, Clarke IJ (2005) Changes in expression of the genes for the leptin receptorand the growth hormone-releasing peptide/ghrelin receptor in the hypothalamicarcuate nucleus with long-term manipulation of adiposity by dietary means. J. Neuroendocrinol. 17: 331–340.

[248] Tung YC, Hewson AK, Carter RN, Dickson SL (2005) Central responsiveness to a ghrelin mimetic (GHRP-6) is rapidly altered by acute changes in nutritional status in rats. J. Neuroendocrinol. 17: 387–393.

[249] Otto B, Cuntz U, Fruehauf E, Wawarta R, Folwaczny C, Riepl RL, Heiman ML, Lehnert P, Fichter M, Tschop M (2001) Weight gain decreases elevated plasma ghrelin concentrations of patients with anorexia nervosa. Europ. J. Endocrinol. 145 669–673.

[250] Hansen TK, Dall R, Hosoda H, Kojima M, Kangawa K, Christiansen JS, Jørgensen JO (2002) Weight loss increases circulating levels of ghrelin in human obesity.Clin. Endocrinol. (Oxf).56 (2): 203-206.

[251] English PJ, Ghatei MA, Malik IA, Bloom SR, Wilding JP (2002) Food fails to suppress ghrelin levels in obese humans. J. Clin. Endocrinol. Metab. 87: 2984-2987.

[252] Cummings DE, Weigle DS, Frayo RS, Breen PA, Ma MK, Dellinger EP, Purnell JQ (2002b) Plasma ghrelin levels after diet-induced weight loss or gastric bypass surgery. N Engl. J. Med. 346: 1623–1630.

[253] Cummings DE, Clement K, Purnell JQ, Vaisse C, Foster KE, Frayo RS, Schwartz MW, Basdevant A, Weigle DS (2002a) Elevated plasma ghrelin levels in PraderWilli syndrome. Nature Med. 8: 643-644.

[254] Erdie-Lalena CR Holm VA, Kelly PC, Frayo RS, Cummings DE (2006) Ghrelin levels in very young children with Prader–Willi syndrome. J. Pediatr. 149, 199–20

[255] Mager U, Lindi V, Lindström J, Eriksson JG, Valle TT, Hämäläinen H, Ilanne-Parikka P, Keinänen-Kiukaanniemi S, Tuomilehto J, Laakso M, Pulkkinen L, Uusitupa M (2006) Association of the Leu72Met polymorphism of the ghrelin gene with the risk of Type 2 diabetes in subjects with impaired glucose tolerance in the finnish diabetes prevention study. Diabet. Med. 23, 685–689

[256] Ishii S, Kamegai J, Tamura H, Shimizu T, Sugihara H, Oikawa S (2002) Role of ghrelin in streptozocin-induced diabetic hyperphagia. Endocrinology 143, 4934–4937

[257] Irako T, Akamizu T, Hosoda H, Iwakura H, Ariyasu H, Tojo K, Tajima N, Kangawa K (2006) Ghrelin prevents development of diabetes at adult age in streptozotocin-treated newborn rats. Diabetologia 249, 1264–1273.

[258] Orbetzova M, Mitkov M, Pehlivanov B (2010) Ghrelin – role in the regulation of body weight, metabolic and reproductive disturbances. Endokrinologiya 4: 212-223 (in Bulgarian).

[259] Barazzoni R, Zanetti M, Ferreira C, Vinci P, Pirulli A, Mucci M, Dore F, Fonda M, Ciocchi B, Cattin L, Guarnieri G (2007) Relationships between desacylated and acylated

ghrelin and insulin sensitivity in the metabolic syndrome. J. Clin. Endocrinol. Metab. 92: 3935–3940.

[260] Ukkola O, S Poykko, M Paivansalo, YA Kesaniemi (2008) Interactions between ghrelin, leptin and IGF-1 affect metabolic syndrome and early atherosclerosis. Annm Med. 40 (6): 465-473.

[261] Lee CC, RP Lee, YM Subeg, CH Wang, TC Fang, BG Hsu (2008) Fasting serum total ghrelin level universly correlates with metabolic syndrome in hemodialysis patients. Arch. Med. Res. 39(8): 785-790

[262] Iantorno M, H Chen, J Kim, Tesauro M, Lauro D, Cardillo C, Quon MJ (2007) Ghrelin has novel vascular actions that mimic PI 3-kinase-dependent actions of insulin to stimulate production of NO from endothelial cells. Am. J. Physiol. Endocrinol. Metab. 292: E756-E764.

[263] Vlasova MA, K Jarvinen, KH Herzig (2009) Cardiovascular effects of ghrelin antagonist in conscious rats. Regul. Pept. 156: 72–76.

[264] Fernandez-Fernandez R, M Tena-Sempere, VM Navarro, ML Barreiro, JM Castellano, E Aguilar, Pinilla L (2006) Effects of Ghrelin upon gonadotropin-releasing hormone and gonadotropin secretion in adult female rats: in vivo and in vitro studies. Neuroendocrinology 82 (5–6): 245–55.

[265] Fernandez-Fernandez R, VM Navarro, ML Barreiro, EM Vigo, S Tovar, AV Sirotkin, Casanueva FF, Aguilar E, Dieguez C, Pinilla L, Tena-Sempere M (2005) Effects of chronic hyperghrelinemia on puberty onset and pregnancy outcome in the rat. Endocrinology 146(7): 3018–3025.

[266] Vulliémoz NR, E Xiao, L Xia-Zhang, M Germond, J Rivier, M Ferin (2004) Decrease in luteinizing hormone pulse frequency during a five-hour peripheral ghrelin infusion in the ovariectomized rhesus monkey. J. Clin. Endocrinol. Metab. 89(11): 5718–5723.

[267] Kluge M, Schüssler P, Schmidt D, Uhr M, Steiger A (2012) Ghrelin suppresses secretion of luteinizing hormone (LH) and follicle-stimulating hormone (FSH) in women. J. Clin. Endocrinol. Metab. 97(3): E448-E451

[268] De Souza MJ, HJ Leidy, E O'Donnell, B Lasley, NI Williams (2004) Fasting ghrelin levels in physically active women: relationship with menstrual disturbances and metabolic hormones. J. Clin. Endocrinol. Metab. 89(7): 3536–3542.

[269] Misra M, KK Miller, K Kuo, K Griffin, V Stewart, E Hunter, Herzog DB, Klibanski A (2005) Secretory dynamics of ghrelin in adolescent girls with anorexia nervosa and healthy adolescents. Am. J. Physiol. Endocrinol. Metab. 289(2): E347–E356.

[270] Garcia JM, M Garcia-Touza, RA Hijazi, G Taffet, D Epner, D Mann, Smith RG, Cunningham GR, Marcelli M (2005) Active ghrelin levels and active to total ghrelin ratio in cancer-induced cachexia. J. Clinlin. Endocrinol. Metab. 90(5): 2920–2926.

[271] Schneider LF, MP Warren (2006) Functional hypothalamic amenorrhea is associated with elevated ghrelin and disordered eating. Fertil. Steril. 86(6): 1744–1749.

[272] Tena-Sempere M, Barreiro ML, Gonzalez LC, Gaytan F, Zhang FP, Caminos JE, Pinilla L, Casanueva FF, Dieguez C and Aguilar E (2002) Novel expression and functional role of ghrelin in rat testis. Endocrinology 143, 711–725

[273] Barreiro ML, Gaytan F, Castellano JM, Suominen JS, Roa J, Gaytan M, Aguilar E, Dieguez C, Toppari J, Tena-Sempere M (2004) Ghrelin inhibits the proliferative activity

of immature Leydig cells in vivo and regulates stem cell factor messenger RNA expression in rat testis. Endocrinology 145, 4825–4834

[274] Pagotto U, Gambineri A, Pelusi C, Genghini S, Cacciari M, Otto B, Castañeda T, Tschöp M, Pasquali R (2003) Testosterone replacement therapy restores normal ghrelin in hypogonadal men. J. Clin. Endocrinol. Metab. 88: 4139–4143.

[275] Pagotto U, Gambineri A, Vicennati V, Heiman ML, Tschop M, Pasquali R (2002) Plasma ghrelin, obesity, and the polycystic ovary syndrome: correlation with insulin resistance and androgen levels. J. Clin. Endocrinol. Metab. 87: 5625-5629.

[276] Schofl C, Horn R, Schill T, Schlosser HW, Müller MJ, Brabant G (2002) Circulating ghrelin levels in patients with polycystic ovary syndrome. J. Clin. Endocrinol. Metab. 87: 4607–4610.

[277] Moran LJ, Noakes M, Clifton PM, Wittert GA, Tomlinson L, Galletly C, Luscombe ND, Norman RJ (2004) Ghrelin and measures of satiety are altered in polycystic ovary syndrome but not differentially affected by diet composition. J. Clin. Endocrinol. Metab. 89: 3337–3344.

[278] Glintborg D, Andersen M, Hagen C, Frystyk J, Hulstrom V, Flyvbjerg A, Hermann AP (2006) Evaluation of metabolic risk markers in polycystic ovary syndrome (PCOS). Adiponectin, ghrelin, leptin and body composition in hirsute PCOS patients and controls. Eur. J. Endocrinol. 155: 337–345.

[279] Micic D, Sumarac-Dumanovic M, Kendereski A, Cvijovic G, Zoric S, Pejkovic D, Micic J, Milic N, Dieguez C, Casanueva FF (2007) Total ghrelin levels during acute insulin infusion in patients with polycystic ovary syndrome. J. Endocrinol. Invest. 30: 820–827.

[280] Orio FJr, Lucidi P, Palomba S, Tauchmanova L, Cascella T, Russo T, Zullo F, Colao A, Lombardi G, De Feo P (2003) Circulating ghrelin concentrations in the polycystic ovary syndrome. J. Clin. Endocrinol. Metab. 88: 942–945.

[281] Kos-Kudla B, Malecka-Mikosz O, Foltyn W, Ostrowska Z, Kudla M, Mazur B (2006) Plasma ghrelin concentrations in patients with polycystic ovary syndrome before and after 6months therapy: correlation with androgen levels. Neuro Endocrinol. Lett. 27: 763–767.

[282] Panidis D, Farmakiotis D, Koliakos G, Rousso D, Kourtis A, Katsikis I, Asteriadis C, Karayannis V, Diamanti-Kandarakis E (2005) Comparative study of plasma ghrelin levels in women with polycystic ovary syndrome, in hyperandrogenic women and in normal controls. Hum. Reprod. 20(8): 2127–2132.

[283] Skommer J, Katulski K, Poreba E, Meczekalski B, Slopień R, Plewa R, Gozdzicka-Józefiak A, Warenik-Szymankiewicz A (2005) Ghrelin expression in women with polycystic ovary syndrome–a preliminary study. Eur. J. Gynaecol. Oncol. 26 : 553–556.

[284] Sağsöz N, Orbak Z, Noyan V, Yücel A, Uçar B, Yildiz L (2009) The effects of oral contraceptives including low-dose estrogen and drospirenone on the concentration of leptin and ghrelin in polycystic ovary syndrome Fertil. Steril. 92(2): 660-666.

[285] Fusco A, Bianchi A, Mancini A, Milardi D, Giampietro A, Cimino V, Porcelli T, Romualdi D, Guido M, Lanzone A, Pontecorvi A, De Marinis L (2007) Effects of ghrelin administration on endocrine and metabolic parameters in obese women with polycystic ovary syndrome. J. Endocrinol. Invest. 30(11): 948-956.

[286] Bik W, Baranowska-Bik A, Wolinska-Witort E, Chmielowska M, Martynska L, Baranowska B (2007) The relationship between metabolic status and levels of adiponectin and ghrelin in lean women with polycystic ovary syndrome. Gynecol. Endocrinol. 23(6): 325-331.

[287] Barber TM, Casanueva FF, Karpe F, Lage M, Franks S, McCarthy MI, Wass JA (2008) Ghrelin levels are suppressed and show a blunted response to oral glucose in women with polycystic ovary syndrome. Eur. J. Endocrinol. 158: 511–516.

[288] Zwirska-Korczala K, Sodowsky K, Konturek SJ, Kuka D, Kukla M, Brzozowski T, Cnota W, Woźniak-Grygiel E, Jaworek J, Bułdak R, Rybus-Kalinowska B, Fryczowski M (2008) Postprandial response of ghrelin and PYY and indices of low-grade chronic inflammation in lean young women with polycystic ovary syndrome. J. Physiol Pharmacol. 59(2): 161-178.

[289] Romualdi D, De Marinis L, Campagna G, Proto C, Lanzone A, Guido M (2008) Alteration of ghrelin-neuropeptide Y network in obese patients with polycystic ovary syndrome: role of hyperinsulinism. Clin. Endocrinol. (Oxf). 69(4): 562-567.

[290] Mitkov M, Pehlivanov B, Orbetzova M (2008) Serum ghrelin level in women with polycystic ovary syndrome and its relationship with endocrine and metabolic parameters. Gynecol. Endocrinol. 24 (11): 625-630.

[291] Mitkov M, Terzieva D, Nonchev B, Orbetzova M (2006) Ghrelin in women with polycystic ovary syndrome and type 2 diabetes mellitus. Endokrinologiya suppl. 3: 101-102 (in Bulgarian).

[292] Panidis D, Asteriadis C, Georgopoulos NA, Katsikis I, Zournatzi V, Karkanaki A, Saltamavros AD, Decavalas G, Diamanti-Kandarakis E (2010) Decreased active, total and altered active to total ghrelin ratio in normal weight women with the more severe form of polycystic ovary syndrome. Eur. J. Obstet. Gynecol. Reprod. Biol. 149: 170–174.

[293] Kamal M, Mohi A, Fawzy M, El-Sawah H (2010) Fasting plasma ghrelin in women with and without PCOS. Middle East Fertil. Soc. J. 15: 91–94.

Chapter 6

Adipose Tissue Inflammation and Insulin Resistance

Francisco L. Torres-Leal, Miriam H. Fonseca-Alaniz, Ariclécio Cunha de Oliveira and Maria Isabel C. Alonso-Vale

Additional information is available at the end of the chapter

http://dx.doi.org/10.5772/53974

1. Introduction

A sustained increase in body mass, particularly fat mass, an unhealthy diet and a sedentary lifestyle trigger metabolic alterations such as metabolic syndrome, obesity, and type 2 diabetes mellitus (2DM). These metabolic conditions increase the cardiovascular disease risks and have become epidemic public health problems (Grundy 2002). Individuals who are overweight and obese are associated with almost 70% of 2DM risk in the U.S. (Sherwin et al., 2004).

2DM is characterized by insulin resistance and hyperglycemia. Insulin resistance – which can be triggered by the presence of metabolic stressors, such as high-fat diets, obesity and high blood non-esterified fatty acids (FA) levels (Phillips et al., 2006; Roche et al., 2005) – is featured as the primary metabolic dysfunction responsible for the development of the metabolic syndrome. With regard to the relationship between high-fat diets, obesity, and 2DM, it is highlighted that the presence of high blood non-esterified FA concentrations compromises insulin sensitivity, reducing the action of this hormone in peripheral tissues, such as the liver, skeletal muscle and adipose tissue. It also impairs glucose and lipid metabolism, with the development of compensatory hyperinsulinemia (Saltiel, 2005) As well as in the obesity, insulin resistance is accompanied by the presence of a chronic low-grade inflammatory state (Dandona et al., 2004; Ghanim et al., 2004; Roche 2004).

The amount of white adipose tissue (WAT) may represent more than 50% of total body mass in obese individuals (body mass index ≥ 30 kg/m^2). The adiposity (and obesity) depends on the size and the number of the adipocytes, the last being regulated by adipogenesis.

The role of WAT as an ordinary tissue responsible for lipid energy storage has been replaced due to studies that demonstrate the central activity of WAT in lipid and glucose metabolism and its ability to secrete factors with endocrine, paracrine and autocrine effects. For example, recent studies suggest that pro-inflammatory and anti-inflammatory substances produced by WAT contribute to the development of insulin resistance (Weisberg et al., 2003; Xu et al., 2004).

2. The White Adipose Tissue (WAT)

The adipose tissue is classified in two major depots distributed throughout the body: WAT and brown adipose tissue (BAT). BAT is implicated in cold- and diet-induced thermogenesis (non-shivering thermogenesis), modulation of body temperature, energy expenditure and adiposity (Saito et al., 2009; Yoneshiro et al., 2011). WAT is specialized in the storage of energy in the form of triacylglycerol (TAG), it protects other organs and tissues from ectopic fat accumulation and, consequently, from lipotoxicity.

Until the 1990s, the functions related to WAT were only associated with passive energy storage (an inert depot for excess metabolic fuel), thermal insulation and organ protection from mechanical damage. The discovery of leptin, a hormone derived from WAT that can "tell" the state of these energy reserves to the central nervous system, introduced a new perspective on the study of adipose tissue role in the body energy homeostasis and metabolism. Subsequently, a number of new substances secreted by WAT have been characterized, which allowed its classification as an endocrine organ, capable of controlling the metabolism of several tissues and organs (Fonseca-Alaniz 2006; 2007).

Besides adipocytes, WAT contains connective tissue matrix (collagen and reticular fibers), nerve fibers, stromovascular cells, lymph nodes, immune cells (e.g., macrophages), fibroblasts and preadipocytes (undifferentiated adipose cells), some of which are also capable of secreting many bioactive products into the bloodstream (Fain et al., 2004; Kershaw et al., 2004).

White adipocytes are responsible for the storage of energy as TAG in a single lipid droplet during periods of abundant energy supply and for the mobilization of TAG when there is a calorie deficit. Adipocytes are capable of changing size according to the metabolic needs of the organism. During the development of obesity, there is an increase in the size (hypertrophy due to excessive lipid storage) and/or in the number (hyperplasia due to preadipocyte differentiation into mature adipocytes) of cells (Drolet et al., 2008).

Adipocytes express receptors for several hormones, cytokines and growth factors and also produce a number of protein/hormones (collectively referred to as "adipokines" or "adipocytokines"), all of which enable adipose tissue to communicate with other tissues and organs, such as skeletal muscle, endothelium and the central nervous system. Through this interaction network, WAT participates in modulating important biological processes, including food intake, energy metabolism, neuroendocrine and immune functions, angiogenesis, regulation of blood pressure and inflammation.

The adipokine secretory profile differs according to adipocyte size. For example, leptin mRNA expression is higher in large adipocytes compared to smaller adipocytes in the same obese individual (Hamilton et al., 1995). Additionally, the cell size of human abdominal subcutaneous adipose tissue correlates with adipose interleukin-6(IL-6) gene expression and its secretion *in vitro* (Sopasakis et al., 2004). Among the adipokines secreted by WAT, there are some pro-inflammatory and anti-inflammatory factors, including cytokines, chemokines, acute-phase proteins and angiogenic factors.

3. Obesity and inflammation in WAT

Obesity is considered a public health problem, as there has been a dramatic increase in the worldwide prevalence of this condition over the past 20 years. According to data from the Centers for Disease Control and Prevention Behavioral Risk Factor Surveillance System, obesity prevalence was under 20% in only one state (Colorado) in the U.S. in 2007, whereas the remaining states saw incidence levels equal to or greater than 25% (in http://www.cdc.gov/brfss/ abourth.htm). Additionally, one study predicted that the incidence of obesity in U.S. adults (above 15 years old) will increase from 32% to 44.2% in men and from 37.8% to 48.3% in women from 2002 to 2010 (Yach et al., 2006).

Obesity, particularly due to excessive accumulation of visceral fat, elevates the risk of developing many health conditions, including respiratory complications, coronary heart disease, 2DM, osteoarthritis and hypertension, and is associated with a nearly 8-year reduction in life expectancy (Kopelman 2000; Trayhurn et al., 2006).

The accumulation of fat mass during the development of obesity is characterized by adipocytes hyperplasia and hypertrophy and is associated with increased angiogenesis, macrophage infiltration, production of extracellular matrix components, endothelial cell activation and production and release of several inflammatory mediators (Bourlier et al., 2008; Henegar et al., 2008). Many of pro-inflammatory molecules are secreted by the adipocytes, whereas others are predominantly derived from WAT infiltrated macrophages. The dysregulation of pro- and anti-inflammatory cytokines/adipokines functions and their production in obese individuals, lead to a state of chronic low-grade inflammation and may promote obesity-linked metabolic disorders and cardiovascular diseases such as insulin resistance, metabolic syndrome and atherosclerosis.

In addition to the enlargement of adipocytes, obesity also promotes WAT macrophage accumulation, which can also contribute to inflammation. Recent studies demonstrated that both genetically obese mice and diet-induced obese mice are characterized by a significant increase in the number of WAT macrophages (Davies et al., 2008; Murano et al., 2008). Macrophage infiltration and the mRNA expression of monocyte chemotactic protein-1 (MCP-1) and colony-stimulating factor-1 (CSF1) was higher in omental visceral fat compared to subcutaneous fat from lean humans and these observations were aggravated in obesity, particularly in intra-abdominal obesity (Harman-Boehm et al., 2007).

Obesity increases the numbers of macrophages and also induces phenotypic switch in the WAT macrophage polarization. It has been demonstrated that in mice with diet-induced obesity there is a shift in the activation state of WAT macrophages from a M2a state, characterized by the expression of anti-inflammatory cytokines (e.g., interleukin-10) to a M1 state, characterized by the production of high levels of anti-inflammatory cytokines [e.g., tumor necrosis factor-alpha (TNF-α) and IL-6] (Lumeng et al., 2008). This obesity-induced switch in WAT macrophage polarization is due to recruitment of inflammatory monocytes from the circulation and not to the conversion of resident M2a macrophages to M1 macrophages in situ (Lumeng et al., 2008).

4. Adipogenesis and inflammation in WAT

Adipocytes derive from multipotent mesenchymal stem cells that reside in the stroma of the adipose tissue (Rosen et al., 2006). These multipotent cells become preadipocytes when they lose their ability to differentiate into other mesenchymal lineages and become committed to the adipocyte lineage. This early stage of adipocyte differentiation is known as determination or commitment and it is still poorly characterized. The next phase of adipogenesis involves activation of a cascade of transcriptional events, including the nuclear hormone receptor PPARγ and CCAAT/enhancer binding protein alpha (C/EBPα), which drive the expression of great importance in WAT, such as genes of glucose and lipid metabolism and adipokines, establishing thus, the differentiated state (Rosen et al., 2006).

The preadipocytes acquire the characteristics of mature adipocytes, such as accumulation of lipid droplets and the ability to respond to hormones such as insulin. The understanding of the events involved in adipogenesis has markedly increased in the last two decades with the use of clonal cells and non-clonal precursors of adipocytes from rodents and humans. Glucocorticoids and insulin-like growth factor 1 (IGF-I) were identified as the most efficient adipogenic agents in *ex vivo* experiments (Aihaud & Hauner, 2004).

As mentioned, the development of obesity results from both, the hypertrophy and the hyperplasia (or adipogenesis) of fat cells. Increase in the size of adipocytes is not an unlimited process. Eventually, the growth reaches a maximum level beyond which the ability of fat storage is exhausted and new cells are being slowly recruited and emerge from this tissue (15-50% of the adipose tissue cells represents a reservoir of mesenchymal stem cells including preadipocytes that can divide and differentiate in response to various extracellular agents). Very large adipocytes get into exhausted ability to store fat and become more lipolytic. This process allows an increase in free FA (FFA) plasma concentration that in turn may impair the function of non-adipose organs, a process called lipotoxicity (DeFronzo, 2004). The excess of circulating FFA is also a strong inducer of peripheral insulin resistance and increases the probability of 2DM and metabolic syndrome development.

The WAT protects other organs and tissues from ectopic fat accumulation and consequently from the lipotoxicity that this phenomenon causes. The lipotoxicity, in turn, is an important cause of insulin resistance. It is important to emphasize that the adipocyte has metabolic features that make itself less susceptible to lipotoxicity due to its high capacity for detoxification of FA (Lundgren & Eriksson, 2004). So, the generation of new fat cells can act as a mechanism to attenuate this by increasing the cellularity without exhausting fat accumulation.

In obese subjects, the WAT appears hypertrophic. In addition, obesity coexists with a high degree of inflammation, especially in the WAT itself. Several pro-inflammatory cytokines generated in the WAT by the infiltration of macrophages or by these hypertrophic adipocytes cause insulin resistance in this tissue limiting its function.

The balance between hyperplasic and hypertrophic activity in the WAT determines the size of the tissue. In obesity, the prevalence of hypertrophied cells causes an imbalance between the tissue mass increase and the unmatched blood flow, which leads ultimately to hypoxia, inflammation and macrophage infiltration in the tissue (Goossens, 2008). Macrophages release factors that affect the adipogenic process in human cells (Permana et al., 2006). There is also a decrease in the capacity of lipid buffering by the WAT with subsequent ectopic deposition of fat in other tissues. This fact coupled with the abnormal production of adipokines causes the disorders associated with obesity, mainly insulin resistance.

Hypertrophic adipocytes are the main producers of pro-inflammatory cytokines, such as, TNFα, IL-6, resistin and MCP1. On the other hand, these cells exhibit a limited ability to synthesize and release an important anti-inflammatory adipokine, adiponectin, which is the most potent endogenous insulin sensitizer. Stimulation of *in vivo* adipogenesis can replace hypertrophic adipocytes by younger and smaller ones with greater ability to produce adiponectin at the expenses of pro-inflammatory adipokines (Figure 1).

The WAT expansion in childhood obesity is recognized to result from the combination of both hypertrophy and hyperplasia of adipocytes. In opposition, for a long time, adults have been thought to present a fixed number of adipocytes and that changes in fat mass were mainly secondary to changes in the volume of fat cell. However, mature adipocytes exhibit remarkably intense and constant renewal (Spalding et al., 2008), and nowadays, it is known that the potential for generating new cells persists throughout the life of the individual in adipose tissue.

5. Perivascular adipose tissue and inflammation

Perivascular adipose tissue (PVAT) is an adipose tissue depot present around the majority of systemic blood vessels and has long been considered serving primarily as a supportive, mechanical purpose. Adipocytes from human PVAT reside at the adventitial border of blood vessels and are not separated from these vessels by a fascial layer or an elastic lamina (Chatterjee et al., 2009). PVAT expresses and secretes a variety of cytokines and chemokines, which may affect vascular physiology and play a pathological role in vascular diseases, like atherosclerosis (Henrichot et al., 2005; Gao et al., 2007).

Atherosclerosis is a disease of large arteries characterized by endothelial cell dysfunction, inflammatory cell recruitment and foam cell formation (Lusis, 2000). A recent study demonstrated that the infiltration of inflammatory cells (accumulation of macrophages and T lymphocytes) was markedly increased at the interface between the PVAT and adventia of atherosclerotic aortas as compared to peripheral arteries, which are not affected by atherosclerotic lesions (Henrichot et al., 2005).

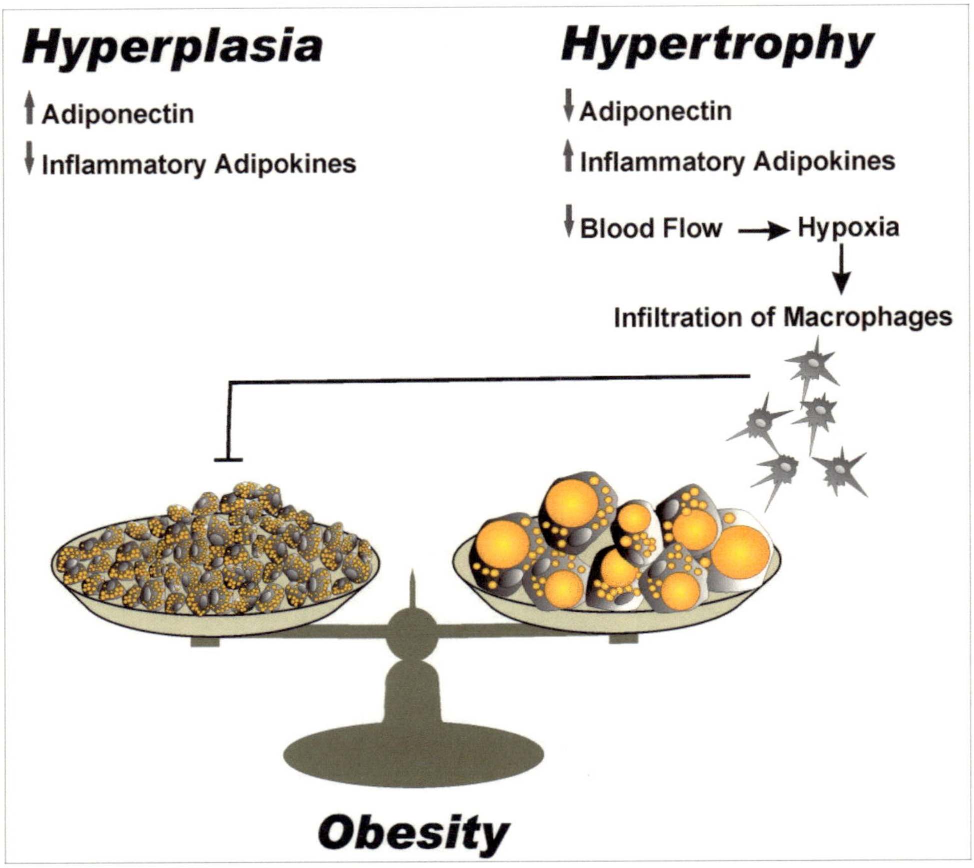

Adapted from: Queiroz et al., 2009.

Figure 1. Physiological balance between hypertrophy and hyperplasia. Obesity is determined by increasing both, the size and number of adipocytes. Adipogenesis can lead to a large number of new adipocytes (hyperplasia) which produce more adiponectin and less inflammatory adipokines. By the other side, hypertrophied adipocytes produce less adiponectin and more inflammatory adipokines. The prevalence of hypertrophied adipocytes in adipose tissue leads to a reduction in blood flow with subsequent hypoxia and macrophage infiltration. In addition, cytokines produced by macrophages inhibit adipogenesis.

Some of PVAT-derived factors are typical proinflammatory cytokines that could influence the chronic inflammation in atherosclerosis. For example, adipocytes surrounding human coronary arteries secrete more IL-6, interleukin-8 (IL-8) and MCP-1 into the culture medium than subcutaneous and visceral (perirenal) adipocytes (Chatterjee et al., 2009). These mediators stimulate the chemotaxis of leucocytes to the vascular endothelium and their migration into the vascular wall, the proliferation of smooth muscle cells and the formation of neo-vessels, contributing, this way, to the atherogenesis (Thalmann, Meyer, 2007). Moreover, feeding mice with high-fat diet increased the amount of PVAT and their local expression of inflammatory genes as compared to mice fed a control diet (Henrichot et al., 2005; Chatterjee et al., 2009).

Besides cytokines, PVAT also secretes classical adipocytokines such as leptin, and visfatin that are able to exert proatherogenic and prothrombotic actions by chemotactively attracting and activating inflammatory cells, producing endothelial dysfunction and stimulating smooth muscle cell proliferation and migration (Wang et al., 2009; Rajsherher et al., 2010). Recently, a study related that leptin and visfatin protein expression in adipose tissue surrounding abdominal aorta (periaortic adipose tissue) was positively correlated with aortic atherosclerotic lesions in humans individuals (Spiroglou et al., 2010)

Taking together, emerging evidences suggest that obesity is accompanied by increase in PVAT mass, hypertrophy of perivascular adipocytes and differential release of cytokines and adipocytokines that could be implicated in the pathogenesis of obesity-associated vascular complications such as atherosclerosis by affecting, among others, the inflammatory process.

6. Adipokines in obesity and inflammation

One of the consequences of the chronic low-grade inflammation state associated with obesity is the development of insulin resistance as well as increased risk of 2DM development.

The mechanisms linking obesity, inflammation and defects in insulin sensitivity seem to involve the contribution of macrophages-derived pro-inflammatory cytokines. For example, it was reported higher expression of macrophage-specific inflammatory-genes such as MCP-1 and macrophage inflammatory protein-1α (MIP-1α), in the fat depot of obese mice preceding accentuated increase in insulin production (Xu et al., 2003). Furthermore, the administration of rosiglitazone, an insulin-sensitizing drug, reduced the expression of these genes (Xu et al., 2003).

WAT produces and secretes a number of substances with a wide range of biological activity. The adipose-derived proteins act both locally in autocrine and paracrine fashions and distally, mediating endocrine effects through the systemic circulation. Among the soluble factors produced by WAT, there are hormones, cytokines and growth factors (adipokines), which include leptin, adiponectin, resistin, visfatin and MCP-1 (see Table 1).

Besides macrophages-derived pro-inflammatory elements, adipocytes also may contribute to development of obesity-related insulin-resistance. Accordingly, hypertrophic adipocytes from humans display elevated expression and secretion of pro-inflammatory adipokines (Skurk et al., 2007). On the other hand, the plasma levels of adiponectin, an insulin-sensitizing adipokine, are reduced in obese individuals and inversely correlate with the degree of insulin resistance and hyperinsulinemia (Arita et al., 1999; Weyer et al., 2001)

The first link between obesity, inflammation and insulin action came from a study developed by Hotamisligil and coworkers (1993). In this study, the authors demonstrated elevate expression of TNF-α mRNA in adipose tissue of obese animals models (*fa/fa* rat and *ob/ob* mouse) and the neutralization of TNF-α in obese *fa/fa* mice increased insulin action on glucose uptake (Hotamisligil et al., 1993). Uysal *et al.* (1997) showed that two different models of murine obesity (ob/ob and high-fat diet fed-mice) had significantly improved insulin sensitivity when TNF-α or TNF-α receptors were lacking and the TNF-α deficient obese mice displayed lower levels of circulating FFA than the obese wild-type counterparts. In addition, the treatment of obese rats with antibodies against TNF-α reduces insulin resistance (XU et al., 2004). These data demonstrate the deleterious effects of TNF-α on insulin action in obesity rodent models and one of the molecular mechanisms underlying TNF-α induced insulin resistance may involve a c-Jun N-terminal kinase (JNK) mediated serine phosphorylation of the insulin receptor substrate (IRS)-1, which inhibits normal tyrosine phosphorylation of IRS-1 and consequently reduces the activation of the insulin signaling cascade (Maury; Brichard, 2010).

Though mature adipocytes secrete TNF- α, majority of its production takes place in macrophages (Maury et al., 2009). In obese humans, serum TNF-α concentration is elevated and decreases after weight loss (Dandona et al., 1998). TNF-α mRNA expression is increased in the adipose depots and correlates with insulin resistant in obese patients (Maury et al., 2009; Kern et al., 2001). However, the treatment of patients with etanercept (a TNF-α inhibitor drug), for a four-week period, in order to neutralize the elevated TNF-α levels, increased circulating resistin and adiponectin levels, reduced muscle fat content, but did not promote improvements in insulin sensitivity (Lo et al., 2007; Bernstein et al., 2006).

TNF-α possesses stimulatory effects on lipolysis by promoting a rise in cAMP levels and by stimulating the activity of hormone sensitive lipase along with perilipin downregulation via mitogen-activated protein kinase (MAPK) activation (Souza et al., 2003) . In WAT, TNF-α reduces the expression and activities of PPAR-γ, lipoprotein lipase and GLUT-4, resulting in diminished glucose uptake, FFA esterification and storage (Imai et al, 2004; Zhang et al, 1996; Stephens et al, 1997). In the liver, TNF-α increases the expression of genes involved in the de novo synthesis of cholesterol and FA and, at the same time, reduces the expression of genes involved in glucose uptake, metabolism and FA oxidation (Guilherme et al, 2008). Thus the effects promoted by this cytokine on lipid metabolism result in high plasma levels of FFA, which also may contribute to the development of peripheral insulin resistance.

IL-6 has been shown to be essential in reducing the inflammatory process by promoting the synthesis of anti-inflammatory cytokines and by negatively regulating inflammatory targets (Xing et al., 1998; Steensberg et al., 2003; Starkie et al., 2003). Thus, this protein has been classified as both a pro-inflammatory and anti-inflammatory adipokine; at some levels it acts as a defense mechanism but in chronic inflammation it is rather pro-inflammatory (Kamimura et al., 2003).

In humans, IL-6 is secreted by a wide variety of cells: endothelial cells, keratinocytes, osteoblasts, myocytes, adipocytes, β pancreatic cells, monocytes, macrophages and a number of other tissues, including a few tumors (Kamimura et al., 2003; Carey et al., 2004).

In healthy humans at resting state, IL-6 level is under 10 pg/mL. High circulating IL-6 levels can be found in several low-level inflammatory conditions such as sepsis, where their levels can reach above 10-1000 pg/mL (Friedland et al., 1992). WAT, especially visceral, may contribute to 10-35% of the basal circulating IL-6 levels in healthy individuals during the resting state (Mohamed-Ali et al., 1997). Adipocytes are capable of producing and secreting IL-6 (Sopasakis et al., 2004; Bastard et al., 2000; Fried et al., 1998; Vicennati et al., 2002; Krogh-Madsen et al., 2004), but contribute to a small fraction of the total IL-6 secreted by this tissue (Sopasakis et al., 2004; Fried et al., 1998), since about 90% of IL-6 expressed in WAT is produced by cells other than adipocytes (Fried et al., 1998).

IL-6 mRNA expression is increased in the obese adipose depots, reduces after weight loss and adipocyte hypertrophy is accompanied by an increase in IL-6 production (Sopasakis et al., 2004; Kern et al., 2001; Bastard et al., 2000; Fried et al., 1998). WAT IL-6 mRNA has been shown to be elevated in insulin resistant obese patients with and without 2DM (Kern et al., 2001; Bastard et al., 2000; Fried et al., 1998; Rotter et al., 2003), which correlates with reduced rates of insulin-stimulated glucose disposal both in vitro (from a glucose uptake assay in adipocytes) and in vivo (from a hyperinsulinemic normoglycemic clamp study) (Bastard et al., 2002).

The cross-talk between IL-6 and insulin-dependent metabolism has been approached by several researchers over the past few years. Adverse effects on insulin action in the liver and WAT have been demonstrated in animals and in cell cultures (Klover et al., 2003; Senn et al., 2002; Rotter et al., 2003; Senn et al., 2003; Sabio et al., 2008). This adipokine reduces insulin-dependent hepatic glycogen synthesis (Klover et al., 2003; Senn et al., 2002) and glucose uptake in adipocytes (Rotter et al., 2003), whose effects could be mediated by the increased expression of suppressor of cytokine signaling (SOCS)-3, a protein that binds and inhibits the insulin receptor and also targets IRS proteins for proteosomal degradation, and by negative regulation of the transcription of IRS-1 (Rotter et al., 2003; Sabio et al., 2008).

IL-6 has lipolytic properties in WAT and adipocyte cultures (Wallenius et al., 2002; van Hall et al., 2003; Trujillo et al., 2004; Petersen et al., 2005). In humans, infusion of IL-6 promotes a rise in FFA levels and stimulates total body fat oxidation (van Hall et al., 2003; Lyngso et al., 2002). Studies in transgenic animals support the effect of IL-6 as a lipolytic factor. A 200% increase was observed in the number of soluble IL-6 receptors (IL-6/sIL-6R) in transgenic mice resulting in reduced body weight (Peters et al., 1997), whereas IL-6 deficiency led to early-onset obesity (Wallenius et al., 2002). However, the obesity phenotype has not been observed in any other study involving IL-6 knockout mice (Di Gregorio et al., 2004).

Circulating MCP-1 levels were increased in animal models of obesity (*ob/ob* mice and diet-induced obesity mice) (Sartipy; Loskutoff, 2003; Takahashi et al., 2003) and in obese subjects (Christiansen et al, 2005; Bruun et al., 2005; Kim et al., 2006), and reduced after weight loss (Christiansen et al, 2005; Takahashi et al., 2003). Furthermore, adipose tissue MCP-1 mRNA expression also was enhanced and correlated with measures of adiposity in obese subjects (Christiansen et al, 2005; Dahlman et al., 2005).

It was reported that adipocytes secrete MCP-1, a factor that is a potent chemoattractant for monocyte/macrophage infiltration (Christiansen et al., 2005; Skurk et al., 2007). Its secretion positively correlates with cell size (Skurk et al., 2007) and although it is produced by both fractions of WAT, it is more expressed in stroma vascular cells than in isolated adipocytes (Fain et al., 2004; Bruun et al., 2005).

Increased MCP-1 levels in 2DM patients compared to non-diabetic subjects were reported in previous studies (Nomura et al., 2000; Ezenwaka et al., 2009). In addition, in a human population-based case-cohort study, elevated serum concentration of MCP-1 was associated with incident of type 2 diabetes (Herder et al., 2006).

Some in vitro and in vivo studies have demonstrated the insulin resistance-inducing effects of MCP-1 and tried to establish the mechanisms by which it may reduce insulin action. Treatment of 3T3-L1 differentiated adipocytes with MCP-1 blunted the insulin-stimulated glucose uptake and reduced the expression of genes such as lipoprotein lipase, GLUT-4 and PPAR-γ (Sartipy and Loskutoff, 2003). In primary human skeletal muscle cells, physiological levels of MCP-1 significantly reduced insulin-stimulated phosphorylation of Akt, GSK3α and GSK3β proteins, impairing insulin signaling and reducing insulin-dependent glucose uptake (Sell et al., 2006). Mice with overexpression of MCP-1 in the WAT displayed normal adiposity, increased macrophage infiltration into fat depot and reduced systemic insulin sensitivity (evaluated by insulin tolerance and hyperinsulinemic-euglycemic clamp tests) (Kamei et al., 2006). Furthermore, MCP-1 overexpression in WAT reduced insulin-stimulated tyrosine phosphorylation of IR and IRS proteins and decreased Akt phosphorylation in skeletal muscle and liver causing insulin resistance in both tissues of these mice (Kamei et al., 2006).

Taken together, the results suggest MCP-1 as an inflammatory link between obesity and the development of insulin resistance.

7. WAT mitochondria in obesity and inflammation

While brown adipose tissue (BAT) converts mitochondrial energy into heat during adaptative thermogenesis, characterization of WAT mitochondria function is still incipient (Forner et al., 2009; De Pauw et al., 2009). A recent *in vivo* proteomics analysis in mice WAT and BAT shows that there are quantitative and qualitative differences between the mitochondria from both tissues: BAT mitochondria are more similar to muscle mitochondria and WAT mitochondria express proteins associated with anabolic functions and proteins involved in the degradation of xenobiotics (Forner et al., 2009). Recent studies suggest that mitochondrial biogenesis and metabolism are implicated in the regulation of various processes in WAT, such as pre-adipocytes proliferation, adipogenesis, carbohydrate and lipid metabolism, adipocyte de-differentiation, TAG accumulation and acquirement of BAT-like characteristics (De Pauw et al., 2009; Forner et al., 2009; Tedesco et al., 2010; Bordicchia et al., 2012; Koponen et al., 2012) and impaired mitochondrial biogenesis contributes to the onset of obesity and related metabolic disorders, such as insulin resistance (Tedesco et al., 2010).WAT mitochondrial biogenesis in mice is correlated with the up-regulation of genes involved in fatty acid oxidation and mitochondrial electron transport activity, boosting WAT catabolism (Granneman et al., 2005). Indeed, it was demonstrated that mitochondrial proliferation and remodeling are enhanced in 3T3-L1 cells during adipogenesis and the use of insulin sensitizers, such as rosiglitazone, leads to significant alterations in mitochondrial morphology and augmentation of the expression of several mitochondrial proteins (Wilson-Fritch et al., 2003). These findings were later proven *in vivo* by the use of white adipocytes from *ob/ob* mice during the development of obesity and after treatment with the insulin-sensitizer rosiglitazone. Adipocytes from rosiglitazone-treated mice displayed increased mitochondrial mass, markedly enhanced oxygen consumption and significantly increased palmitate oxidation, suggesting that WAT enhanced lipid utilization may affect whole-body energy homeostasis and insulin sensitivity (Wilson-Fritch et al., 2004). Mitochondria are now considered as a target to improve whole-body sensitivity to insulin, mainly via enhanced WAT mitochondrial biogenesis, augmented FA uptake and FA oxidation which, in turn, may protect against adipocyte hypertrophy. Compounds with the potential to boost mitochondrial biogenesis are being investigated and, besides rosiglitazone and β3-adrenergic receptor activation, the combined use of R-α-lipoic acid and acetyl-L-carnitine to treat 3T3L1 adipocytes seems to enhance WAT mitochondrial population (Granneman et al., 2005; Shen et al., 2008). Accordingly, it was recently demonstrated that mice WAT mitochondria activation leads to the augmentation of both glucose sensitivity and serum adiponectin levels via the upregulation of genes involved in lipid metabolism and mitochondrial functioning (Duivenvoorde et al., 2011). Noteworthy, mitochondria mild uncoupling reduces TAG content in 3T3-L1 adipocytes, suggesting that WAT mitochondria modulation is a potential target for the development of therapies against obesity (Si et al., 2009; Tejerina et al., 2009).

WAT inflammation induces cytokine-mediated insulin resistance in adipocytes, triggering lipolysis and FAs release in the cytosol (Maassen et al., 2007). FAs play a pivotal role in the cell acting as an energetic substrate as well as a component of biomolecules. Nevertheless, elevated plasma levels of FFA are observed in conditions such as 2DM, obesity and sepsis, conditions associated with impaired immune function and a high prevalence of infections (Takahashi et al., 2012).

Apart from ATP synthesis, one of the most important functions of mitochondria is the removal of circulating FFA through β-oxidation, which occurs in tissues where glucose homeostasis is relevant, such as liver, muscle and adipose tissue (Maassen et al., 2007). In WAT, an impairment in mitochondrial fatty acid β-oxidation with increased glucose uptake might result in TAG accumulation in preadipocytes (Vankoningsloo et al., 2005) and muscle (Schereurs et al., 2010), hepatic insulin resistance (Zhang et al., 2007) and pancreatic beta cells lipotoxicity (Maassen et al., 2007). Accordingly, an increase in WAT oxidative capacity is correlated to the reduction of local inflammatory responses (Granneman et al., 2005). Curiously, marine-derived eicosapentaenoic (EPA) and docosahexaenoic (DHA) acids have an antiadipogenic effect via a metabolic switch in adipocytes, enhancing β-oxidation and upregulating mitochondrial biogenesis (Flachs et al., 2005).

Thus, WAT oxidative capacity was recently unveiled and it is implicated in the regulation of FFA concentration and the prevention of TAG accumulation in many tissues. An enhancement of WAT mitochondrial β-oxidation and, consequently, fatty acid catabolism is considered as a subject for prevention and treatment of obesity, insulin resistance and lipotoxicity (Granneman et al., 2005; Maassen et al., 2007; De Pauw et al., 2009; Schreurs et al., 2010; Gaidhu et al., 2011).

8. Conclusion

The chronic inflammatory state associated with obesity, particularly visceral obesity, favors the development of insulin resistance, metabolic syndrome, DM2, atherosclerosis, arterial hypertension and other cardiovascular diseases. In addition to its active role in energy metabolism, WAT secretes a number of substances with autocrine, paracrine and endocrine effects. Some WAT-derived factors contribute to the activation and infiltration of macrophages into fat depots. These macrophages, when activated, secrete cytokines that increase cell infiltration and inflammatory process. During this process, WAT turns into an inflamed organ that releases large amounts of FFA, which contributes to the lipid accumulation in non-adipose tissues, including liver and skeletal muscle. Inadequate lipid storage in these tissues is strongly associated with insulin resistance.

WAT also secretes a large numbers of proteins that participate in the inflammatory response. Several recent studies suggest that cytokines secreted by both adipocytes and infiltrated macrophages impair insulin signaling in peripheral tissues and then, may represent an important link between WAT inflammation in obesity and the pathogenesis of insulin resistance and DM2.

Moreover, the investigation of WAT mitochondrial function (and dysfunction) is recent and promising for a better understanding of WAT plasticity and metabolism and, consequently, for the development of new therapies to improve insulin sensitivity and treat obesity and related diseases.

Author details

Francisco L. Torres-Leal*
Department of Physiology and Biophysics, Institute of Biomedical Sciences, University of Sao Paulo, Sao Paulo, Brazil
Department of Biophysics and Physiology, Federal University of Piauí, Teresina, Brazil

Miriam H. Fonseca-Alaniz
Laboratory of Genetics and Molecular Cardiology, Heart Institute, University of São Paulo Medical School, Sao Paulo, Brazil

Ariclécio Cunha de Oliveira
Department of Physiology and Biophysics, Institute of Biomedical Sciences, University of Sao Paulo, Sao Paulo, Brazil
Superior Institute of Biomedical Sciences, State University of Ceará, Fortaleza, Ceará, Brazil

* Corresponding Author

Maria Isabel C. Alonso-Vale
Department of Biological Sciences, Institute of Environmental Sciences, Chemical and Pharmaceutical, University of São Paulo, Diadema, Sao Paulo, Brazil

9. References

[CDC - Centers for Disease Control and Prevention. Behavioral Risk Factor Surveillance System – BRFSS. Abouth the BRFSS http://www.cdc.gov/brfss/ abourth.htm]

Ailhaud G, Hauner H. Development of white adipose tissue. In: Bray AGB, editor. Handbook of obesity: Etiology and pathophysiology. New York, USA: Marcel Dekker, Inc.; 2004.

Arita Y, Kihara S, Ouchi N, Takahashi M, Maeda K, Miyagawa J, et al. Paradoxical decrease of an adipose-specific protein, adiponectin, in obesity. Biochem Biophys Res Commun 1999; 257(1):79-83.

Bastard JP, Jardel C, Bruckert E, Blondy P, Capeau J, Laville M, et al. Elevated levels of interleukin 6 are reduced in serum and subcutaneous adipose tissue of obese women after weight loss. J Clin Endocrinol Metab 2000; 85(9):3338-42.

Bastard JP, Maachi M, Van Nhieu JT, Jardel C, Bruckert E, Grimaldi A, et al. Adipose tissue IL-6 content correlates with resistance to insulin activation of glucose uptake both in vivo and in vitro. J Clin Endocrinol Metab 2002; 87(5):2084-9.

Bernstein LE, Berry J, Kim S, Canavan B, Grinspoon SK. Effects of etanercept in patients with the metabolic syndrome. Arch Intern Med 2006; 166(8):902-8.

Bordicchia M, Liu D, Amri EZ, Ailhaud G, DessÏ-Fulgheri P, Zhang C, et al. Cardiac natriuretic peptides act via p38 MAPK to induce the brown fat thermogenic program in mouse and human adipocytes. J Clin Invest 2012; 122(3):1022-36.

Bourlier V, Zakaroff-Girard A, Miranville A, De Barros S, Maumus M, Sengenes C, et al. Remodeling phenotype of human subcutaneous adipose tissue macrophages. Circulation 2008; 117(6):806-15.

Bruun JM, Lihn AS, Pedersen SB, Richelsen B. Monocyte chemoattractant protein-1 release is higher in visceral than subcutaneous human adipose tissue (AT): implication of macrophages resident in the AT. J Clin Endocrinol Metab 2005; 90(4):2282-9.

Carey AL, Febbraio MA. Interleukin-6 and insulin sensitivity: friend or foe? Diabetologia 2004; 47(7):1135-42.

Chatterjee TK, Stoll LL, Denning GM, Harrelson A, Blomkalns AL, Idelman G, et al. Proinflammatory phenotype of perivascular adipocytes: influence of high-fat feeding. Circ Res 2009; 104(4):541-9.

Christiansen T, Richelsen B, Bruun JM. Monocyte chemoattractant protein-1 is produced in isolated adipocytes, associated with adiposity and reduced after weight loss in morbid obese subjects. Int J Obes (Lond) 2005; 29(1):146-50.

Dahlman I, Kaaman M, Olsson T, Tan GD, Bickerton AS, Wåhlén K, et al. A unique role of monocyte chemoattractant protein 1 among chemokines in adipose tissue of obese subjects. J Clin Endocrinol Metab 2005; 90(10):5834-40.

Dandona P, Aljada A, Bandyopadhyay A. Inflammation: the link between insulin resistance, obesity and diabetes. Trends Immunol 2004; 25(1):4-7.

Dandona P, Weinstock R, Thusu K, Abdel-Rahman E, Aljada A, Wadden T. Tumor necrosis factor-alpha in sera of obese patients: fall with weight loss. J Clin Endocrinol Metab 1998; 83(8):2907-10.

Davis JE, Gabler NK, Walker-Daniels J, Spurlock ME. Tlr-4 deficiency selectively protects against obesity induced by diets high in saturated fat. Obesity (Silver Spring) 2008; 16(6):1248-55.

De Pauw A, Tejerina S, Raes M, Keijer J, Arnould T. Mitochondrial (dys)function in adipocyte (de)differentiation and systemic metabolic alterations. Am J Pathol 2009; 175(3):927-39.

DeFronzo RA. Dysfunctional fat cells, lipotoxicity and type 2 diabetes. Int J Clin Pract Suppl 2004; 143:9-21.

Di Gregorio GB, Hensley L, Lu T, Ranganathan G, Kern PA. Lipid and carbohydrate metabolism in mice with a targeted mutation in the IL-6 gene: absence of development of age-related obesity. Am J Physiol Endocrinol Metab 2004; 287(1):E182-7.

Drolet R, Richard C, Sniderman AD, Mailloux J, Fortier M, Huot C, Rheaume C, Tchernof A. Hypertrophy and hyperplasia of abdominal adipose tissues in women. Int J Obes (Lond) 2008; 32(2):283-91.

Duivenvoorde LP, van Schothorst EM, Bunschoten A, Keijer J. Dietary restriction of mice on a high-fat diet induces substrate efficiency and improves metabolic health. J Mol Endocrinol 2011; 47(1):81-97.

Ezenwaka CE, Nwagbara E, Seales D, Okali F, Sell H, Eckel J. Insulin resistance, leptin and monocyte chemotactic protein-1 levels in diabetic and non-diabetic Afro-Caribbean subjects. Arch Physiol Biochem 2009; 115(1):22-7.

Fain JN, Madan AK, Hiler ML, Cheema P, Bahouth SW. Comparison of the release of adipokines by adipose tissue, adipose tissue matrix, and adipocytes from visceral and subcutaneous abdominal adipose tissues of obese humans. Endocrinology 2004; 145(5):2273-82.

Fain JN, Madan AK, Hiler ML, Cheema P, Bahouth SW. Comparison of the release of adipokines by adipose tissue, adipose tissue matrix, and adipocytes from visceral and subcutaneous abdominal adipose tissues of obese humans. Endocrinology 2004; 145(5):2273-82.

Flachs P, Horakova O, Brauner P, Rossmeisl M, Pecina P, Franssen-van Hal N, et al. Polyunsaturated fatty acids of marine origin upregulate mitochondrial biogenesis and induce beta-oxidation in white fat. Diabetologia 2005; 48(11):2365-75.

Fonseca-Alaniz MH, Takada J, Alonso-Vale MI, Lima FB. Adipose tissue as an endocrine organ: from theory to practice. J Pediatr 2007; 83(5 Suppl):S192-203.

Fonseca-Alaniz MH, Takada J, Alonso-Vale MI, Lima FB. The adipose tissue as a regulatory center of the metabolism. Arq Bras Endocrinol Metabol 2006; 50(2):216-29.

Forner F, Kumar C, Luber CA, Fromme T, Klingenspor M, Mann M. Proteome differences between brown and white fat mitochondria reveal specialized metabolic functions. Cell Metab 2009; 10(4):324-35.

Fried SK, Bunkin DA, Greenberg AS. Omental and subcutaneous adipose tissues of obese subjects release interleukin-6: depot difference and regulation by glucocorticoid. J Clin Endocrinol Metab 1998; 83(3):847-50.

Friedland JS, Suputtamongkol Y, Remick DG, Chaowagul W, Strieter RM, Kunkel SL, et al. Prolonged elevation of interleukin-8 and interleukin-6 concentrations in plasma and of leukocyte interleukin-8 mRNA levels during septicemic and localized Pseudomonas pseudomallei infection. Infect Immun 1992; 60(6):2402-8.

Gaidhu MP, Frontini A, Hung S, Pistor K, Cinti S, Ceddia RB. Chronic AMP-kinase activation with AICAR reduces adiposity by remodeling adipocyte metabolism and increasing leptin sensitivity. J Lipid Res 2011; 52(9):1702-11.

Gao YJ, Lu C, Su LY, Sharma AM, Lee RM. Modulation of vascular function by perivascular adipose tissue: the role of endothelium and hydrogen peroxide. Br J Pharmacol 2007; 151(3):323-31.

Ghanim H, Aljada A, Hofmeyer D, Syed T, Mohanty P, Dandona P. Circulating mononuclear cells in the obese are in a proinflammatory state. Circulation 2004; 110(12):1564-71.

Goossens GH. The role of adipose tissue dysfunction in the pathogenesis of obesity-related insulin resistance. Physiology & Behavior 2008; 94(2):206-18.

Granneman JG, Li P, Zhu Z, Lu Y. Metabolic and cellular plasticity in white adipose tissue I: effects of beta3-adrenergic receptor activation. Am J Physiol Endocrinol Metab 2005; 289(4):E608-16.

Grundy SM: Obesity, metabolic syndrome, and coronary atherosclerosis. Circulation 2002; 105(23):2696-8.

Guilherme A, Virbasius JV, Puri V, Czech MP. Adipocyte dysfunctions linking obesity to insulin resistance and type 2 diabetes. Nat Rev Mol Cell Biol 2008; 9(5):367-77.

Hamilton BS, Paglia D, Kwan AY, Deitel M: Increased obese mRNA expression in omental fat cells from massively obese humans. Nat Med 1995; 1(9):953-6.

Harman-Boehm I, Bluher M, Redel H, Sion-Vardy N, Ovadia S, Avinoach E, et al. Macrophage infiltration into omental versus subcutaneous fat across different populations: effect of regional adiposity and the comorbidities of obesity. J Clin Endocrinol Metab 2007; 92(6):2240-7.

Henegar C, Tordjman J, Achard V, Lacasa D, Cremer I, Guerre-Millo M, et al. Adipose tissue transcriptomic signature highlights the pathological relevance of extracellular matrix in human obesity. Genome Biol 2008; 9(1):R14.

Henrichot E, Juge-Aubry CE, Pernin A, et al. Production of chemokines by perivascular adipose tissue: a role in the pathogenesis of atherosclerosis? Arterioscler Thromb Vasc Biol 2005; 25(12):2594–9.

Herder C, Müller-Scholze S, Rating P, Koenig W, Thorand B, Haastert B, et al. Systemic monocyte chemoattractant protein-1 concentrations are independent of type 2 diabetes or parameters of obesity: results from the Cooperative Health Research in the Region of Augsburg Survey S4 (KORA S4). Eur J Endocrinol 2006; 154(2):311-7.

Hotamisligil GS, Shargill NS, Spiegelman BM. Adipose expression of tumor necrosis factor-alpha: direct role in obesity-linked insulin resistance. Science 1993; 259(5091):87-91.

Imai T, Takakuwa R, Marchand S, Dentz E, Bornert JM, Messaddeq N, et al. Peroxisome proliferator-activated receptor gamma is required in mature white and brown adipocytes for their survival in the mouse. Proc Natl Acad Sci USA 2004; 101(13):4543-7.

Kamei N, Tobe K, Suzuki R, Ohsugi M, Watanabe T, Kubota N, et al. Overexpression of monocyte chemoattractant protein-1 in adipose tissues causes macrophage recruitment and insulin resistance. J Biol Chem 2006; 281(36):26602-14.

Kamimura D, Ishihara K, Hirano T. IL-6 signal transduction and its physiological roles: the signal orchestration model. Rev Physiol Biochem Pharmacol 2003; 149:1-38.

Kern PA, Ranganathan S, Li C, Wood L, Ranganathan G. Adipose tissue tumor necrosis factor and interleukin-6 expression in human obesity and insulin resistance. Am J Physiol Endocrinol Metab 2001; 280(5):E745-51.

Kershaw EE, Flier JS. Adipose tissue as an endocrine organ. J Clin Endocrinol Metab 2004; 89(6):2548-56.

Kim CS, Park HS, Kawada T, Kim JH, Lim D, Hubbard NE, et al. Circulating levels of MCP-1 and IL-8 are elevated in human obese subjects and associated with obesity-related parameters. Int J Obes (Lond) 2006; 30(9):1347-55.

Klover PJ, Zimmers TA, Koniaris LG, Mooney RA. Chronic exposure to interleukin-6 causes hepatic insulin resistance in mice. Diabetes 2003; 52(11):2784-9.

Kopelman PG. Obesity as a medical problem. Nature 2000; 404(6778):635-43.

Koponen T, Cerrada-Gimenez M, Pirinen E, Hohtola E, Paananen J, Vuohelainen S, et al. The activation of hepatic and muscle polyamine catabolism improves glucose homeostasis. Amino Acids 2012; 42(2-3):427-40.

Krogh-Madsen R, Plomgaard P, Keller P, Keller C, Pedersen BK. Insulin stimulates interleukin-6 and tumor necrosis factor-alpha gene expression in human subcutaneous adipose tissue. Am J Physiol Endocrinol Metab 2004; 286(2):E234-8.

Lo J, Bernstein LE, Canavan B, Torriani M, Jackson MB, Ahima RS, et al. Effects of TNF-alpha neutralization on adipocytokines and skeletal muscle adiposity in the metabolic syndrome. Am J Physiol Endocrinol Metab 2007; 293(1):E102-9.

Lumeng CN, DelProposto JB, Westcott DJ, Saltiel AR. Phenotypic switching of adipose tissue macrophages with obesity is generated by spatiotemporal differences in macrophage subtypes. Diabetes 2008; 57(12):3239-46.

Lundgren M, Eriksson JW. No in vitro effects of fatty acids on glucose uptake, lipolysis or insulin signaling in rat adipocytes. Horm Metab Res 2004; 36(4):203-9.

Lusis AJ. Atherosclerosis. Nature 2000; 407(6801):233-41.

Lyngsø D, Simonsen L, Bülow J. Metabolic effects of interleukin-6 in human splanchnic and adipose tissue. J Physiol 2002; 543(Pt 1):379-86.

Maassen JA, Romijn JA, Heine RJ. Fatty acid-induced mitochondrial uncoupling in adipocytes as a key protective factor against insulin resistance and beta cell dysfunction: a new concept in the pathogenesis of obesity-associated type 2 diabetes mellitus. Diabetologia 2007; 50(10):2036-41.

Maury E, Brichard SM. Adipokine dysregulation, adipose tissue inflammation and metabolic syndrome. Mol Cell Endocrinol 2010; 314(1):1-16.

Maury E, Noël L, Detry R, Brichard SM. In vitro hyperresponsiveness to tumor necrosis factor-alpha contributes to adipokine dysregulation in omental adipocytes of obese subjects. J Clin Endocrinol Metab 2009; 94(4):1393-400.

Mohamed-Ali V, Goodrick S, Rawesh A, Katz DR, Miles JM, Yudkin JS, et al. Subcutaneous adipose tissue releases interleukin-6, but not tumor necrosis factor-alpha, in vivo. J Clin Endocrinol Metab 1997; 82(12):4196-200.

Murano I, Barbatelli G, Parisani V, Latini C, Muzzonigro G, Castellucci M, Cinti S. Dead adipocytes, detected as crown-like structures, are prevalent in visceral fat depots of genetically obese mice. J Lipid Res 2008; 49(7):1562-68.

Nomura S, Shouzu A, Omoto S, Nishikawa M, Fukuhara S. Significance of chemokines and activated platelets in patients with diabetes. Clin Exp Immunol 2000; 121(3):437-43.

Peters M, Schirmacher P, Goldschmitt J, Odenthal M, Peschel C, Fattori E, et al. Extramedullary expansion of hematopoietic progenitor cells in interleukin (IL)-6-sIL-6R double transgenic mice. J Exp Med 1997; 185(4):755-66.

Petersen EW, Carey AL, Sacchetti M, Steinberg GR, Macaulay SL, Febbraio MA, et al. Acute IL-6 treatment increases fatty acid turnover in elderly humans in vivo and in tissue culture in vitro. Am J Physiol Endocrinol Metab 2005; 288(1):E155-62.

Phillips C, Lopez-Miranda J, Perez-Jimenez F, McManus R, Roche HM: Genetic and nutrient determinants of the metabolic syndrome. Curr Opin Cardiol 2006; 21(3)185-93.

Queiroz JC, Alonso-Vale MI, Curi R, Lima FB. Control of adipogenesis by fatty acids. Arq Bras Endocrinol Metabol 2009; 53(5):582-94.

Rajsheker S, Manka D, Blomkalns AL, Chatterjee TK, Stoll LL, Weintraub NL. Crosstalk between perivascular adipose tissue and blood vessels. Curr Opin Pharmacol 2010; 10(2):191-6.

Roche HM, Phillips C, Gibney MJ. The metabolic syndrome: the crossroads of diet and genetics. Proc Nutr Soc 2005; 64(3):371-7.

Roche HM. Dietary lipids and gene expression. Biochem Soc Trans 2004; 32(Pt6):999-1002.

Rosen ED, MacDougald OA. Adipocyte differentiation from the inside out. Nat Rev Mol Cell Biol 2006; 7(12):885-96.

Rotter V, Nagaev I, Smith U. Interleukin-6 (IL-6) induces insulin resistance in 3T3-L1 adipocytes and is, like IL-8 and tumor necrosis factor-alpha, overexpressed in human fat cells from insulin-resistant subjects. J Biol Chem 2003; 278(46):45777-84.

Sabio G, Das M, Mora A, Zhang Z, Jun JY, Ko HJ, et al. A stress signaling pathway in adipose tissue regulates hepatic insulin resistance. Science 2008; 322(5907):1539-43.

Saito M, Okamatsu-Ogura Y, Matsushita M, Watanabe K, Yoneshiro T, Nio-Kobayashi J, et al. High incidence of metabolically active brown adipose tissue in healthy adult humans: effects of cold exposure and adiposity. Diabetes 2009; 58(7):1526-31

Saltiel AR. Series introduction: the molecular and physiological basis of insulin resistance: emerging implications for metabolic and cardiovascular diseases. J Clin Invest 2000; 106(2):163-4.

Sartipy P, Loskutoff DJ. Expression profiling identifies genes that continue to respond to insulin in adipocytes made insulin-resistant by treatment with tumor necrosis factor-alpha. J Biol Chem 2003; 278(52):52298-306.

Sartipy P, Loskutoff DJ. Monocyte chemoattractant protein 1 in obesity and insulin resistance. Proc Natl Acad Sci USA 2003; 100(12):7265-70.

Schreurs M, Kuipers F, van der Leij FR. Regulatory enzymes of mitochondrial beta-oxidation as targets for treatment of the metabolic syndrome. Obes Rev 2010; 11(5):380-8.

Sell H, Dietze-Schroeder D, Kaiser U, Eckel J. Monocyte chemotactic protein-1 is a potential player in the negative cross-talk between adipose tissue and skeletal muscle. Endocrinology 2006; 147(5):2458-67.

Senn JJ, Klover PJ, Nowak IA, Mooney RA. Interleukin-6 induces cellular insulin resistance in hepatocytes. Diabetes 2002; 51(12):3391-9.

Senn JJ, Klover PJ, Nowak IA, Zimmers TA, Koniaris LG, Furlanetto RW, et al. Suppressor of cytokine signaling-3 (SOCS-3), a potential mediator of interleukin-6-dependent insulin resistance in hepatocytes. J Biol Chem 2003; 278(16):13740-6.

Shen W, Liu K, Tian C, Yang L, Li X, Ren J, et al. R-alpha-lipoic acid and acetyl-L-carnitine complementarily promote mitochondrial biogenesis in murine 3T3-L1 adipocytes. Diabetologia 2008; 51(1):165-74.

Sherwin RS, Anderson RM, Buse JB, Chin MH, Eddy D, Fradkin J, et al. American Diabetes Association; National Institute of Diabetes and Digestive and Kidney Diseases. Prevention or delay of type 2 diabetes. Diabetes Care 2004; 27 Suppl 1:S47-54.

Si Y, Shi H, Lee K. Metabolic flux analysis of mitochondrial uncoupling in 3T3-L1 adipocytes. PLoS One 2009; 4(9):e7000.

Skurk T, Alberti-Huber C, Herder C, Hauner H. Relationship between adipocyte size and adipokine expression and secretion. J Clin Endocrinol Metab 2007; 92(3):1023-33.

Sopasakis VR, Sandqvist M, Gustafson B, Hammarstedt A, Schmelz M, Yang X, et al. High local concentrations and effects on differentiation implicate interleukin-6 as a paracrine regulator. Obes Res 2004; 12(3):454-60.

Souza SC, Palmer HJ, Kang YH, Yamamoto MT, Muliro KV, Paulson KE, et al. TNF-alpha induction of lipolysis is mediated through activation of the extracellular signal related kinase pathway in 3T3-L1 adipocytes. J Cell Biochem 2003; 89(6):1077-86.

Spalding KL, Arner E, Westermark PO, Bernard S, Buchholz BA, Bergmann O, et al. Dynamics of fat cell turnover in humans. Nature 2008; 453:783-7.

Spiroglou SG, Kostopoulos CG, Varakis JN, Papadaki HH. Adipokines in periaortic and epicardial adipose tissue: differential expression and relation to atherosclerosis. J Atheroscler Thromb 2010; 17(2):115-30.

Starkie R, Ostrowski SR, Jauffred S, Febbraio M, Pedersen BK. Exercise and IL-6 infusion inhibit endotoxin-induced TNF-alpha production in humans. FASEB J 2003; 17(8):884-6.

Steensberg A, Fischer CP, Keller C, Møller K, Pedersen BK. IL-6 enhances plasma IL-1ra, IL-10, and cortisol in humans. Am J Physiol Endocrinol Metab 2003; 285(2):E433-7.

Takahashi HK, Cambiaghi TD, Luchessi AD, Hirabara SM, Vinolo MA, Newsholme P, et al. Activation of survival and apoptotic signaling pathways in lymphocytes exposed to palmitic acid. J Cell Physiol 2012; 227(1):339-50.

Takahashi K, Mizuarai S, Araki H, Mashiko S, Ishihara A, Kanatani A, et al. Adiposity elevates plasma MCP-1 levels leading to the increased CD11b-positive monocytes in mice. J Biol Chem 2003; 278(47):46654-60.

Tedesco L, Valerio A, Dossena M, Cardile A, Ragni M, Pagano C, et al. Cannabinoid receptor stimulation impairs mitochondrial biogenesis in mouse white adipose tissue, muscle, and liver: the role of eNOS, p38 MAPK, and AMPK pathways. Diabetes 2010; 59(11):2826-36.

Tejerina S, De Pauw A, Vankoningsloo S, Houbion A, Renard P, De Longueville F, et al. Mild mitochondrial uncoupling induces 3T3-L1 adipocyte de-differentiation by a PPARgamma-independent mechanism, whereas TNFalpha-induced de-differentiation is PPARgamma dependent. J Cell Sci 2009; 122(Pt 1):145-55.

Thalmann S, Meier CA. Local adipose tissue depots as cardiovascular risk factors. Cardiovasc Res 2007; 75(4):690-701.

Trayhurn P, Bing C, Wood IS. Adipose tissue and adipokines-energy regulation from the human perspective. J Nutr 2006; 136(7 Suppl):1935-9S.

Trujillo ME, Sullivan S, Harten I, Schneider SH, Greenberg AS, Fried SK. Interleukin-6 regulates human adipose tissue lipid metabolism and leptin production in vitro. J Clin Endocrinol Metab 2004; 89(11):5577-82.

van Hall G, Steensberg A, Sacchetti M, Fischer C, Keller C, Schjerling P, et al. Interleukin-6 stimulates lipolysis and fat oxidation in humans. J Clin Endocrinol Metab 2003; 88(7):3005-10.

Vankoningsloo S, Piens M, Lecocq C, Gilson A, De Pauw A, Renard P, et al. Mitochondrial dysfunction induces triglyceride accumulation in 3T3-L1 cells: role of fatty acid beta-oxidation and glucose. J Lipid Res 2005; 46(6):1133-49.

Vicennati V, Vottero A, Friedman C, Papanicolaou DA. Hormonal regulation of interleukin-6 production in human adipocytes. Int J Obes Relat Metab Disord 2002; 26(7):905-11.

Wallenius K, Wallenius V, Sunter D, Dickson SL, Jansson JO. Intracerebroventricular interleukin-6 treatment decreases body fat in rats. Biochem Biophys Res Commun 2002; 293(1):560-5.

Wallenius V, Wallenius K, Ahrén B, Rudling M, Carlsten H, Dickson SL, et al. Interleukin-6-deficient mice develop mature-onset obesity. Nat Med 2002; 8(1):75-9.

Wang P, Xu TY, Guan YF, Su DF, Fan GR, Miao CY. Perivascular adipose tissue-derived visfatin is a vascular smooth muscle cell growth factor: role of nicotinamide mononucleotide. Cardiovasc Res 2009; 81(2):370-80.

Weisberg SP, McCann D, Desai M, Rosenbaum M, Leibel RL, Ferrante AW Jr. Obesity is associated with macrophage accumulation in adipose tissue. J Clin Invest 2003; 112(12):1796-808.

Weyer C, Funahashi T, Tanaka S, Hotta K, Matsuzawa Y, Pratley RE, et al. Hypoadiponectinemia in obesity and type 2 diabetes: close association with insulin resistance and hyperinsulinemia. J Clin Endocrinol Metab 2001; 86(5):1930-5.

Wilson-Fritch L, Burkart A, Bell G, Mendelson K, Leszyk J, Nicoloro S, et al. Mitochondrial biogenesis and remodeling during adipogenesis and in response to the insulin sensitizer rosiglitazone. Mol Cell Biol 2003; 23(3):1085-94.

Wilson-Fritch L, Nicoloro S, Chouinard M, Lazar MA, Chui PC, Leszyk J, et al. Mitochondrial remodeling in adipose tissue associated with obesity and treatment with rosiglitazone. J Clin Invest 2004; 114(9):1281-9.

Xing Z, Gauldie J, Cox G, Baumann H, Jordana M, Lei XF, et al. IL-6 is an antiinflammatory cytokine required for controlling local or systemic acute inflammatory responses. J Clin Invest 1998; 101(2):311-20.

Xu FP, Chen MS, Wang YZ, Yi Q, Lin SB, Chen AF, et al. Leptin induces hypertrophy via endothelin-1-reactive oxygen species pathway in cultured neonatal rat cardiomyocytes. Circulation 2004; 110(10):1269-75.

Xu FP, Chen MS, Wang YZ, Yi Q, Lin SB, Chen AF, Luo JD. Leptin induces hypertrophy via endothelin-1-reactive oxygen species pathway in cultured neonatal rat cardiomyocytes. Circulation 2004; 110(10):1269-75.

Xu H, Barnes GT, Yang Q, Tan G, Yang D, Chou CJ, et al. Chronic inflammation in fat plays a crucial role in the development of obesity-related insulin resistance. J Clin Invest 2003; 112(12):1821-30.

Yach D, Stuckler D, Brownell KD. Epidemiologic and economic consequences of the global epidemics of obesity and diabetes. Nat Med 2006; 12(1):62-6.

Yoneshiro T, Aita S, Matsushita M, Okamatsu-Ogura Y, Kameya T, Kawai Y, et al. Age-related decrease in cold-activated brown adipose tissue and accumulation of body fat in healthy humans. Obesity 2011; 19(9):1755-60.

Zhang B, Berger J, Zhou G, Elbrecht A, Biswas S, White-Carrington S, et al. Insulin- and mitogen-activated protein kinase-mediated phosphorylation and activation of peroxisome proliferator-activated receptor gamma. J Biol Chem 1996; 271(50):31771-4.

Zhang D, Liu ZX, Choi CS, Tian L, Kibbey R, Dong J, et al. Mitochondrial dysfunction due to long-chain Acyl-CoA dehydrogenase deficiency causes hepatic steatosis and hepatic insulin resistance. Proc Natl Acad Sci USA 2007; 104(43):17075-80.

Section 4

Systemic Effects of Insulin Resistance

Chapter 7

Cardiovascular and Renal Complications in Obesity and Obesity-Related Medical Conditions: Role of Sympathetic Nervous Activity and Insulin Resistance

Kazuko Masuo and Gavin W. Lambert

Additional information is available at the end of the chapter

http://dx.doi.org/10.5772/50523

1. Introduction

Elevated sympathetic activation, as assessed using a variety of indices, has been observed in lean hypertensive and diabetic patients, and obese individuals [Huggett *et al.* 2006; Masuo *et al.* 2000]. Similarly, many epidemiological studies have shown that hypertensive patients, even those without increased adiposity, display a higher prevalence of insulin resistance, thereby indicating the possible association between sympathetic activation and insulin resistance in the pathogenesis of hypertension [Esler *et al.* 2006; Masuo *et al.* 2002; de Silva *et al.* 2009]. Overweight and obesity is a growing problem across the globe and has reached "epidemic" proportions. The prevalence of diabetes, especially type 2 diabetes, and hypertension are significantly increased with the prevalence of obesity. Obesity, itself, and type 2 diabetes and hypertension associated with obesity are known to be more closely linked with insulin resistance and elevated sympathetic nervous activity. It has been well documented that obesity, hypertension, and diabetes are risk factors for subsequent cardiovascular and renal complications. Many patients are both diabetic and hypertensive while they are obese, but not all diabetic patients have hypertension, indicating that insulin resistance is not the only mechanism for blood pressure elevation in diabetic-hypertensive patients. Several investigators have reported that sympathetic nervous activation plays an important role in cardiovascular complications in patients with hypertension, diabetes, and obesity.

Sympathetic nervous activation accompanying insulin resistance is closely linked with left ventricular hypertrophy in otherwise healthy subjects [Masuo, *et al.* 2008]. In addition, sympathetic activation may predict the development of renal injury in healthy normotensive subjects [Masuo, *et al.* 2010]. Weight loss associated suppression of sympathetic nervous activity is associated with improvement of insulin sensitivity and resultant improvement in renal function in obese patients [Masuo, *et al.* 2011b; Straznicky, *et al.* 2009b & 2011]. Furthermore, weight loss improved the prevalence of left ventricular hypertrophy [Masuo, *et al.* 2008], which is one of the predictors for future cardiac complications, renal complications (injury) [Masuo, *et al.* 2007] and hyperuricacidemia [Straznicky, *et al.* 2011].These findings suggest that elevated sympathetic nerve activity associated with insulin resistance may contribute to the onset and maintenance of cardiovascular and renal complications in diabetes, and hypertension in obesity.

Furthermore, genetic polymorphisms of the β2- and β3-adrenoceptor gene have been associated with obesity [Masuo, *et al.* 2005 & 2011a; Kawaguchi, *et al.* 2006], hypertension [Masuo, et al. 2005b & 2010b; Kawaguchi, et al. 2006], type-2 diabetes and insulin resistance [Masuo, et al. 2005 & 2010} in epidemiological studies and may also be implicit in the close relationship between insulin resistance and sympathetic nerve activation. Recently, Masuo *et al.* reported that β2-adrenoceptor polymorphisms (Arg16Gly) accompanying high plasma norepinephrine levels may contribute to the prevalence of left ventricular hypertrophy and renal dysfunction [Masuo, *et al.* 2010a, b & 2011b]. These investigations suggest that β2-adrenoceptor polymorphisms are related to sympathetic activation and insulin resistance and may contribute to cardiovascular- and renal complications in obesity and obesity-related hypertension or type 2 diabetes.

This chapter will provide a synthesis of the current findings on the mechanisms of the onset and maintenance of cardiovascular and renal complications in obesity, hypertension and type 2 diabetes, with a particular focus on sympathetic nervous activity and insulin resistance. A better understanding of the relationships between sympathetic nervous activity and insulin resistance in these important clinical conditions might help with the clinical treatment of diabetes and hypertension in obesity and prevent further cardiovascular and renal complications in this at risk group.

2. Prevalence of type 2 diabetes and hypertension in obesity

The clustering of cardiovascular risk factors associated with obesity, in particular abdominal obesity, is well established [Athyrus, *et al.* 2011]. The prevalence of obesity and overweight increased in the United States between 1978 and 1991 [Mokdad, *et al.* 2001], and recent reports have suggested continuing increases [Ogden, et al. 2004]. The National Health and Nutrition Examination Survey (NHANES) I (1971-1974), NHANES II (1976-1980), and NAHNES III (1988-1994) were conducted by the National Center for Health Statistics, Centers for Disease Control and Prevention (CDC). These data from the continuous NHANES studies have showed that the prevalence of obesity and overweight people increased significantly in the United States between 1960 and 2003 [Preis, *et al.* 2009; Ogden, *et al.* 2004; Flegal, *et al.* 2012]. Evidence from several studies indicates that obesity and weight gain are associated with an increased risk of hypertension [Masuo, *et al.* 2000 &

2005a, b, c] and diabetes [Resnick, *et al.* 2000; Ford, *et al.* 1997], and that intentional weight loss reduces the risk that overweight individuals will develop hypertension [Masuo, *et al.* 2001b; Straznicky, *et al.* 2009b] or diabetes [Will, *et al.* 2002].

Recent large cohort studies have showed an increasing prevalence of obesity in children and, importantly, obesity in children is strongly associated with several major health risk factors, including type 2 diabetes mellitus and hypertension [Hedley, *et al.* 2004].

Focusing on the close associations between obesity, hypertension and diabetes, the NHANES and the Behavioural Risk Factor Surveillance System (BRFSS) investigations [Mokdad, *et al.* 2003] showed very close relationships between the prevalence of obesity, hypertension, and diabetes. Further, the Framingham Heart Study [Preis, et al. 2009] showed that diabetic subjects had a 2-fold higher mortality risk consisting of cardiovascular and non-cardiovascular mortality.

3. Sympathetic nervous activity in obesity, hypertension and diabetes

The sympathetic nervous system represents a major pathophysiological hallmark of both hypertension and renal failure, and is an important target of the therapeutic intervention [Grassi, *et al.* 2012; Schlaich, *et al.* 2009]. The sympathetic nervous system participates in regulating the energy balance through thermogenesis. Reduced energy expenditure and resting metabolic rate are predictive of weight gain (obesity). It is also widely recognized that insulin resistance or hyperinsulinemia relates to obesity [Minicardi, *et al.* 1996; Farrannini, *et al.* 1995; Ward, *et al.* 1996]. Many epidemiological and clinical studies have shown a close relationship between sympathetic nervous system activity and insulin levels in obesity [Masuo. *et al.* 2002]. Several studies of longitudinal design have examined the effect of body weight changes (weight loss or weight gain) on sympathetic nervous system activity and insulin sensitivity (fasting plasma insulin levels and the (homeostasis model assessment of insulin resistance, HOMA-IR). Elevations of sympathetic nervous system activity and insulin levels during weight gain [Masuo, *et al.* 2000; Gentale, *et al.* 2007; Barms, *et al.* 2003], and reductions of sympathetic activity and insulin levels during weight loss [Anderson, *et al.* 1991; Straznicky, et al. 2009], are typically observed. While these longitudinal studies have clearly shown that heightened sympathetic nerve activity and insulin resistance are closely linked to obesity (weight gain), the onset of obesity and the maintenance of obesity, it remains to be elucidated, whether sympathetic hyperactivity or insulin resistance is the prime mover.

The response of the sympathetic nervous system to change in plasma insulin levels after oral glucose loading (oral glucose tolerance test) are different between subjects with and without insulin resistance [Masuo, *et al.* 2005], between nonobese and obese subjects [Straznicky, *et al.* 2009a], and between subjects with and without the metabolic syndrome [Straznicky. 2009b]. Recently, changes in the sympathetic nerve firing pattern were observed with sympatho-inhibition during weight loss [Lambert, *et al.* 2011]. In addition, different regulation by insulin of regional (i.e. hind limb, kidney and brown adipose tissue) sympathetic outflow to peripheral tissue was observed in agouti obese mice compared to lean control mice [Morgani, *et al.* 2010]. These observations provide the evidence of a strong linkage between the activity of the sympathetic nervous system and insulin levels. Huggett *et al.* [Huggett, *et al.* 2003] examined muscle sympathetic nerve activity (MSNA) in four groups of subjects, patients with essential hypertension and type 2 diabetes, patients with type 2 diabetes alone, patients with essential hypertension alone, and healthy normotensive controls. They found higher MSNA in the hypertensive-type 2 diabetic patients as compared with hypertensive alone patients or type 2 diabetic alone patients, and higher MSNA in hypertensive alone patients or type 2 diabetic alone patients as compared with healthy normotensive controls. Fasting insulin levels were greater in hypertensive-type 2 diabetic patients and type 2 diabetic patients compared to hypertensive patients or healthy normotensive subjects. These findings, although obtained in patients still under medication, provided evidence that type 2 diabetic patients had elevated sympathetic nerve activity regardless of the prevailing blood pressure levels, and that the combination of hypertension and type 2 diabetes resulted in an augmentation in sympathetic nerve activity and levels of plasma insulin.

Several investigations on the contributions of β2- and β3-adrenoceptor polymorphisms to type 2 diabetes also support a strong relationship between sympathetic nerve hyperactivity and insulin resistance in type 2 diabetes [Masuo, *et al.* 2004 & 2005a, b; Ikarashi, *et al.* 2004].

Figure 1 summarizes the relationships between sympathetic nerve activity and insulin resistance in obesity and type 2 diabetes mellitus (**Figure 1**).

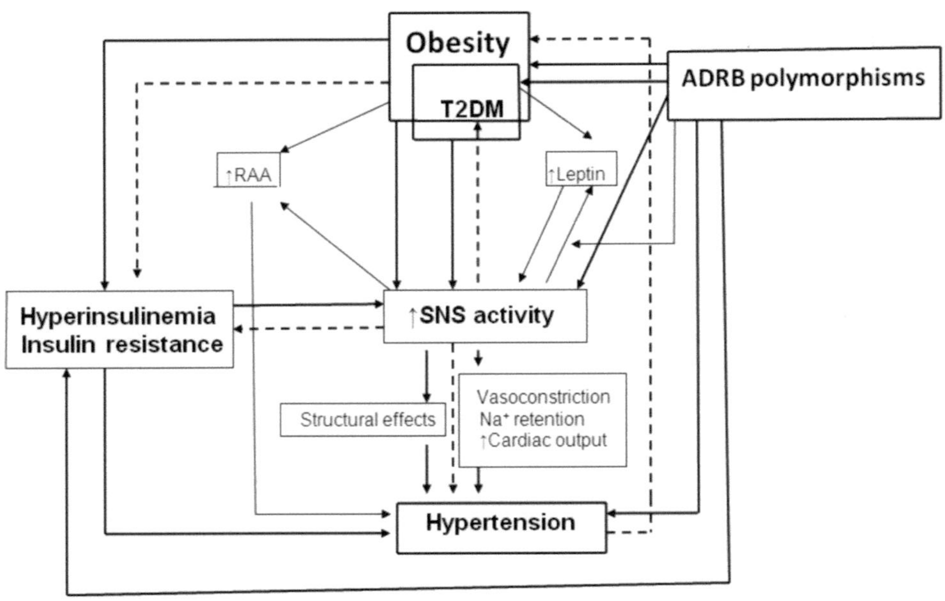

Obesity causes both insulin resistance/hyperinsulinemia and sympathetic nervous activation, and both link closely each other. Many investigations have shown that insulin resistance, sympathetic nervous activation, and adrenoceptor polymorphisms play important roles in the onset and maintenance of obesity, type 2 diabetes and hypertension. T2DM, type 2 diabetes, RAA, renin-angiotensin-aldosterone system; ADRB polymorphisms, adrenoceptor polymorphisms; SNS, sympathetic nervous system.

Figure 1. Potential pathophysiological mechanisms in obesity, hypertension and type2diabetes (T2DM)

4. Insulin resistance in obesity, hypertension and type 2 diabetes

Insulin resistance [Ferrannini, *et al.* 1998] is one of the criteria underpinning the development of the metabolic syndrome. The clinical evaluation of insulin resistance is growing interest because it is a strong predictor and plays an important role in the development of the metabolic syndrome, type 2 diabetes mellitus and hypertension. **Table 1** shows the criteria for metabolic syndrome characterisation, as can be seen insulin resistance is prominent [Alberti, *et al.* 1998; Grundy, *et al.* 2004] (**Table 1**). Measuring insulin sensitivity is important to define insulin resistance. **Table 2** summarizes the methods usually used in clinical and epidemiological studies (**Table 2**). The hyperinsulinemic-euglycemic glucose clamp method is the gold standard and may be suitable for research investigations in specialized laboratories, but the homeostasis model assessment of insulin resistance (HOMA-IR) or fasting plasma insulin concentrations is more practical for epidemiological studies comprising a large number of subjects.

4.1. Hyperinsulinemia as a marker of insulin resistance

Insulin is an exceptional hormone in that its action is regulated not only by changes in concentration but also by changes in the sensitivity of target tissues. Inadequate insulin action can be the consequence of: (*i*) insufficient insulin concentration at the site of action, (*ii*) decreased tissue (effectors) responses to insulin, or (*iii*) a combination of low concentration and a decreased response. Regulation of circulating insulin levels is mainly (but not exclusively) achieved by changes in secretory rates. Nevertheless, the major determinant of insulin secretion, and therefore of plasma insulin concentration, is glucose. Any change in glucose concentration from the narrow normal range results in an insulin response appropriate to restore homeostasis. Thus, changes in insulin sensitivity occur in various physiological states and pathological conditions.

For any amount of insulin secreted by the pancreas, the biological response of a given effector is dependent on its insulin sensitivity. The term insulin resistance customarily refers to glucose metabolism. Any decrease in insulin sensitivity (insulin resistance) is immediately translated into minute increases in blood glucose concentrations that will in turn act on the β-cell to produce a compensatory stimulus of insulin secretion, leading to a degree of hyperinsulinemia that is approximately proportional to the degree of effector resistance. Therefore, hyperinsulinemia may be responsible for insulin resistance. In steady-state conditions, this compensatory hyperinsulinemia prevents a more exaggerated hyperglycaemia. The inability of β-cells to enhance insulin secretion means that blood glucose will keep increasing until the level of hyperglycaemia produces an adequate β-cell stimulus to attain the required insulin response. When the β-cell is unable to compensate for the prevalent insulin resistant state by further augmenting insulin secretion, hyperglycaemia continues to increase, producing impaired fasting glucose, impaired glucose tolerance and diabetes mellitus development.

	WHO (51)	**EGIR** (52, 53)	**NCEP AT III (Expert Panel on Detection Evaluation and Treatment of High Blood Cholesterol in Adults)** (54)	**American Heart Association Updated NCEP III** (55)
Insulin resistance	Top 25% of population Distribution	Top 25% of population distribution	Not considered	Not considered
Hyperinsulinemia	Not considered	Top 25% of population distribution	Not considered	Not considered
Fasting glucose (mmol/L) hyperglycemia	impaired fasting glucose, or impaired glucose tolerance or diabetes	>6.1, but not diabetic	≥6.1	≥5.6 (100 mg/dL) or medications for
Hypertension (mmHg)	≥160/≥ 90	≥140/≥ 90 or on medications for hypertension	≥130/85	≥130/85 or medications for hypertension
Central obesity	waist/hip ratio >0.9 (men), >0.85 (women) and/or BMI≥30kg/m^2	---	---	---
Waist circumference (cm)	Not considered	≥94 (men), ≥ 80 (women)	>102 (men), >88 (women)	≥102 (men), ≥88 (women)
HDL-cholesterol (mmol/L)	<1.0 or medications for dyslipidemia	<1.0 or medications for dyslipidemia	<1.07 (40 mg/dL, men), <1.25 (50 mg/dL , women)	<1.07 (40 mg/dL, men) <1.25 (50 mg/dL, women)
Triglyceride (mmol/L)	<1.0 or medications for Dyslipidemia	>2.0 or medications for dyslipidemia	≥1.695 (150 mg/dL)	≥1.695 (150 mg/dL)
Micro-albuminemia	Present	Not considered	Not considered	Not considered
Criteria	1 of the first two + 2 of other features	1of the first two + 2 of other features	3 of above	3 of above

BMI, body mass index; EGIR, European Group of the study of Insulin Resistance; NCEP ATPIII, 3rd Recommendations of the Adult Treatment Panel of the National Cholesterol Education Program; HDL-cholesterol, high-density lipoprotein cholesterol. Values in NECP definition and American Heart Association/Updated NCEP are approximations of values in mg/dL.

Table 1. Criteria for Metabolic Syndrome including Insulin Resistance (50)

Methods	Summary/Comments (reference number)
Plasma insulin concentrations	Measurement of insulin concentrations under physiological concentrations (i.e. fasting, postprandial) correlates with IR Useful especially in epidemiological studies including a large number of subjects.
Oral glucose tolerance test (OGTT)	The OGTT contains critical information regarding insulin secretion and sensitivity. (1) The AUC of plasma insulin or C-peptide provides some indication of insulin secretion. The AUCIns/AUCGluc appears to be a good parameter to assess beta-cell function from an OGTT in either diabetic or non-diabetic subjects. (2) ISI provides a reasonable approximation of whole-body insulin sensitivity that represents a composite of hepatic and peripheral tissues and considers insulin sensitivity both in the basal state (fasting glucose · fasting insulin) and after the ingestion of a glucose load (mean glucose · mean insulin). ISIcomp = 10,000/square root of [fasting glucose · fasting insulin] · [mean glucose · mean insulin during OGTT]. (56)
HOMA-IR (homeostasis model assessment of insulin resistance)	Index based on fasting glucose and insulin concentration. Fasting insulin (U/mL) x fasting glucose (mmol/L)/22.5. HOMA-IR correlates strongly with the results of clamping studies. (57, 58)
QUICKI (quantitative insulin sensitivity check index)	QUICKI is said to provide a reproducible and robust estimate of insulin sensitivity that shows excellent linear correlation with the gold standard clamp measurement and has similar variability and discriminative power QUICKI=1/[log (fasting insulin)+log (fasting glucose)], thus QUICKI is the logarithm of the values from one of the HOMA equations. (59)
HOMA-B (homeostasis model assessment of insulin secretion)	HOMA-B allows the beta-cell function (HOMA-B) to be deduced for a given subject from pairs of fasting glucose and insulin (or C-peptide) measurements. HOMA-B=insulin (U/mL) x 20/[glucose (mmol)-3.5].
Minimal model	Estimating IR from results of frequent blood samples during intravenous glucose tolerance test (IVGTT)
Insulin tolerance test	High dose insulin is given intravenously and the decline of glucose concentration measured.
Steady state plasma glucose (SSPG)	A sophisticated method but currently little used. Subjects are infused continuously with an intravenous infusion of somatostatin to suppress endogenous insulin and glucose secretion for 150 min, and determined the steady state plasma glucose levels. Subjects with SSPG>150 mg/dL are considered to be IR. (60) shows the insulin secretary index rather than insulin sensitivity.

Methods	Summary/Comments (reference number)
Clamp methods	
Hyperinsulinemic, euglycemic clamp	The gold standard for investigating and quantifying IR. The amount of glucose necessary to compensate for an increased insulin level without hypoglycemia and to maintain blood glucose level (5.0-5.5 mmol/dL) is determined by continuously glucose infusion. Low dose insulin infusion is more useful for assessing the response of liver, whereas high dose insulin infusion are useful for assessing peripheral (i.e. fat, muscle) insulin action. Required glucose infusion rate ≤4.0 mg/min=insulin resistance, 4.0-7.5 mg/min=impaired glucose tolerance, ≥7.5 mg/min=insulin sensitive.
Hyperglycemic clamp	Sustained hyperglycemia can cause peripheral IR, pancreatic beta-cell dysfunction, and resultant glucose toxicity or glucose desensitization. The amount of insulin necessary to maintain a steady high blood glucose level (220 mg/dL)

IR, insulin resistance; AUS, the area under the curve; ISI, insulin sensitivity index

Table 2. Methods for Measuring Insulin Sensitivity

4.2. Relationships between sympathetic nervous activity and insulin resistance in obesity, hypertension, and type 2 diabetes

It is widely recognized that insulin resistance or hyperinsulinemia relates to obesity [Ferrannini, *et al.* 1991 & 1995; Ward, *et al.* 1996], but the precise relationships linking those factors remain controversial. Many epidemiological and clinical studies have shown a close relationship between sympathetic nervous system activity and insulin levels in obesity [Anderson, *et al.* 1991; Ward, *et al.* 1996; Masuo, *et al.* 2002]. Several studies of longitudinal design have examined the effect of body weight changes (weight loss or weight gain) on sympathetic nervous system activity and insulin sensitivity (fasting plasma insulin levels and HOMA-IR). Elevations of sympathetic nervous system activity and insulin levels during weight gain [Masuo, *et al.* 2000; Bernes, *et al.* 2003; Gentle, et al. 2007} and reductions of sympathetic nerve activity and insulin levels during weight loss [Masuo, *et al.* 2001; Andersson, *et al.* 1991; Straznicky, *et al,* 2010] have been observed. These longitudinal studies have shown that heightened sympathetic nerve activity and insulin resistance are closely linked to obesity (weight gain), the onset of obesity and the maintenance of obesity. In addition, a calorie restricted diet and exercise may have different mechanism on weight loss-induced blood pressure reduction. **Figure 2** shows changes in neurohormonal parameters over a 24-week period weight loss regimens with a mild calorie restricted diet alone, mild exercise alone, or a combination with a mild calorie restricted diet and mild exercise. This study showed that a calorie restricted diet contributed strongly to normalization/suppression of sympathetic activation, and exercise related to insulin resistance. In addition, calorie restricted diet and exercise may have different mechanisms on weight loss-induced blood pressure reduction [Masuo, et al. 2012a].

Reduced energy expenditure and resting metabolic rate are predictive of weight gain and obesity development. The sympathetic nervous system participates in regulating energy balance through thermogenesis **(Figure 1)**. Landsberg and other investigators hypothesized that energy intake stimulates hyperinsulinemia and sympathetic nerve activity resulting in blood pressure elevations in a cycle in order to inhibit thermogenesis. Insulin-mediated sympathetic nerve stimulation in obese subjects is therefore considered part of a compensatory mechanism aimed at restoring the energy balance by increasing the metabolic rate [Landsberg. 2001]. Hyperinsulinemia and insulin resistance in obese subjects are all part of a response to limit further weight gain via stimulating sympathetic nerve activity and thermogenesis [Landsberg, 2001].

On the other hand, Julius and Masuo generated a hypothesis based on data from their longitudinal studies that increased sympathetic nerve activity in skeletal muscle causes neurogenic vasoconstriction, thereby reducing blood flow to muscle and consequently inducing a state of insulin resistance by lowering glucose delivery and uptake in hypertension and obesity. Both blood pressure elevations and weight gain may reflect a primary increase in sympathetic nervous tone. Masuo *et al.* [Masuo, *et al.* 1997, 2000, and 2003] demonstrated that high plasma norepinephrine could predict future blood pressure elevations accompanying deterioration in insulin resistance. This was observed in HOMA-

IR (homeostasis model assessments of insulin resistance) in nonobese, normotensive subjects using longitudinal studies. Rocchini *et al.* [Rocchini, *et al.* 1990] reported that clonidine prevented insulin resistance development in obese dogs over a 6-week period, suggesting that sympathetic nervous activity might play a major role in the development of insulin resistance accompanying blood pressure elevation. The longitudinal studies [Straznicky, *et al.* 2005, 2009b & 2012. Masuo, *et al.* 2000, 2001b, 2003, 2005a, 2012] might provide strong evidence for a close linkage of high sympathetic nervous activity accompanying insulin resistance with the onset of hypertension. Heightened sympathetic nerve activity might play a major role in blood pressure elevations, and insulin resistance might play an ancillary mechanism for blood pressure elevation and genesis of hypertension. In hypertensive patients who already have heightened sympathetic nerve activity and insulin resistance, both heightened sympathetic nerve activity and insulin resistance are related to further blood pressure elevations.

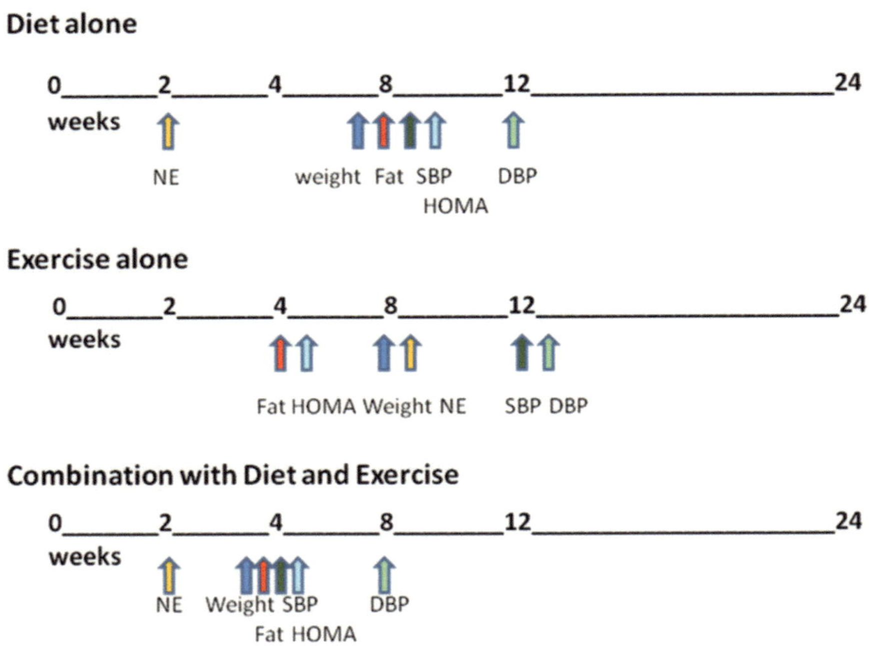

During weight loss with a mild calorie restricted diet, normalization of sympathetic activation measured by plasma norepinephrine was observed following significant weight loss and normalization of insulin resistance (HOMA-IR). On the other hand, in exercise alone group, normalization of insulin resistance was observed, and then weight loss and suppression of sympathetic activation. A low caloric diet and exercise may exert different effects on weight loss. NE, plasma norepinephrine levels; Fat, total body fat-mass; SBP, systolic blood pressure; DBP, diastolic blood pressure; HOMA, homeostasis model of assessment of insulin resistance. [Masuo, et al. 2012]

Figure 2. When significant changes were observed comparisons between a calorie restricted diet vs. mild exercise alone vs. combination with diet + exercise over 24 weeks

Very recently, Masuo *et al.* [Masuo, *et al.* 2012} showed the differences in mechanisms of weight loss-induced blood pressure reductions with neurohormonal parameters changes over 24 weeks with loss regimens **(Figure 2)**. A calorie restricted diet caused suppression/normalization of sympathetic activation measured with plasma norepinephrine levels followed by improvements of insulin resistance, whereas exercise improved insulin resistance followed by normalization of norepinephrine levels. BMI and blood pressure decreased after significant reductions in both plasma norepinephrine and HOMA-IR **(Figure 2)**. Their investigations may help to explain why discordant results have been observed. However, at least their hypotheses showed a strong linkage between sympathetic activation, insulin resistance, obesity and hypertension.

Valentine *et al.* [Valentine, *et al.* 2004] reported attenuation of hemodynamic and energy expenditure responses to isoproterenol infusion in hypertensive patients. Their findings that a generalized decrease of β-adrenergic responsiveness in hypertension supports the hypothesis that heightened sympathetic nerve activity through down-regulation of β-adrenoceptor-mediated thermogenesis, may facilitate the development of obesity in hypertension. Their results suggested that sympathetic nerve activity-induced hypertension may subsequently lead to the development of obesity.

Hoffmann *et al.* [Hoffmann, *et al.* 1999] investigated the effects of the acute induction of hyperglycemia on sympathetic nervous activity and vascular function in eight young normal control subjects. Muscle sympathetic nerve activity (MSNA) and forearm vascular resistance were measured before and during systemic infusion of 20% dextrose with low dose insulin with 60 min of hyperglycemia. Acute hyperglycemia caused sympathetic activation and peripheral vasodilation. Moreover, both acute and chronic hyperglycemia and hyperinsulinemia may enhance adrenergic vasoconstriction and decrease vasodilation in animal models (pithed rats) [Takatori, *et al.* 2006; Zamai, *et al.* 2008]. Insulin causes forearm vasoconstriction in obese, insulin resistant hypertensive humans [Gudbjornsdotti, *et al.* 1998]. On the other hand, van Veen *et al.* [van Veen, *et al.* 1999] found that hyperglycemia induced vasodilation in the forearm, but this vasodilation was not modified by hyperinsulinemia.

4.3. Sympathetic nervous activity and leptin in obesity and the metabolic syndrome

Interactions between the sympathetic nervous system and leptin are widely acknowledged with each being able to influence the other. Indeed, the leptin system mediates some of its action through the sympathetic nervous system [Haynes, et al. 1997; Kuo, et al. 2003]. Trayhurn *et al.* [Trayhurn, *et al.* 1995; Hardie, *et al.* 1996] investigated the effect of acute sympathetic nerve activation caused by exposure to cold on the expression of the leptin gene in white adipose tissue of lean mice, but not in obese mice. In addition, Masuo *et al.* reported the blunted linkage between the sympathetic nervous system and leptin in obese subjects [Masuo, *et al.* 2006; Kawaguchi, *et al.* 2006]. These studies, together with others, indicate that both insulin resistance and leptin may be regulated by the sympathetic nervous system.

Masuo *et al.* [Masuo, *et al.* 2008] showed during oral glucose loading that plasma insulin and plasma norepinephrine increased in both insulin-sensitive and insulin-resistant subjects, but plasma leptin levels decreased in insulin-sensitive nonobese subjects and increased in insulin- resistant nonobese subjects. Straznicky *et al.* [Straznicky, *et al.* 2005] also reported the blunted responses of whole-body norepinephrine spillover, insulin, and plasma leptin during oral glucose loading in obese subjects with insulin resistance as compared to insulin sensitive subjects. In subjects with the metabolic syndrome, weight loss with a low caloric diet diminished the whole-body and regional sympathetic nerve activity, as indicated by determinants of the whole-body norepinephrine spillover to plasma and muscle sympathetic nerve activity. Of interest, the decrease in norepinephrine spillover to plasma after weight loss was positively and independently associated with the decrease in plasma leptin, but not with insulin sensitivity in overweight insulin resistant subjects, while in overweight subjects without insulin resistance, the decrease in plasma norepinephrine after weight loss correlated with the improvement of insulin sensitivity.

4.4. Sympathetic nervous activity and insulin resistance in the metabolic syndrome

The metabolic syndrome is a cluster of abnormalities with basic characteristics being insulin resistance and visceral obesity. The criteria/definitions of metabolic syndrome are shown in **Table 1**. Importantly, obesity and the metabolic syndrome are associated with significant co-morbidities, such as type 2 diabetes, cardiovascular disease, stroke, and certain types of cancers.

Huggett *et a*l. [Huggett, *et al.* 2003 % 2004] demonstrated in a series of studies using microneurography (muscle sympathetic nerve activity, MSNA) that type 2 diabetic patients had elevated sympathetic nerve activity regardless of the prevailing level of blood pressure, and that the combination of hypertension and type 2 diabetes resulted in an augmentation in sympathetic nerve activity and levels of plasma insulin. They also compared MSNA and insulin levels in 23 non-diabetic offspring of type 2 diabetic patients and 23 normal control individuals [Huggett, *et al.* 2006]. In non-diabetic offspring of type 2 diabetic patients, the fasting plasma levels of insulin and MSNA were greater ($p<0.009$ and $p<0.003$) than control subjects. Sympathetic nerve activity was significantly correlated to insulin levels ($p<0.0002$) and resistance ($p<0.0001$) in offspring of type 2 diabetic patients, but not in control subjects. Sympathetic activation occurred in not only subjects with the metabolic syndrome, diabetic patients, but also in normotensive non-diabetic offspring of patients with type 2 diabetes with the degree of activation being in proportion to their plasma insulin levels. This series of studies indicates the presence of a mechanistic link between hyperinsulinemia and sympathetic activation, both of which could play a role in the subsequent development of cardiovascular risk factors.

5. Cardiovascular and renal complications in obesity, obesity-related hypertension and diabetes

It has been documented that patients with obesity, hypertension and type 2 diabetes frequently have cardiovascular and renal complications. Obesity was closely associated with an increase in blood pressure, left ventricular mass, and with early signs of disturbed left ventricular diastolic function [Wikstrand, *et al.* 1993], and changes in left ventricular morphology and diastolic function [Alpert, *et al.* 2012]. It is well known that sudden cardiac death is the most common cause of death in dialysis patients and is usually preceded by sudden cardiac arrest due to ventricular tachycardia or ventricular fibrillation [Alpert, *et al.* 2011]. Left ventricular (LV) mass and loading conditions that may affect LV mass are important determinants of corrected QT intervals (QTc) in normotensive severely obese subjects [Mukergi, *et al.* 2011]. The RICARHD study (Cardiovascular risk in patients with arterial hypertension and type 2 diabetes study), was a multicenter and cross-sectional study, conducted in Spain and included 2,339 patients who were 55 years or more with hypertension and type 2 diabetes of greater than 6 months duration. Left ventricular hypertrophy (LVH) or renal damage (GFR<60 ml/min/1.73 m2 and/or albumin/creatinine ratio ≥0 mg/g or an urinary albumin excretion ≥30 mg/24 hours) were compared between these hypertensive and type 2 diabetes patients and healthy controls. The combined presence of both hypertension and type 2 diabetes were associated with an increased prevalence of established cardiovascular diseases. Similarly, the presence of both cardiac and renal damage was associated to the higher prevalence of cardiovascular diseases [Cea-Calvo, *et al.* 2006].

The Lifestyle Interventions and Independence for Elders (LIFE) study in 8,029 patients with stage II-III hypertension with LVH on ECG showed high prevalence of co-existence of LVH and albuminuria [Wachtell, *et al.* 2002]. In patients with moderately severe hypertension, LVH on two consecutive ECGs is associated with increased prevalence of micro- and macro-albuminuria compared to patients without persistent LVH on ECG. High albumin excretion was related to LVH independent of age, blood pressure, diabetes, race, serum creatinine or smoking, suggesting parallel cardiac damage and albuminuria.

5.1. Hyperglycemia and insulin resistance as risk factors of cardiovascular complications in type 2 diabetes

Hyperglycemia and hyperinsulinemia or insulin resistance that is a characteristic of type 2 diabetes and obesity play major roles in the cardiovascular complications of type 2 diabetes mellitus and obesity. Hyperglycemia is the major risk factor for microvascular complications (retinopathy, neuropathy, and nephropathy) in type 2 diabetes, however 70% or 80% of patients with type 2 diabetes die of macrovascular disease. Atherogenic dyslipidemia (elevated triglyceride levels, low HDL-cholesterol levels, high LDL-cholesterol levels) is the major cause of atherosclerosis in patients with type 2 diabetes [Reasner, *et al.* 2008].

Several investigators have demonstrated that insulin resistance could predict future type 2 diabetes even in nonobese individuals [Morrison, *et al.* 2008], and even in children [Koska, *et al.* 2007; Morrison, *et al.* 2008] Insulin resistance accompanying sympathetic nerve activation may also predict future hypertension development [Masuo, *et al.* 1997, 1998, 2003, & 2005]. Insulin resistance coexisting with inflammation may predict cardiac disease but, interestingly, not stroke in the Japanese diabetic population [Matsumoto, *et al.* 2006].

Hyperglycemia (*i.e.* elevated plasma glucose levels) can also predict hospitalization for congestive heart failure in patients at high cardiovascular risk [Held, *et al.* 2007]. Hyperglycemia and insulin resistance are risk factors of cardiovascular complications.

5.2. Sympathetic nervous activity as a risk factor for cardiovascular complications and renal complications

Heightened sympathetic nerve activity plays an important role in cardiovascular complications and cardiac risk in humans [Esler, *et al.* 2000]. There is consistent evidence that high plasma norepinephrine level, as an index of heightened sympathetic nerve activity, predicts mortality in cardiovascular diseases such as chronic congestive heart failure [Cohn *et al.* 1984; Brum, *et al.* 2006], left ventricular dysfunction [Grassi, *et al.* 2009], remodelling [Abel, et al. 2010], structural changes in obesity {Benedict, 1996}, and end-stage renal disease (ESRD) [Masuo, *et al.* 2007; Grassi, *et al.* 2012; Benedict, *et al.* 1996; Ksiazck, *et al.* 2008]. Renal injury also predicts the development of cardiovascular disease [Masuo, *et al.* 2007; Joles, *et al.* 2009].

Hogarth *et al.* [Hogarth, *et al.* 2001] reported that acute myocardial infarction (AMI) in hypertensive patients resulted in greater sympathetic nervous activity, persisting for at least 6 months longer than in normotensive subjects, indicating that AMI further augmented the sympathetic nerve hyperactivity of hypertension. Sympathetic nerve hyperactivity could be one mechanism involved in the reported worse prognosis in AMI in hypertensive patients [Hogarth, *et al.* 2001]. The sympathetic activation that follows AMI has been associated with increased morbidity and mortality in both anterior-AMI and inferior-AMI, with a similar magnitude of sympathetic nerve hyperactivity [Graham, et al. 2004]. Patients with congenital long-QT syndrome are susceptible to life-threatening arrhythmias, and the sympathetic nervous system may have an important triggering role for cardiovascular events this condition [Shamsuzzaman, *et al.* 2001].

Changes in heart rates during exercise and recovery from exercise are mediated by the balance between sympathetic and vagal activity, and changes in heart rates were evaluated in a total of 5,713 asymptomatic working men cohort (between the ages of 42 and 53 years) in whom there was no evidence of the presence or history of cardiac disease over the preceding 23 years. Baseline heart rates, changes in heart rates during exercise and recovery were strongly related to an increased risk of sudden death from myocardial infarction [Jeuven, *et al.* 2005].

Zoccali *et al.* [Zoccali, *et al.* 2002 & 2004] examined the relationships between sympathetic nerve activity (plasma norepinephrine levels) and mortality and cardiovascular events in 228 patients undergoing chronic hemodialysis originally without heart failure. They found 45% of dialysis subjects had significantly high plasma norepinephrine levels located in the upper limit of the normal range. One-hundred and twenty four (124) fatal and nonfatal cardiovascular events occurred in 85 patients during the follow-up period (34±15 months). Plasma norepinephrine levels proved to be an independent predictor of fatal and nonfatal cardiovascular events in a multivariate Cox regression model. Recently, Joles *et al.* reported that sympathetic nerve stimulation contributes to the progression of renal disease [Joles, *et al.* 2004]. Masuo *et al.* reported that plasma norepinephrine levels predicted future renal injury in normotensive healthy subjects over a 5-year follow up study in a Japanese cohort [Masuo, *et al.* 2007]. They also found that plasma norepinephrine levels were associated with concentric left ventricular hypertrophy in these patients [Zoccali, *et al.* 2002 a & 2002b].

Petersson *et al.* [Petersson, *et al.* 2002] showed that increased cardiac sympathetic nervous activity in renovascular hypertension might lead to high cardiovascular mortality and morbidity. Prolonged sympathetic nerve stimulation and elevated circulating norepinephrine levels can induce changes in intra-renal blood vessels. Catecholamines can induce proliferation of smooth muscle cells and adventitial fibroblasts in vascular wall.

The association between hypertension, obesity and chronic kidney disease (CKD) is well recognized [White, *et al.* 2005; Hall, *et al.* 2001; Zoccali, *et al.* 2002]. Obesity and hypertension also leads to an increase in the incidence of metabolic diseases such a type 2 diabetes mellitus, which is frequently associated with renal injury (proteinuria/microalbuminuria). In the majority of cases, ESRD occurs as a result of complication of diabetes or hypertension [WHO. 1995]. Obesity, hypertension and type 2 diabetes are characterized as stimulated sympathetic nervous activity and insulin resistance states, indicating renal injury and ESRD are strongly related to sympathetic nervous activity and insulin resistance. Masuo *et al.* reported that significant weight loss resulted in significant amelioration on renal function following suppression on sympathetic activation and hyperinsulinemia (insulin resistance) [Masuo, *et al.* 2012]. The findings suggest that strong linkage between sympathetic nervous activity, insulin resistance and renal function.

Joles *et al.* reported that sympathetic nerve stimulation contributes to the progression of renal disease [Joles, *et al.* 2004]. The 40-minute infusion of NE into the renal artery of dogs produced a reversible ischemic model of acute renal failure [Bulger, et al. 1982]. Another study demonstrated renal protection by β-adrenergic receptor blockade in a nephrectomized rat experiment without any BP changes [Amam, *et al.* 2001]. There is consistent evidence that high plasma norepinephrine levels, as an index of heightened sympathetic nervous activity, predicts mortality in cardiovascular disease, such as chronic congestive heart failure [Cohn, et al. 1984; Brum, et al. 2006], left ventricular dysfunction [Benedict, *et al.* 1996] and end-stage renal disease (ESRD) [Masuo, *et al.* 2007; Ksiazek, *et al.* 2008]. Renal injury also predicts the development of cardiovascular disease [Joles, *et al.* 2004; Masuo, *et al.* 2007].

These investigations have shown strong associations between sympathetic nervous activation, cardiovascular complications and renal complications. Given these observations it may be of importance to aim antihypertensive treatments or anti-diabetic treatment not only at the reduction of raised blood pressure or blood glucose but also at the excessive sympathetic activation and insulin resistance that may underpin these effects.

5.3. Sympathetic nerve hyperactivity in patients with ESRD

Evidence now strongly indicates a role for the sympathetic nervous system in the pathogenesis of hypertension in renal failure (ESRD) [Hausberg, et al. 2002; Schlaich, et al. 2009; Masuo, *et al.* 2010a]. Hypertension occurs commonly and early in renal disease and is paralleled by increases in sympathetic nerve activity, as indicated by increased muscle sympathetic nerve activity and circulating norepinephrine. This appears to be driven by the diseased kidneys, because nephrectomy or denervation has been shown to correct blood pressure and sympathetic nerve activity both in human and animal studies [Jacob, *et al.* 2003].

Masuo *et al.* [Masuo, *et al.* 1995 & 2010] showed that plasma norepinephrine levels were significantly higher in patients with ESRD regardless of hemodialysis compared with those in blood pressure- and body mass index-matched hypertensive patients or healthy normotensive subjects **(Figure 3)**. Further, this was recognized significantly in subjects with a shorter duration of ESRD with hemodialysis compared with those with longer duration, suggesting that sympathetic nerve hyperactivity may be of particular importance in the onset or the early development of ESRD or, alternatively, be influenced by long-term renal replacement therapy (hemodialysis). In the normal state, interactions between the kidney and sympathetic nervous system serve to maintain blood pressure and glomerular filtration rate within tightly controlled levels, but in renal failure, a defect in renal sodium excretory function leads to an abnormal pressure natriuresis relationship and activation of the renin-angiotensin system (RAS), contributing to the development of hypertension and progression of kidney disease [Hall, *et al.* 1997; Lohmeier, *et al.* 2001]. Another mechanism could involve the sympathetic nervous modulation of baroreflex regulation and vasculature tone through the central nervous system and angiotensin II [Burke, *et al.* 2008]. Afferent signals from the kidney, detected by chemoreceptors and mechanoreceptors, feed directly into central nuclei regulating sympathetic nerve activity by circulating and brain-derived angiotensin II [Philips, *et al.* 2005]. Therefore, the pathogenesis of hypertension in renal failure (ESRD) is complex and arises most likely from the interaction of hemodynamic and neuroendocrine factors. Sympathetic nerve activity has strong relationships with regards to increased risk of cardiovascular disease including hypertension [Zoccali, *et al.* 2002a & 2002b] in patients with ESRD and the mortality and morbidity of cardiovascular disease, suggesting that we have to pay much attention to sympathetic nerve activation in our attempts to adequately treat patients with ESRD.

Sympathetic nerve activity is consistently elevated in patients with ESRD, and in obese subjects and hypertensive patients in cross-sectional studies [Masuo, et al. 1995, 2011a & 2011b). The sympathetic nerve hyperactivity is at least in part independent of increased blood pressure levels or obesity. Further, patients with early-ESRD without hemodialysis had already significantly higher plasma norepinephrine levels compared with hypertensive subjects as well as normotensive subjects. Therefore, sympathetic nervous activation in ESRD patients may be independent from obesity or hypertension.

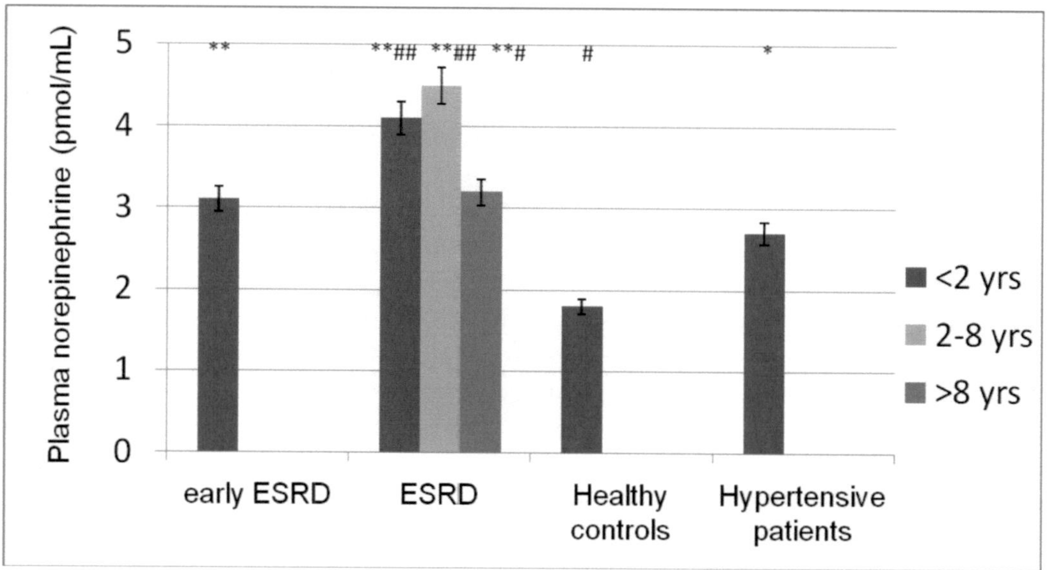

ESRD, end-stage renal disease; *P<0.05 versus healthy controls; **P<0.01 versus healthy controls; #P<0.05 versus hypertensive patients with normal renal function; ##P<0.01 versus hypertensive patients with normal renal function. [Masuo, *et al.* 2010a]

Figure 3. Figure 3. Comparisons of plasma norepinephrine levels between patients with patients with ESRD, hypertensive patients with normal renal function and normal healthy controls.

The amount of norepinephrine in plasma is only a fraction of the amount released into the synaptic cleft, and plasma norepinephrine levels are affected by dialysis therapy, so it is difficult to discount that the elevated plasma norepinephrine levels did not derive in part from reduced plasma norepinephrine clearance rather than solely from elevated sympathetic nerve activity. Grassi *et al.* [Grassi, *et al.* 2009] however, reported similar results using microneurography. In addition, plasma norepinephrine levels did not change between before- and after-hemodialysis therapy (data was not shown), and between after-hemodialysis therapy and before-next hemodialysis therapy. Thus, one could speculate that plasma norepinephrine levels in ESRD patients are reflective of the degree of sympathetic nerve activity.

5.4. β2-adrenoceptor polymorphisms accompanying sympathetic nervous activation may relate to renal injury

Rao *et al.* [Rao, *et al.* 2007] and Masuo *et al.* [Masuo, *et al.* 2007] have shown strong associations between β2-adrenoceptor polymorphisms, elevated plasma norepinephrine levels and elevated HOMA-IR (insulin resistance) or future renal injury, suggesting that stimulated sympathetic nerve activity associated with insulin resistance, may independently play a major role in the onset and development of ESRD without obesity or hypertension. However, the precise mechanisms underlying sympathetic activation in CKD and ESRD have not been clarified.

Furthermore, Masuo *et al.* [Masuo, *et al.* 2011b] measured renal function (creatinine, BUN and creatinine clearance), plasma norepinephrine levels and HOMA-IR (insulin sensitivity) annually over a 5-year period in nonobese, normotensive men with normal renal function. Subjects who had a significant deterioration of renal function (more than 10% increases from baseline of creatinine and BUN or decrease in creatinine clearance) over a 5-year period had higher plasma norepinephrine at the entry period, and greater increases in plasma norepinephrine over 5 years [Masuo, *et al.* 2011b]. In this study, subjects who had significant changes in body weight or blood pressure were excluded, indicating the contributions of obesity or hypertension might be excluded. Further, subjects who had significantly higher levels of plasma norepinephrine had a higher frequency of the Gly16 allele of the β2-adrenoceptor polymorphism [Masuo, *et al.* 2007] (**Figure 4**). The Gly16 allele of the β2-adrenoceptor polymorphism has been shown to be related to obesity [Masuo, *et al.* 2005, 2005a, 2005b], hypertension [Masuo, *et al.* 2005a, 2005b, 2010b, 2011c] and metabolic syndrome development [Masuo, *et al.* 2005b]. Thus, high plasma norepinephrine levels appear to be a predictor that is determined genetically by the β2-adrenoceptor polymorphism (Arg16Gly) for renal injury, obesity, hypertension and metabolic syndrome.

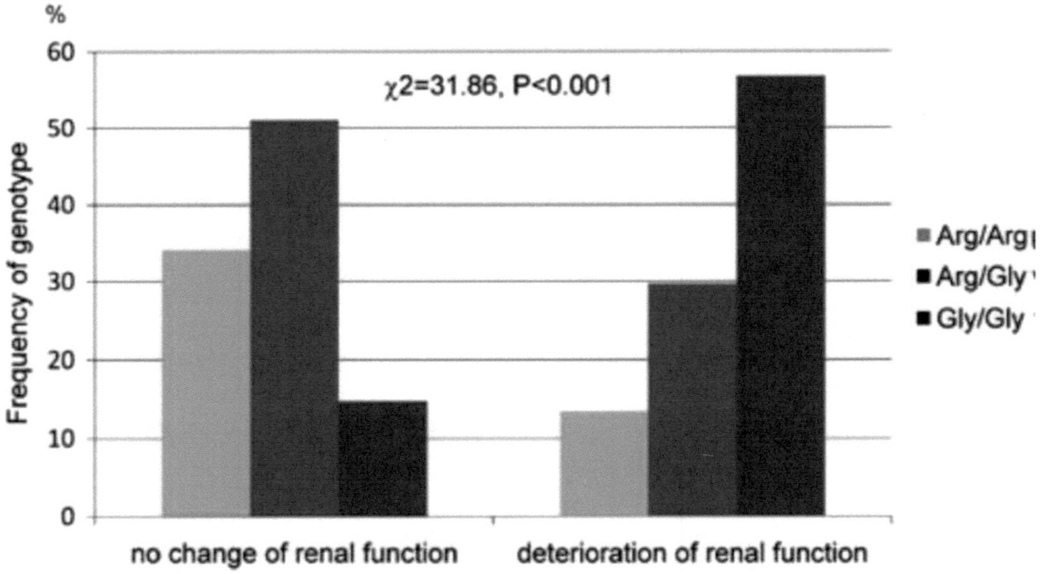

In 154 nonobese, normotensive subjects, renal function (creatinine clearance) was measured over a 5-year period. The deterioration of renal function was defined as >10% decreases in creatinine clearance over a 5-year period. Subjects with deterioration of renal function had higher frequency of Gly allele or Gly homozygous compared to those without changes in renal function. [Masuo, *et al.* 2011b]

Figure 4. Subjects with deteriorations of renal function (creatinine clearance) carried higher frequency of the Gly16 allele of Arg16Gly, the β2-adrenoceptor polymorphisms

These observations show that plasma norepinephrine levels associated with insulin resistance are strongly linked with the onset and development of renal injury.

6. Other medical conditions in obesity

6.1. Obstructive sleep apnea in obesity is a risk factor for cardiovascular diseases

Vozoris [Vozoris. 2012] investigated the relationships between prevalence of obstructive sleep apnea (OSA), obesity, and hypertension, diabetes, congestive heart failure, myocardial infarction, and stroke using a population-based multi-year cross-sectional study design including 12,593 individuals with data from the 2005-2008 United States National Health and Nutrition Examination Surveys (NHANES). They found individuals with OSA had elevated rates of cardiovascular diseases compared to the general population [Vozoris. 2012]. OSA is a common disorder that has been associated with many cardiovascular disease processes, including hypertension and arrhythmias. OSA has also been identified as an independent risk factor for stroke and all-cause mortality. OSA is highly prevalent in patients with transient ischemic attacks and stroke [Das, *et al.* 2012]. Indeed, the majority of patients with OSA suffer from hypertension [Ziegler, *et al.* 2011]. The mechanisms underlying the link between OSA and cardiovascular disease are not completely established. However, there is increasing evidence that autonomic mechanisms are implicated. A number of studies have consistently shown that patients with OSA have high levels of sympathetic nerve traffic [Narkiewicz, *et al.* 2003]. In animal studies, intermittent hypoxia that simulates changes seen in OSA leads to chemoreceptor and chromaffin cell stimulation of sympathetic nerve activity, endothelial damage and impaired blood pressure modulation. Human studies reveal activation of sympathetic nerves, endothelial damage and exaggerated pressor responses to sympathetic neurotransmitters and endothelin [Ziegler, *et al.* 2011]. OSA is also frequently observed in obese individuals [Dos, *et al.* 201].2

6.2. Gout and hyperuricacidemia in obesity

Gout is a growing worldwide health problem, and is associated with increased prevalence of obesity. Gout and hyperuricacidemia are associated with the metabolic syndrome, diabetes mellitus, obesity and hypertension. Masuo *et al.* observed the importance of serum uric acid levels as a predictor for future obesity and hypertension [Masuo, et al. 2003]. Several epidemiological studies have shown the close linkage between hyperuricemia, obesity and hypertension [Robinson, *et al.* 2012]. Recently Robinson, *et al.* [Robinson, *et al.* 2012] reviewed prevalence of hyperuricemia in Australia in 25 articles and 5 reports using a systematic journal search method. From 1968 to 1995/6, the prevalence of gout increased from 0.5% to 1.7% of the population. Especially in the Australian indigenous population a significant rise in the prevalence of gout from 0% in 1965 to 9.7% in 2002 in males, and 0% to 2.9% in females were observed. Those elevations were strongly synchronized with the prevalence of obesity [Chang, *et al.* 2001]. Similar result has been reported in Taiwanese populations that, using a multivariate analysis, showed that BMI (obesity) was an important factor associated with hyperuricemia in both males and females, whereas age was associated with hyperuricemia only in males. In addition, the associations of basic and repeated measures of uric acid level with treatments for uric acid over a 11-year period, and risk of coronary heart disease (CHD) and stroke events were assessed in Taiwanese populations

[Chien, *et al.* 2005]. The study showed that uric acid had significant risk only in hypertension and metabolic syndrome subgroups, but not in their counterparts. They also observed that uric acid, in the baseline and time-dependent variables, could predict cardiovascular events in the community of relatively low CHD but high stroke risk.

Straznicky *et al.* examined the effects of weight loss on serum uric acid levels, and showed that it had ameliorative effects on uric acid levels in the obese subjects with the metabolic syndrome [Straznicky, *et al.* 2011]. Furthermore, they compared these effects between a mild calorie restricted diet alone, combination with a low calorie diet and exercise and control groups. Interestingly, moderate weight loss in obese patients with metabolic syndrome is associated with a reduction in serum uric acid levels, albuminuria and an improvement in eGFR which is augmented by exercise co-intervention [Straznicky, *et al.* 2011]. Improvement of insulin resistance and sympathetic activation were synchronized with a reduction in serum uric acid levels.

7. Conclusion

The role of the sympathetic nervous activity and insulin resistance plays important roles in the etiology of obesity, hypertension, and type 2 diabetes. Several investigations have demonstrated that the sympathetic nervous activation and insulin resistance are strongly related to cardiovascular complication (*i.e.* LVH, congestive heart failure) and the onset and development of ESRD (renal injury). Interestingly, relevant investigations of sympathetic nervous activity and β2-adrenoceptor polymorphisms indicate their contribution to the onset and maintenance of renal injury and LVH in healthy subjects and in patients with chronic renal failure and cardiovascular events in ESRD patients. Interestingly, the prevalence of OSA and hyperuricemia (gout) are significantly linked with increases in obesity, and both states are connected with the cardiovascular risks associated with sympathetic nervous activation. Serum uric acid, which may be affected strongly by sympathetic nervous activity, may be a predictor for future hypertension and renal injury (ESRD) development.

Recently, it has been demonstrated that renal sympathetic nerve denervation provides promising results in patients with refractory hypertension [Krum, *et al.* 2009; Symplicity HTN-1 Investigators. 2011]. Besides the demonstrable effect on reducing blood pressure, renal denervation significantly and favourably influences LV mass and improves diastolic function, which might have important prognostic implications in patients with resistant hypertension at high cardiovascular risk [Brandt, *et al.* 2012]. Further, renal denervations showed an accompanying improvements in insulin resistance [Mahfoud, *et al.* 2011,: Witkowski, *et al.* 2012] and OSA [Brandt, *et al.* 2011]. Renal sympathetic denervation may conceivably be a potentially useful option for patients with co-morbid refractory hypertension, glucose intolerance, and obstructive sleep apnea.

A better understanding of the relationships between sympathetic nervous activity, insulin resistance, cardiovascular complications, and renal complications, will help to develop appropriate treatment strategies targeting renal injury or cardiac risk in hypertensive and diabetes patients with and without ESRD or LVH.

Author details

Kazuko Masuo*
Human Neurotransmitters Laboratory, Australia
Nucleus Network Ltd., Baker ID Heart & Diabetes Institute, Australia

Gavin W. Lambert
Human Neurotransmitters Laboratory, Australia
Faculty of Medicine, Nursing and Health Science, Monash University, Melbourne, Australia

8. References

Abel AD, Litwin SE, Sweeney G. (2010) Cardiac remodelling in obesity. Physiol Rev. Vol 88, No. 2, p389-419.

Alberi KG, Zimmet PZ, (1998) Definition, diagnosis and classification of diabetes mellitus and its complications. Part 1: diagnosis and classification of diabetes mellitus provisional report of a WHO consultation. Diabet Med. Vol. 15, No. 7, p539-553.

Alpert MA, Chan EJ. (2012) Left ventricular morphology and diastolic function in severe obesity: current views. Rev. Esp Cardiol. Vol. 65, No. 1, p1-3.

Alpert MA. (2011) Sudden cardiac arrest and sudden cardiac death on dialysis: Epidemiology, evaluation, treatment, and prevention. Hemodial Int. Vol. 15, No. Suppl 1, pS22-S29.

Amann K, Koch A, Hofstetter J, Gross ML., et al. (2001). Glomerulosclerosis and progression: Effect of sub-antihypertensive doses of alpha and beta blockers. Kidney Int. Vol. 60, No. 4, p309-323.

Anderson EA, Hoffman RP, Balon TW, Sinkey CA, Mark AL. (1991) Hyperinsulinemia produces both sympathetic neural activation and vasodilation in normal humans. J Clin Invest. Vol. 87, No. 6, p2246-2252.

Andersson B, Elam M, Wallin BG, Bjorntorp P, Andersson OK. (1991) Effect of energy-restricted diet on sympathetic muscle nerve activity in obese women. Hypertension. Vol. 18, No. 6, p783-789.

Athyros VG, Eisaf MS, Alexandrides T, Achimastos AM, et al. (2011) Long-term impact of multifactorial treatment on new-onset diabetes and related cardiovascular events in metabolic syndrome: A Post Hoc ATTEMPT analysis. Angiology. 2011 Oct 17 [Epub ahead of print].

Barnes MJ, Lapanowski K, Conley A, Rafols JA, Jen KL, Dunbar JC. (2003) High fat feeding is associated with increased blood pressure, sympathetic nerve activity and hypothalamic mu opiod receptors. Brain Res Bull. Vol. 61, No. 5, P511-516.

* Corresponding Author

Benedict CR, Shelton B, Johnstone DR, Francis G, et al. (1996) Prognostic significance of plasma norepinephrine in patients with asymptomatic left ventricular dysfunction. Circulation. Vol. 94, No. 4, p690-697.

Brandt MC, Mahfoud F, Reda S, Schimer SH, et al. (2012) Renal sympathetic denervation reduces left ventricular hypertrophy and improves cardiac function in patients with resistant hypertension. J Am Coll Cardiol. Vol. 59, No. 110, p901-909.

Brum PC, Rolim NP, Bacurau AV, Medeiros A. (2006) Neurohormonal activation in heart failure: the role of adrenergic receptors. An Acad Bras Cienc. Vol. 78, NO. 3, p485-503.

Bulger RE, Burjke TJ, Cronin RE, Schrier RW, Dabyan DC. (1986) Morphology of norepinephrine-induced acute renal failure in the dog. Anat Rev. Vol. 214, No. 4, p341-347.

Burke SL, Evans RG, Moretti JL, Head GA. (2008) Levels of renal and extra-renal sympathetic drive in angiotensin II-induced hypertension. Hypertension. Vol 51, No. 4, p878-883.

Burm PC, Rolim NP, Bacurau AV, Medeiros A. (2006) Neurohormonal activation in heart failure: the role of adrenergic receptors. An Acad Bras Cienc. Vol. 78, No. 3, p485-503.

Cea-Calvo L, Conthe P, Gomez-Fernandez P, de Alvaro F, Fernandez-Perez C. RICHARHD investigators. (2006) Target organ damage and cardiovascular complications in patients with hypertension and type 2 diabetes in Spain: a cross-sectional study. Cardiovasc Diabetol. Vol. 3, No. 5, p23.

Chang HY, Pan WH, Yeh WT, Tsai KS. (2001) Hyperuricemia and gout in Taiwan: results from the nutritional and health survey in Taiwan (1993-96). J Rheumatol. Vol. 28, No. 7, 1640-1646.

Chien KL, Hsu HC, Sung FC, Su TC, Chen MF, Lee YT. (2005) Hyperuricemia as a risk factor on cardiovascular events in Taiwan: The Chin-Shan community cardiovascular cohort study. Atherosclerosis. Vol. 183, No. 1, p147-155,

Cohn JN, Levine TB, Olivari MT, Garberg V, et al. (1984) Plasma norepinephrine and a guide to prognosis in patients with chronic congestion heart failure. N Engl J Med. Vol. 31, No 13, p819-823.

Cohn JN, Rolim NP, Bacurau AV, et al. (2006) Plasma norepinephrine as a guide to prognosis in patients with chronic congestive heart failure. N Engl J Med. Vol. 31, No. 13, p819-823.

Das AM, Khan M. (2012) Obstructive sleep apnea and stroke. Expert Rev Cardiovasc Ther. Vol. 10, No. 4, p525-535.

de Silva A, do Carmo J, Dubinion J, Hall JE. Role of sympathetic nervous system in obesity related hypertension. (2009) Curr Hypertens Rep. vol. 11, No. 3, p206-215. .

Esler M, Kaye D. (2000) Sympathetic nervous system activation in essential hypertension, cardiac failure and psychosomatic heart failure disease. J Cardiovasc Pharmacol. Vol. 15, No. 7 (Supple 4), p51-57.

Esler M, Straznicky N, Eikelis N, Masuo K, Lambert G, Lambert E. (2006) Mechanism of sympathetic activation in obesity-related hypertension. Hypertension. Vol. 48, No. 5, P787-796.

Ferrannini E, Haffner SM, Mitchell BD, Stern MD. (1991) Hyperinsulinemia: the key feature of a cardiovascular and metabolic syndrome. Diabetologia. Vol. 34, No. 6, p416-423.

Ferrannini E, Mari A. (1998) How to measure insulin sensitivity. J Hypertens. Vol. 16, No. 7, p895-901.

Ferrannini E. (1995) Physiologic and metabolic consequence of obesity. Metabolism. Vol. 44, No. 9 Suppl 3, p15-17.

Flegal KM, Carroll MD, Kit BK, Ogden CL. (2012) Prevalence of obesity and trends in the distribution of body mass index among US adults, 1999-2010. JAMA. Vol. 307, No. 5, p491-497.

Ford ES, Williamson DF, Liu S. (1997) Weight change and diabetes incidence: finding from a national cohort of US adults. Am J Epidemiol. Vol. 146, No. 3, p214-222.

Gentile CL, Orr JS, Davy BM, Davy KP. (2007) Modest weight gain is associated with sympathetic neural activation in nonobese humans. Am J Physiol Regul Interg Comp Physiol. Vol. 292, No. 5, pR1834-R1838.

Graham LN, Smith PA, Huggett RJ, Stokeer JB, Mackintosh AF, Mary DA. (2004) Sympathetic drive in anterior and inferior uncomplicated acute myocardial infarction. Circulation. Vol. 109, No. 7, p2285-2289.

Grassi G, Seravalle G, Colombo M, Bolla G, et al. (1998) Body weight reduction, sympathetic nerve traffic, and arterial baroreflex in obese normotensive humans. Circulation. Vol. 97, No. 26, p2037-2042.

Grassi G, Seravalle G, Arenare F, Buccianti G, et al. (2009a) Behaviour of regional adrenergic outflows in mild-to-moderate renal failure. J Hypertens. Vol. 27, No. 3, p562-566.

Grassi G, Seravalle G, Quarti-Trevano F, Dell'Oro R, et al. (2009b) Sympathetic and baroreflex cardiovascular control in hypertension-related left ventricular dysfunction. Hypertension. Vol. 53, No. 2, p205-209.

Grassi G, Bertoli S, Seravalle G. (2012) Sympathetic nervous system: role in hypertension and in chronic kidney disease. (2012) Curr Opin Nephrrol Hypertens. Vol. 21, No. 1, p46-51.

Grundy SM, Brewer HB Jr., Cleeman JL, Smith SC Jr., Lenfant C. (2004). The American Heart Association, National Heart Lung and Blood Institute/American Heart Association Conference on scientific issue related to definition. Circulation. Vol. 109, No. 3, p433-438.

Gudbjornsdottir S, Elanm M, Sellgren J, Anderson EA. (1996) Insulin increases forearm vascular resistance in obese, insulin-resistant hypertensives. J Hypertens. Vol. 14, No. 1, p91-97.

Hall JE, Jones DW, Kuo JJ, de Silva A, Tallam LS, Liu J. (2005) Impact of the obesity epidemic on hypertension and renal disease. Curr Hypertens Rep. Vol. 5, No. 5, p386-392.

Hall JE. (1997) Mechanisms of abnormal renal sodium handling in obesity hypertension. Am J Hypertens. Vol. 10, No. 5 (Pt 2), p495-555.
Hall JE. (2003) The kidney, hypertension, and obesity. Hypertension. Vol. 41, No. 3 (Part 2), p625-633.
Hardie LJ, Rayner DV, Holmes S, Tryhurn P. (1996) Circulating leptin levels are modulated by fasting, cold exposure and insulin administration in lean but not Zuker (fa/fa) rats measured by ELISA. Biochemi Biophy Res Commun. Vol. 25, No. 223 (3), p660-665.
Hausberg M, Kosch M, Hamelink P, Barenbrock M, et al. (2002) Sympathetic nerve activity in end-stage renal disease. Circulation. Vol. 106, No. 15, p1974-1979.
Haynes WG, Morgan DA, Walsh SA, Mark AL, Sivitz WI. (1997) Receptor-mediated regional sympathetic nerve activation by leptin. J Clin Invest. Vol. 15, No. 100 (2), p270-279.
Hedley AA, Ogden CT, Johnson CL, Carroll MD, Curtin LR, Flegal KM. (2004) Prevalence of overweight and obesity among US Children, adolescents, and adults. 1999-2002. JAPA. Vol. 291, No. 23, p2847-2850.
Held C, Cerstein HC, Yusuf S, Zhao F, et al. the ONTARGET/TRANSCEND investigators. (2007) Glucose levels predict hospitalization for congestive heart failure in patients at high cardiovascular risk. Circulation. Vol. 115, No. 11, p1371-1375.
Hoffman RP, Hausberg M, Sinkey CA, Anderson EA. (1999) Hyperglycemia without hyperinsulinemia produces both sympathetic neural activation and vasodilation in normal humans. J Diabetes Complications. Vol. 13, No. 1, p17-22.
Hogarth AJ, Mackintosh AF, Mary DA. (2006) The sympathetic drive after acute myocardial infarction in hypertensive patients. Am J Hypertens. Vol. 19, No. 10, p1070-1076.
Huggett RJ, Scott EM, Gilbey SG, Stoker JB, Mackintosh AF, Mary DA. (2003) Impact of type 2 diabetes mellitus on sympathetic neural mechanisms in hypertension. Circulation. Vol. 108, No. 15, p3097-3101.
Huggett RJ, Burns J, Mackintosh AF, Mary DA. (2004) Sympathetic neural activation in nondiabetic metabolic syndrome and its further augmentation by hypertension. Hypertension. Vol. 44, No. 6, p847-852.
Huggett RJ, Hogarth AJ, Mackintosh AF, Mary DA. (2006) Sympathetic nerve hyperactivity in non-diabetic offspring of patients with type 2 diabetes mellitus. Diabetologia. Vol.49. No 11. p2741-2744.
Ikarashi T, Hanyu O, Maruyama S, Souda S, et al. (2004). Genotype Gly/Gly of the Arg16Gly polymorphism of the beta2-adrenergic receptor is associated with elevated fasting serum insulin concentrations, but not with acute insulin response to glucose in type 2 diabetc patients. Diabetes Res Clin Pract. Vol. 63, No. 1, p11-18.
Jacob F, Ariza P, Osborn JW. (2003) Renal denervation chronically lower arterial pressure independent of dietary sodium intake in normal rats. Am J Physiol Heart Circ Physiol. Vol. 284, No. 8, H2302-H2310.
Joles JA, Koomans HA. (2004) Causes and consequence of increased sympathetic activity in renal disease. Hypertension. Vol 43, No. 5, p469-706.

Jouven X, Empana JP, Schwartz PJ, Desnos M, Courbon D, Ducimetiere P. (2005) Heart-rate profile during exercise as a predictor of sudden death. N Engl J Med. Vol. 352, No. 19, p1951-1958.

Kawaguchi H, Masuo K, Katsuya T, Sugimoto K, et al. (2006) Beta2- and beta3-adrenoceptor polymorphisms relate to subsequent weight gain and blood pressure elevation in obese, normotensive individuals. Hypertens Res. Vol. 29, No. 12, p951-959.

Koska J, Ortega E, Bogardus C, Krakoff J, Bunt JC. (2007) The effect of insulin on net lipid oxidation predicts worsen of insulin resistance and development of type 2 diabetes. Am J Physiol Endocrinol Metab. Vol. 293, No. 1, pE264-E269.

Krum H, Schlaich M, Whitboum R, Sobotka PA, et al. (2009) Catheter-based renal sympathetic denervation for resistant hypertension: a multicentre safety and proof-of-principle cohort study. Lancet. Vol. 373, No. 9671, p1275-1281.

Ksiazek A, Zatuska W. (2008) Sympathetic overactivity in uremia. J Ren Nutr. Vol. 18, No. 1, p118-121.

Kuo JJ, Jones OB, Hall JE. (2003) Chronic cardiovascular and renal actions of leptin during hyperinsulinemia. Am J Physiol Regul Integr Comp Physiol. Vol. 284, No. 4, pR1037-R1042.

Lambert E, Straznicky NE, Dawood T, Ika-Sari C, et al. (2011) Changes in sympathetic nerve firing pattern associated with dietary weight loss in the metabolic syndrome. Frontiers in Physiology. Doi: 10.3389/fphys.2011.00052.

Landsberg L. (2001). Insulin-mediated sympathetic stimulation: role in the pathogenesis of obesity-related hypertension (or, how insulin affects blood pressure, and why. J Hypertens. Vol. 19, No. 3 Pt2, p523-528.

Libropoulos EN, Mikhailidis DP, Elisaf MS. (2005) Diagnosis and management of the metabolic syndrome in obesity. Obs Rev. Vol. 6, No. 4, p283-296.

Lohmeier TE, Lohmeier JR, Reckelhoff JF, Hildebrandt DA. (2001) Sustained influence of the renal nerves to attenuate sodium intake retention in angiotensin hypertension. Am J Physiol Regul Interg Comp Physiol. Vol. 281, No. 2, R434-443.

Mahfoud F, Schlaich M, Kindermann I, Ukena I, et al. (2011) Effect of renal sympathetic denervation on glucose metabolism in patients with essential hypertension: a pilot study. Circulation. Vol. 123, No. 18, p1940-1946.

Manicardi V, Camellini L, Bellodi G, Coscelli C, et al. (1986) Evidence for and association of high blood pressure and hyperinsulinemia in obese men. J Clin Endocrinol Metab. Vol. 62, No. 6, p1302-1304.

Manicardi V, Camellini L, Bellodi G, Coscelli C, Ferrannini E. (1986) Evidence for and association of high blood pressure and hyperinsulinemia in obese men. J Clin Endocrinol Metab. Vol 62, No. 6, p1302-1304.

Masuo K, Ogihara T, Kumahara Y, Yamatodani A, Wada H. (1983). Plasma norepinephrine and dietary sodium intake in normal subjects and patients with essential hypertension. Hypertension. Vol. 5, No. 5, p767-771.

Masuo K, Mikami H, Ogihara T, Tuck ML. (1995) Hormonal mechanisms in blood pressure reduction during hemodialysis in patients with chronic renal failure. Hypertens Res. Vol. 18, No. Suppl 1, S201-S203.

Masuo K, Mikami H, Ogihara T, Tuck ML. (1997) Sympathetic nerve hyperactivity precedes hyperinsulinemia and blood pressure elevation in a young, nonobese, Japanese population. Am J Hypertens. Vol. 10, No. 1, p77-83.

Masuo K, Mikami H, Ogihara T, Tuck ML. (2000) Weigh gain-induced blood pressure elevation. Hypertension. Vol. 35, No. 111, p1135-1140.

Masuo K, Mikami H, Ogihara T, Tuck ML. (2001a) Familial hypertension, insulin, sympathetic activity, and blood pressure elevation. Hypertension. Vol. 32, No. 1, p98-100.

Masuo K, Mikami H, Ogihara T, Tuck ML. (2001b) Weight reduction and pharmacological treatment in obese hypertensives. Am J Hypertens. Vol. 14, No. 6 Pt 1, p530-538.

Masuo K, Mikami H, Ogihara T, Tuck ML. (2001c). Differences in mechanisms between weight loss-sensitive and -resistant blood pressure reduction in obese subjects. Hypertens Res. Vol. 24, No. 4, p371-376.

Masuo K. (2002) Obesity-related hypertension: Role of sympathetic nervous system, insulin, and leptin. Curr Hypertens Rep. Vol. 4, No. 2, p112-118.

Masuo K, Kawaguchi H, Mikami H, Ogihara , Tuck ML. (2003) Serum uric acid and plasma norepinephrine concentrations predict subsequent weigh gain and blood pressure elevation. Hypertension. Vol. 42, No. 4, p474-480.

Masuo K, Katsuya T, Fu Y, Rakugi H, Ogihara T, Tuck ML. (2005a) Beta2- and beta3-adrenergic receptor polymorphisms are related to the onset of weight gain and blood pressure elevation over 5 years. Circulation. Vol. 111, No. 25, p3429-3434.

Masuo K, Katsuya T, Fu Y, Rakugi H, Ogihara T. (2005b) Beta2- adrenoceptor polymorphisms relate to insulin resistance and sympathetic overactivity as early markers of metabolic disease in nonobese, normotensive individuals. Am J Hypertens. Vol. 18, No, 7, p1009-1014.

Masuo K, Katsuya T, Ogihara T, Tuck ML. (2005c) Acute hyperinsulinemia reduces plasma leptin levels in insulin sensitive men. Am J Hypertens. Vol. 18, No. 2 (Pt 1), p235-243.

Masuo K, Katsuya T, Kawaguchi H, Fu Y, Rakugi H, Ogihara T, Tuck ML. (2006) Beta2-adrenoceptor polymorphisms relate to obesity through blunted leptin-mediated sympathetic activation. Am J Hypertens. Vol. 19, No,. 10, P1084-1091.

Masuo K, Katsuya T, Sugimoto K, Kawaguchi H, et al. (2007) High plasma norepinephrine levels associated with beta2-adrenoceptor polymorphisms predict future renal damage in nonobese normotensive individuals. Hypertens Res. Vol 30, No. 6, p503-511.

Masuo K, Katsuya T, Sugimoto K, Rakugi H, et al. (2008). Beta1 (Arg389Gly, Ser49Gly)- and beta2 (Arg16Gly)-adrenoceptor polymorphisms are related to left ventricular hypertrophy in middle aged nonobese, normotensive men, but through different mechanism. Circulation. Vol. 118, No. 18, S1154.

Masuo K, Lambert GW, Esler MD, Rakugi H, et al. (2010a) The role of sympathetic nervous activation in renal injury and end-stage renal disease. Hypertens Res. Vol. 33, No. 6, p521-524.

Masuo K. (2010b) Roles of beta2- and beta3-adrenoceptor polymorphisms in hypertension and metabolic syndrome. Int J Hypertens. DOI: 2010. Oct 21; 2010:832821.

Masuo K, Rakugi H, Ogihara T, Esler MD, Lambert GW. (2011a) The effects of weight loss on renal function in overweight Japanese men. Hypertens Res. Vol. 34, No. 8, p915-921.

Masuo K, Rakugi H, Ogiharas T, Lambert GW. (2011b) Beta2-adrenoceptor polymorphisms (Arg16Gly) accompanying with plasma norepinephrine is related to cardiac and renal complications in obese subjects. Hypertension. Vol 58, Suppl. p146.

Masuo K, Lambert GW. (2011c) Relationships of adrenoceptor polymorphisms with obesity. J Obes. Doi: 2011;2011.609485.

Masuo K, Rakugi H, Ogihara T, Lambert GW. (2012) Different mechanisms in weight loss-induced blood pressure reduction between a calorie-restricted diet and exercise. Hypertens Res. Vol. 35, No. 1, p41-47.

Matsumoto K, Fujita N, Ozaki M, Tominaga T, Ueki Y, Miyake S. (2006) Coexistence of insulin resistance and inflamation effectively predicts cardiac disease but not stroke in Japanese patients with type 2 diabetes mellitus. Diabetes Res Clin Pract. Vol. 74, No. 3, p316-321.

Mokdad AH, Ford ES, Bowman BA, Dietz WH, et al. (2001) Prevalence of obesity, diabetes, and obesity-related health risk factors. JAPA. Vol. 289, No. 1, p76079.

Morgan DA, Rahmouni K. (2010) Different effects of insulin on sympathetic nerve activity in Agouti obese mice. J Hypertens. Vol. 28, No. 9, p1913-1919.

Morrison JA, Glueck CJ, Horn PS, Schreiber GBm, Wang P. (2008) Preteen insulin resistance predicts weight gain, impaired fasting glucose, and type 2 diabetes at age 18-19y: a 10-y prospective study of blood and white girls. Am J Clin Nutr. Vok 88, No. 137, P778-788.

Mukerji R, Terry BE, Fresen JL, Petruc M, Govindarajan G, Alpert MA. (2011) Relation of left ventricular mass to QTc in normotensive severely obese patients. Obesity (Silver Spring). Vol. 4, doi. 10.1038/oby 2011.255

Narkiewicz K, Somers VK. (2003) Sympathetic nerve activity in obstructive sleep apnea. Acta Physiol Scand. Vol. 17, No. 3, p385-390.

Ogden CL, Carroll MD, Curtin LR, McDowell MA, Tabak CJ, Flegal KM. (2006) Prevalence of overweight and obesity in the United States. 1999-2004. JAMA. Vol. 295, No. 13, p1549-1555.

Ogden CL, Fryar SC, Carroll MD, Flegal KM. (2004) Advance data from vital and health statics. CDC. Vol. 27, No. 347, p1-17.

Petersson MJ, Rundqvist B, Johansson M, Eisenhofer G, et al. (2002). Increased cardiac sympathetic drive in renovascular hypertension. J Hypertens. Vol. 20, No. 6, p1181-1187.

Philips JK. (2004) Pathogenesis of hypertension in renal failure: role of the sympathetic nervous system and renal afferents. Clin Exp Pharmacol Physiol. Vol. 32, No. 5-6, p415-418.

Preis SR, Hwang SJ, Coady S, Pencina MJ, D'Agostino RB Sr, et al. (2009) Trends in all-cause and cardiovascular disease mortality among women and men with and without diabetes mellitus in the Framingham Heart Study. 1950 to 2005. Circulation. Vol. 119, No. 13, p1728-1735.

Rao F, Wessel J, Wen G, Ahang L, et al. (2007) Renal albumin excretion. Twin studies identify influence of heredity, environment, and adrenergic pathway polymorphism. Hypertension. Vol. 49, No. 5, p1015-1031.

Reasner CA. (2008) Reducing cardiovascular complications of type 2 diabetes by targeting multiple risk factors. J Cardiovasc Pharmacol. Vol. 52, No. 123, p136-144.

Report of a WHO Expert Committee. (1995) Physiological status: the use and interpretation of anthropometry. World Health Organ Tech Rep Ser. Vol.854, p1-452.

Resnick HE, Valsania P, Halter JB, Lin X. (2000) Relation of weight gain and weight loss on subsequent diabetes risk in overweight adults. J Epidemiol Community Health. Vol. 54, No. 8, p596-602.

Rocchini AP, Mao HZ, Babu K, Marker P, Rocchini AI. (1999). Clonidine prevents insulin resistance and hypertension in obese dogs. Hypertension. Vol. 33, No. 1 (Pt 2), p548-553.

Schlaich MP, Socratous F, Hennebry S, Eikelis N, et al. (2009) Sympathetic activation in chronic renal failure. J Am Soc Nephrol. Vol. 20, No. 5, p933-939.

Shamsuzzaman AS, Ackerman MJ, Kara T, Lanfran P, Somers VK. (2003) Sympathetic nerve activity in the congenital long-QT syndrome. Circulation. Vol. 107, No. 14, p1844-1847.

Straznicky NE, Lambert EA, Lambert GW, Masuo K, Esler MD, Nestel PJ. (2005) Effects of dietary weight loss on sympathetic activity and cardiac risk factors associated with the metabolic syndrome. J Clin Endocrinol Metab. Vol. 90, No. 11, p5998-6005.

Straznicky NE, Lambert GW, Masuo K, Dawood T, et al. (2009a) Blunted sympathetic neural response to oral glucose in obese subjects with the insulin-resistant metabolic syndrome. Am J Clin Nutr. Vol. 89, No. 1, p27-36.

Straznicky NE, Lambert GW, McGrane MT, Masuo K, et al. (2009b) Weight loss may reverse blunted sympathetic neural responsiveness to glucose ingestion in obese subjects with metabolic syndrome. Diabetes. Vol. 58, No. 5, p1126-1132.

Straznicky NE, Lambert EA, Nestel PJ, McGrane MT, et al. (2010) Sympathetic neural adaptation to hypocaloric diet with or without exercise training in obese metabolic syndrome subjects. Diabetes. Vol. 59, No. 1, p71-79.

Straznicky NE, Grima MT, Lambert EA, Masuo K, et al. (2011) Exercise augments weight loss induced improvement in renal function in obese metabolic syndrome individuals. J Hypertens. Vol, 29, No. 3, p553-564.

Straznicky NE, Lambert EA, Grima MT, Eikelis N, et al. (2012). The effects of dietary weight loss with or without exercise training on liver enzymes in obese metabolic syndrome subjects. Diabetes Obes Metab. Vol. 14, No. 2, p139-146.

Symplicity HTN-1 Investigators. (2011) Cather-based renal sympathetic denervation for resistant hypertension: durability of blood pressure reduction out to 24 months. Hypertension. Vol. 57, No. 5, p911-917.

Takatori S, Zamami Y, Mio M, Lurosaki Y, Kawasaki H. (2006) Chronic hyperinsulinemia enhances adrenergic vasoconstriction and decreases calcitonin gene-related peptide-containing nerve-mediated vasodilation in pithed rats. Hypertens Res. Vol. 29, No. 5, p361-365.

Tryhurn P, Duncan JS, Rayner DV. (1995) Acute cold induced suppression of ob (obese) gene expression in white adipose tissue of mice: mediation by the sympathetic system. Biochem J. Vol. 1, no. 311 (Pt 3)), p729-733.

Tuck ML, Sowers JR, Dornfeld L, Whitefield L, Maxwell M. (1983) Reductions in plasma catecholamines and blood pressure during weight loss in obese subjects. Acta Endocrinol (Copenh). Vol. 10, No. 2, p252-257.

Valentini M, Julius S, Palatini P, Brook RD, et al. (2004) Attenuation of haemodynamic, metabolic and energy exopenditure responses to isoproterenol in patients with hypertension. J Hypertens. Vol. 22, No. 10, p1999-2006.

van Veen S, Frolich M, Chang PC. (1999) Acute hyperglycemia in the forearm induces vasodilation that is not modified by hyperinsulinemia. J Hyman Hypertens. Vol. 13, No. 4, p263-268.

Vozoris NT. (2012) Sleep apnea-plus: Prevalence, risk factors, and association with cardiovascular disease using United States population-level data. Sleep Med. Vol. Apr 2 [Epub ahead]

Wachtell K, Olsen MH, Dahlof B, Devereux RB, Kjeldsen SE, et al. (2002) Microalbumiuria in hypertensive patients with electriocardiographic left ventricular hypertrophy: the LIFE study. J Hypertens. Vol. 20, No. 3, p405-412.

Ward KD, Sparrow D, Landsberg L, Young JB, Vokonas PS, Weiss ST. (1996) Influence of insulin, sympathetic nervous system activity, and obesity on blood pressure: the Normative Aging Study. J Hypertension. Vol. 14, No. 4, p301-308.

White SL, Cass A, Atkins RC, Chadban SJ. (2005) Chronic kidney disease in the general population. Adv Chronic Dis. Vol. 12, No. 1, p5-13.

Wikstrand J, Pettersson P, Biorntorp P. (1993) Body fat distribution and left ventricular morphology and function in obese females. J Hypertens. Vol. 11, No. 1, p1259-1268.

Will JC, Williamson DF, Ford ES, Calle EE, Thun MJ. International weight loss and 13-year diabetes uincidence in overweight adults. Am J Public Health. Vol. 92, No. 8, p1245-1248.

Witkowski A, Prejbisz A, Florczak E, Kadziela J, et al. (2011) Effects of renal sympathetic denervation on blood pressure, sleep apnea course, and glycemic control in patients with resistant hypertension and sleep apnea. Hypertension. Vol. 58, No. 4, p559-565.

Zamami Y, Takatori S, Yamawaki K, Miyashita S, et al. (2008) Acute hyperglycemia and hyperinsulinemia enhance adrenergic vasoconstriction and decrease calcitonin gene-related peptide-containing nerve-mediated vasoconstriction in pithed rats. Hypertens Res. Vol. 31, No. 5, p1033-1044.

Ziefler MG, Milic M, Elavan H, (2011) Cardiovascular regulation in obstructive sleep apnea. Drug Discov Today Dis Models. Vol. 8, No. 4, p155-160.

Zoccali C, Benedetto FA, Mallamaci F, Tripepi G, et al. (2004) Left ventricular mass monitoring in the follow-up of dialysis patients: prognostic value of left ventricular hypertrophy progression. Kidney Int. Vol. 65, No. 4, p1492-1498.

Zoccali C, Mallamaci F, Parlongo S, Cutrupi S, et al. (2002a). Plasma norepinephrine predicts survivcal and incident cardiovascular events in patients with end-stage renal disease. Circulation. Vol. 105, No. 11, p1354-1369.

Zoccali C, Mallamaci F, Tripepi G, Parlongo S, et al. (2002b) Norepinephrine and concentric hypertrophy in patients with end-stage renal disease. Hypertension. Vol. 40, No. 1, p41-46.

Chapter 8

Myocardial Insulin Resistance: An Overview of Its Causes, Effects, and Potential Therapy

Eugene F. du Toit and Daniel G. Donner

Additional information is available at the end of the chapter

http://dx.doi.org/10.5772/50619

1. Introduction

Normal insulin sensitivity is essential for the maintenance of normal circulating carbohydrate and lipid levels and their metabolism. In healthy individuals elevated blood glucose levels stimulate the pancreas to release insulin which lowers blood glucose levels by stimulating glucose uptake and metabolism in muscle, adipose tissue and several other insulin sensitive organs. Blood glucose increases are not only countered by increased tissue glucose uptake but also by insulin induced suppression of hepatic glycogenolysis and gluconeogenesis. Besides its effects on blood glucose, insulin also affects circulating lipid levels by reducing hepatic very low density lipoprotein cholesterol (VLDL-cholesterol) formation from free fatty acids (FFAs). This is primarily due to the reduced free fatty acid supply to the liver caused by insulin induced suppression of lipogenesis in adipose tissue [1]. In addition to its effects on lipogenesis, insulin also reduces lipolysis in adipose tissue by inhibiting hormone sensitive lipase. The latter hydrolyses adipocyte triglycerides to release free fatty acids and glycerol into the circulation. When delivered acutely, insulin inhibits fatty acid synthase while chronic hyperinsulinaemia (as occurs in insulin resistance) may induce fatty acid synthase activity and increase fatty acid synthesis [2]. The net effect of elevated insulin in normal healthy individuals is to reduce circulating glucose and free fatty acid levels.

When an individual becomes insulin resistant, control of circulating lipid and blood glucose levels is compromised. Insulin resistance ensues when normal physiological concentrations of insulin are unable to induce effective uptake of glucose by insulin sensitive tissue. As a compensatory mechanism aimed at maintaining euglycaemia, pancreatic insulin secretion increases leading to a state of hyperinsulinaemia. If the elevated insulin levels are inadequate to fully compensate for the insulin insensitivity glucose intolerance ensues. The degree of glucose intolerance in insulin resistant individuals is thus dependent on the extent of the loss of the *in vivo* function of insulin, and the ability of the pancreas to adjust for this by secreting more insulin [3, 4]. Once elevated circulating levels of insulin are no longer able to maintain euglycaemia, and glucose levels deviate beyond normal physiological ranges an individual is considered to be frankly diabetic.

Myocardial insulin resistance translates to compromised intracellular insulin signalling and reduced glucose oxidation rates in animal models of obesity [5] and adversely affects myocardial mechanical function and tolerance to ischaemia and reperfusion. In this chapter we will review the mechanisms implicated in the aetiology of insulin resistance (skeletal and heart muscle) and discuss the effects of insulin resistance on cardiac metabolism, mechanical function and tolerance to ischaemia and reperfusion. We will also briefly review therapies used to prevent or counter insulin resistance and its associated adverse effects on the cardiovascular system.

2. Myocardial insulin signalling

Insulin induced activation of the insulin receptor (IR) invokes a cascade of events which ultimately enhances myocardial glucose uptake and metabolism. Insulin binding to its receptor results in autophosphorylation and activation of the insulin receptors (IRs) intrinsic tyrosine kinases. Following phosphorylation the insulin receptor phosphorylates insulin receptor substrate (IRS) [6] which subsequently associates with phosphoinositide 3-kinase (PI3K) via its p85 subunit [7, 8]. These events are vital for initiating insulin's effects on glucose metabolism [6, 9, 10]. Activated PI3K will induce (via various signalling mechanisms) protein kinase B (PKB/Akt)[11] which plays a pivotal role in glucose metabolism by regulating the translocation of the cytosolic glucose transporter type 4 (GLUT4), to the sarcolemma [12, 13]. Inhibition of PI3K and/or PKB/Akt attenuates sarcolemmal GLUT4 translocation, effectively reducing insulin stimulated signalling and glucose uptake [14, 15]. Besides facilitating glucose uptake via GLUT4, insulin stimulation also increases glycolytic flux rates through activation of phosphofructosekinase 2 (PFK-2) which promotes the production of fructose-2,6-bisphosphate from fructose-6-phosphate [16-18]. Fructose-2,6-bisphosphate stimulates PFK-1 activity, which will also enhance glycolysis (see review by Hue *et al.* [18]).

Although insulin increases long chain fatty acid (LCFA) uptake into the cardiomyocyte by increasing sarcolemmal fatty acid translocase/cluster of differentiation 36 (FAT/CD36) [19], elevated insulin levels also suppress tissue fatty acid β-oxidation rates. This suppression is most likely due to the effects of by-products of elevated glucose oxidation on malonyl-CoA levels [20]. As acetyl-CoA levels increase, acetyl-CoA carboxylase (ACC) is activated which increases malonyl-CoA induced inhibition of fatty acid oxidation.

3. The role of obesity or a high fructose diet in the aetiology of insulin resistance

Insulin resistance is strongly associated with both obesity and the consumption of high fructose containing diets [21-25]. Although not all obese individual are insulin resistant, there is a strong association between obesity and insulin resistance [21, 25]. Adipose tissue is not only a storage organ but also a metabolically active organ synthesising and secreting a large range of substances that include fatty acids, pro-inflammatory cytokines, angiotensin II, leptin, resistin, visfatin and other adipocytokines [26] that can all influence tissue metabolism. Obesity and high fructose diets both induce increases in: 1) circulating FFAs [27, 28], 2) renin-angiotensin system (RAS) activity [29, 30], and 3) inflammation (caused by tissue and macrophage derived pro-inflammatory cytokines) [31] that are all associated with, and implicated in insulin resistance.

Besides the negative impact of obesity on circulating lipids, recent studies provide convincing evidence for a role for high fructose diets in dyslipidaemia and insulin resistance [24, 27, 32]. These lipid profile altering effects of high fructose diets are primarily caused by fructose induced alterations in hepatic lipid metabolism [22-24]. Hepatic fructose metabolism differs significantly from glucose metabolism with fructose being a lipogenic sugar that promotes the deposition of triglycerides in adipose tissue and ectopic organs such as the liver and muscle. This tissue triglyceride accumulation eventually contributes to dyslipidaemia and insulin resistance [22, 27, 33].

Increasing dietary fructose consumption increases plasma triglyceride levels through stimulation of hepatic lipogenesis [34] and decreased VLDL-triglyceride removal from the plasma by adipose tissue [35]. Fructose evidently also activates genes involved in hepatic *de novo* lipogenesis [36, 37] which causes increased hepatic fatty acid generation. These fatty acids are incorporated into hepatic triglycerides which promotes VLDL-triglyceride synthesis and release from the liver (Figure 1)[38].

A recent review highlights the possible effects of high fructose diets on hepatic insulin resistance [22]. These authors propose that high fructose diets promote hepatic inflammation by increasing fatty acid β-oxidation (secondary to hepatic lipid accumulation) which generates peroxidation products that stimulate inhibitor of nuclear factor kappa-B kinase subunit beta (IKKβ) and activate nuclear factor kappa-light-chain-enhancer of activated B cells (NFκB). The NFκB then enters the nucleus and induces the transcription of genes that encode for pro-inflammatory cytokines that include tumour necrosis factor alpha (TNFα) and interleukin-6 (IL-6). These cytokines potentially activate c-Jun N-terminal kinase-1 (JNK-1) which will increase inhibitory serine^{307} phosphorylation of IRS-1 and contribute to hepatic insulin resistance [22] (Figure 2).

Because of its lipogenic effects, fructose causes more marked changes in 24 hour lipid profiles than does the consumption of glucose while also favouring visceral rather than subcutaneous fat deposition [33]. This fat deposition pattern differs from that of glucose which promotes subcutaneous adipose tissue deposition rather that visceral fat deposition in men [39]. In rodents, a high fructose diet increases intrahepatic fat content and serum VLDL-triglyceride concentrations within 6 weeks of feeding. In the same study intramuscular fat content was increased within 3 months of initiating the high fructose feeding with these changes being closely followed by hepatic and muscle insulin resistance [32]. Another animal based study supports a role for high fructose diets in increased hepatic VLDL-triglyceride secretion [40]. In humans increasing fructose content in the diet increases plasma triglycerides [34, 41], decreases VLDL-triglyceride clearance [35] and increases triglyceride deposition in hepatocytes and skeletal muscle within a week of increasing dietary fructose content [41].

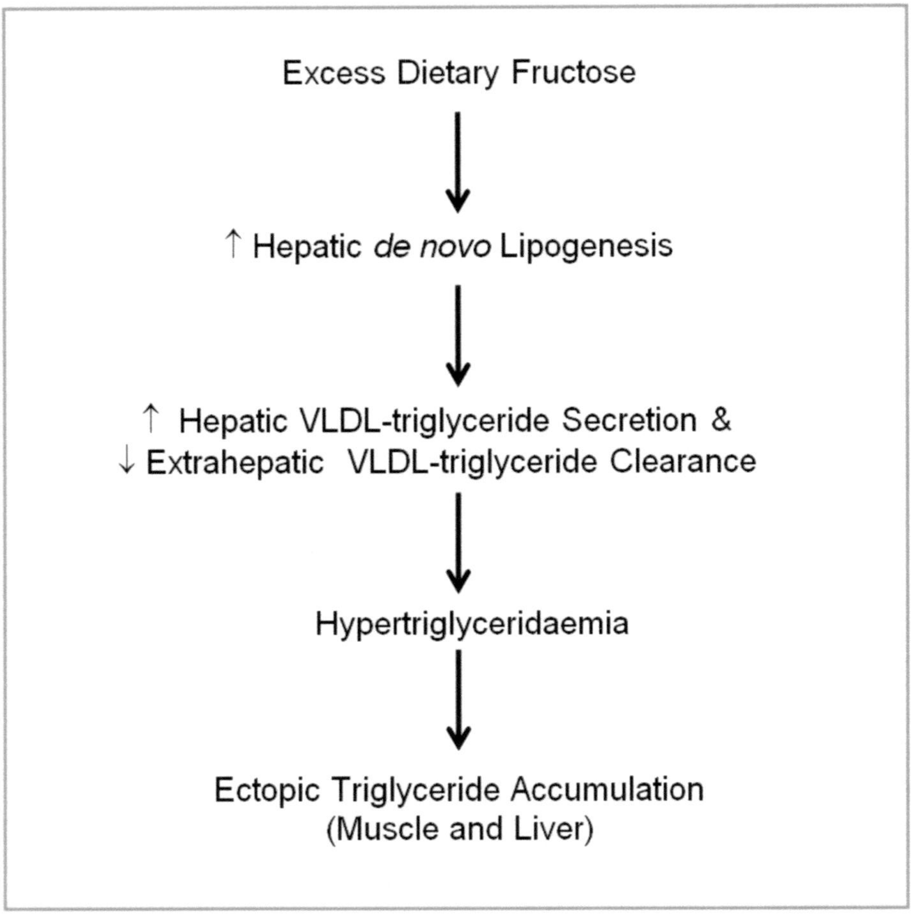

Figure 1. Mechanism for high fructose diet induced dyslipidaemia and ectopic lipid accumulation. High fructose diets promote hepatic *de novo* lipogenesis and lipid accumulation and reduce extra-hepatic VLDL-triglyceride clearance. The associated hypertriglyceridaemia promotes adipose tissue expansion (obesity) and muscle lipid accumulation which induces insulin resistance.

Since high fructose diets are often also associated with obesity, it is difficult to differentiate between the effects of the changes in dietary fructose content and the effects of obesity on tissue insulin sensitivity. Data from studies demonstrating that some individuals are obese but metabolically healthy [42] and metabolic syndrome appears to be more closely linked to intrahepatic fat content than obesity *per se* [1, 41, 43], suggests that hepatic lipid metabolism and circulating lipid levels play a critical role in the induction of insulin resistance in response to obesity and high fructose diets. Tappy and co-workers [23, 24] recently proposed that fructose increases hepatic *de novo* lipogenesis which leads to intrahepatic lipid deposition, hepatic insulin resistance and increased VLDL-triglyceride secretion. This potentially leads to increased visceral fat deposition while the elevated VLDL-triglyceride and inhibition of lipid oxidation (induced by fructose) may promote ectopic fat deposition in muscle with lipotoxicity leading to systemic insulin resistance (Figure 1) [22-24]

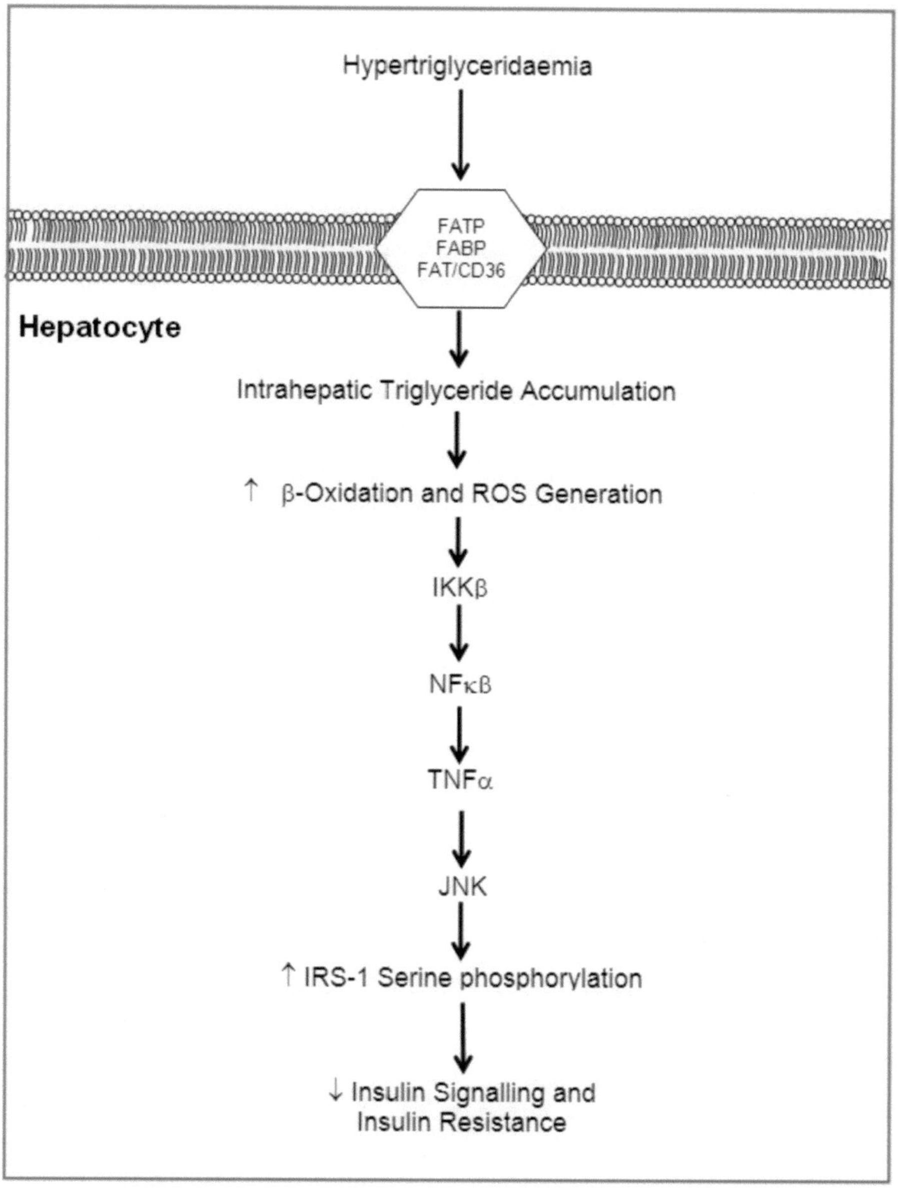

Figure 2. The proposed mechanism for intrahepatic lipid accumulation induced stimulation of β-oxidation and ROS generation. ROS induced increases in cytokine (TNFα and possibly other cytokines) expression and synthesis activates JNK which phosphorylates IRS-1 (insulin receptor substrate) at the serine^{307} residue. This inhibitory phosphorylation of IRS-1 prevents its tyrosine phosphorylation by the insulin receptor and interferes with the normal insulin signalling cascade (Illustration modified from review by Rutledge and Adeli [22].

The experimental evidence implicating inflammation/pro-inflammatory cytokines and overactive renin-angiotensin systems (organ and systemic) in the aetiology of insulin resistance will be discussed later. We will first review the evidence for a role for elevated circulating free fatty acids, and tissue triglycerides and lipid intermediates accumulation in the aetiology of insulin resistance in skeletal and heart muscle.

4. The role of free fatty acids and intracellular lipid accumulation in insulin resistance

A prevalent metabolic change associated with obesity [44-49] and high fructose feeding [22-24] is the increase in the circulating free fatty acids and triglycerides. Under conditions of over-nutrition and dyslipidaemia, not all fatty acids entering the cell are utilized for oxidative purposes. Long chain fatty acyl-CoA accumulation provides substrates for non-oxidative processes such as triglyceride, diacylglycerol (DAG) and ceramide synthesis [50, 51]. In the myocardium lipid accumulation is a direct result of a mismatch between fatty acid uptake and oxidation by the cell [47, 52]. What is not clear is whether this accumulation is due to: 1) increased FFA uptake by the heart 2) compromised FFA oxidation, or, 3) a combination of the two.

There is a strong link between increased circulating free fatty acids, myocardial triglyceride accumulation and insulin resistance. Increased circulating free fatty acids increase the expression of sarcolemmal fatty acid transporters and increases fatty acid uptake into the myocyte. Obese Zucker rats [46, 48] and *db/db* mice [53] with insulin resistance have increased FAT/CD36 localised to the sarcolemma. The exact mechanism for the increased localisation of FAT/CD36 in the sarcolemma is not clear but may relate to the chronic hyperinsulinaemia associated with insulin resistance. It is well established that insulin stimulates FAT/CD36 translocation to the sarcolemma [54, 55]. This increased sarcolemmal FAT/CD36 content increases fatty acid uptake in cardiac myocytes and possibly leads to tissue fatty acyl-CoA accumulation if not metabolised through concomitant increased β-oxidation [56]. Besides its adverse effects on insulin signalling and glucose metabolism, excessive intramyocellular lipid accumulation may also have direct lipotoxic effects [50, 57]. Both altered substrate utilization and excess intramyocardial lipid accumulation which is characteristic of obesity, dyslipidaemia and insulin resistance may have serious cardiac consequences that ultimately lead to compromised cardiac metabolism, morphology and mechanical function.

Lipid intermediates may adversely influence insulin signalling and contribute to insulin resistance [5, 58, 59]. The accumulation of triglycerides, diacylglycerol (DAG) and ceramide is known to activate kinases that down-regulate insulin signalling [60-62]. These kinases include JNK, IKK and protein kinase C (PKC) that is known to inhibit insulin signalling via serine phosphorylation of IRS-1 [5, 63].

Ceramide accumulation occurs through *de novo* synthesis from saturated fatty acids [64] or hydrolysis of sphingomyelin [65]. It has been shown to cause insulin resistance by inhibiting Akt phosphorylation in skeletal muscle [66-68] and adipocytes [69] with the pharmacological inhibition of ceramide synthesis being effective in preventing lipid induced insulin resistance in rats [67, 70].

Models of lipotoxicity have also demonstrated that elevated myocardial ceramide levels are associated with increases in indices of apoptosis [52, 71]. Rat neonatal cardiomyocytes incubated with physiological concentrations of palmitate have increased intracellular triglycerides, increased ceramide levels and increased indices of apoptosis [72]. The mechanism implicated in ceramide induced apoptosis may involve activation of NFκB which in turn up regulates inducible nitric oxide synthase (iNOS) expression [73]. The resulting increase in nitric oxide production [74] may cause a subsequent rise in the formation of peroxynitrite, which induces mitochondrial cytochrome C release [75] and subsequent apoptosis. In addition, ceramide has been shown to directly induce the generation of damaging reactive oxygen species in the mitochondria [76]. Obese insulin resistant (prediabetic) Zucker rats also have elevated intramyocardial triglycerides which are accompanied by increased myocardial ceramide levels and cardiomyocyte apoptosis. These cellular alterations are present before the onset of diabetes and cardiac dysfunction [71]. Reducing myocardial lipid levels by treating the rats with peroxisome proliferator-activated receptor gamma (PPARγ) agonists lead to reduced cardiac ceramide levels and apoptosis and prevented cardiac dysfunction [71]. In a similar study, mice over-expressing cardiac specific long chain acyl-CoA synthase display high intramyocardial triglycerides and ceramide levels. These changes were accompanied by increased DNA fragmentation and cytochrome C release with the mice developing cardiac hypertrophy and left-ventricular dysfunction [52].

Lipid infusion increases intracellular DAG and causes skeletal muscle insulin resistance in rodents [60]. This association between intracellular DAG levels and skeletal muscle insulin resistance has been confirmed in several rodent and human studies [77-79]. Increased muscle DAG is associated with increased activation of protein kinase C theta (PKC-θ) in obese and diabetic patients [80, 81]. Increased PKC-θ activation interferes with insulin signalling by increasing IRS-1 serine[307] phosphorylation (Figure 3)[60, 81]. Accelerating fatty acid oxidation rates potentially prevents fatty acid, acetyl-CoA and subsequent DAG accumulation and may improve insulin sensitivity. This proposal was recently supported by a study showing that carnitine palmitoyltransferase I (CPT-1) over-expression in L6E9 myotubes increases mitochondrial fatty acid uptake, decreased intracellular DAG concentrations and protects against elevated fatty acid induced insulin resistance [82].

4.1. Evidence for lipid accumulation in skeletal muscle insulin resistance

An inverse correlation exists between intramuscular lipid content and insulin sensitivity. Measurements of insulin sensitivity (120 min euglycaemic hyperinsulinaemic clamp) in skeletal muscle from healthy subjects demonstrated that high intramuscular lipid content was associated with lower whole body insulin stimulated glucose uptake. These subjects also exhibited elevated circulating free fatty acids, reduced tyrosine phosphorylation of the insulin receptor (IR) and lower (insulin receptor substrate) IRS-1 mediated PI3K activation during hyperinsulinaemia than subjects with low intramuscular lipids [83]. Studies comparing lean and obese individuals have made similar observations linking intracellular lipid accumulation to skeletal muscle insulin resistance [84, 85]. Boden and colleagues [86] reported a strong association between serum free fatty acid levels, intramuscular lipid content and insulin resistance after lipid injection in healthy subjects. Elevated circulating free fatty acid levels, induced by lipid injection, was associated with a gradual increase in intramuscular lipid content and a 40% increase in insulin resistance. These observations also corroborated earlier studies demonstrating that elevated fatty acids reduced skeletal muscle glucose uptake in humans [87].

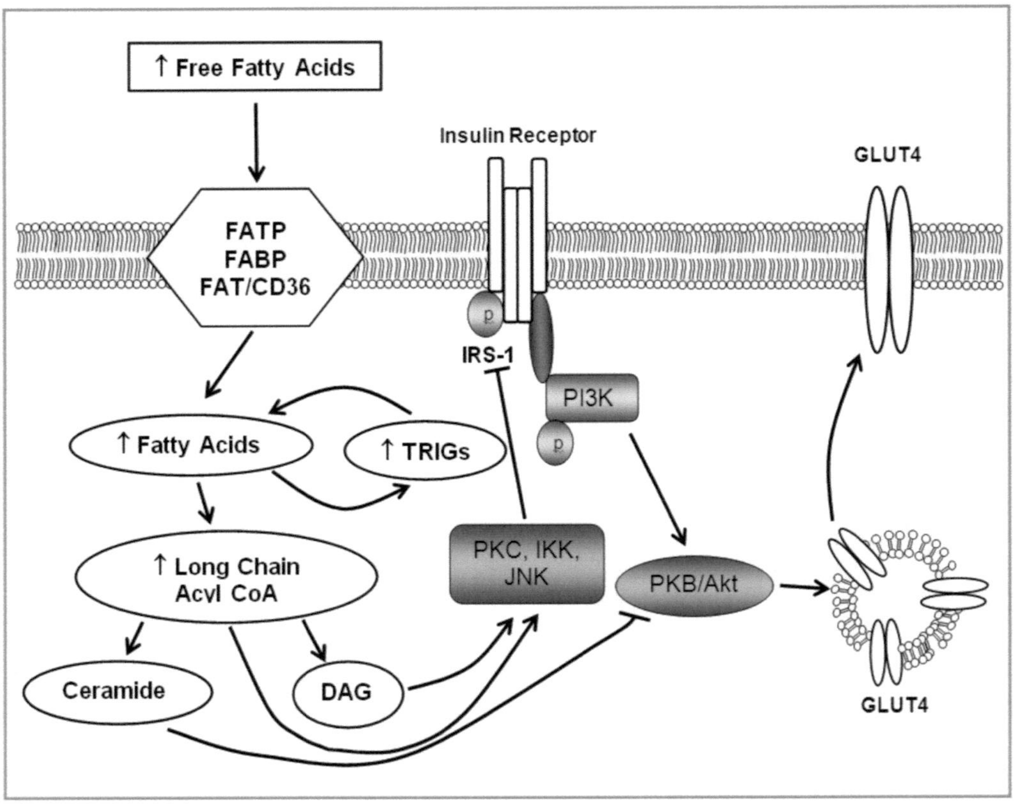

Figure 3. The proposed mechanism for dyslipidaemia induced insulin resistance. Increased circulating free fatty acids as occurs during overfeeding/obesity and/or high fructose diet feeding will increase fatty acid uptake. Long chain acetyl CoA not oxidised can be used in non-oxidative pathways with the generation of triglycerides, diacylglycerol (DAG) and ceramide. Both the latter lipid metabolites have been implicated in aetiology of insulin resistance through the activation of PKC, IKK and JNK.

In rodent skeletal muscle, experimentally elevated circulating free fatty acids increased intracellular acetyl-CoA and DAG levels which was coupled to increased active protein kinase C (PKC) theta. These changes were accompanied by increased IRS-1 serine phosphorylation, reduced IRS-1 tyrosine phosphorylation and reduced IRS-1 associated PI3K activity [60, 88]. Phosphorylation of IRS-1 at serine^{307} evidently hinders IRS-1's interaction with PI3K and therefore interferes with normal insulin signalling.

4.2. Evidence for lipid accumulation in cardiac muscle insulin resistance

Similar associations between increased intracellular lipid accumulation and reduced insulin sensitivity have been observed in cardiac muscle from obese insulin resistant animals [47, 71, 89, 90]. In obese insulin resistant JCR:LA-cp rats, the increased supply of circulating free fatty acids was associated with a 50% increase in myocardial triglyceride content and a 50% reduction in myocardial glycolytic flux rates [89].

In humans, plasma free fatty acid levels correlate with intramyocardial triglyceride levels [91]. This association is also evident in obese [91, 92], obese glucose intolerant [93] and diabetic [93, 94] individuals. Excessive intramyocardial triglyceride accumulation precedes the development of type-2 diabetes and tends to increase linearly with the degree of systemic insulin resistance [93]. Obese insulin resistant humans do not always have elevated serum free fatty acid levels but do appear to maintain higher rates of free fatty acid uptake, utilization and subsequent oxidation than lean controls [95].

5. The role of cytokines and chronic inflammation in insulin resistance

Obesity and insulin resistance is associated with chronic systemic inflammation caused by activation of the intrinsic immune systems in organs and the macrophages that infiltrate them [96]. The most prominent pro-inflammatory mediators involved in this inflammation are TNFα and IL-6 that originate from: 1) macrophages in adipose tissue and the liver [97], 2) the adipocytes themselves [97], and, 3) several other cytokine synthesising tissues in the body [97-99].

Elevated free fatty acids may increase pro-inflammatory cytokine expression and synthesis since studies inducing acute increases in plasma free fatty acids have observed activation of NFκB in skeletal muscle in humans [79] and increases hepatic TNFα, IL-1β and IL-6 and circulating monocyte chemotactic protein-1 (MCP-1) in rats [100, 101]. How elevated fatty acid cause NFκB activation is unknown but may involve DAG and PKC [102] or the Toll-like receptor 4 (TLR-4) [103]. MCP-1 is also known to regulate recruitment of macrophages to sites of inflammation and may be involved in the recruitment and differentiation of monocytes to macrophages that produce pro-inflammatory cytokines in conditions such as obesity and dyslipidaemia [97, 104].

TNFα causes insulin resistance by suppressing IRS-1 associated insulin signalling and glucose transport in skeletal muscle while IL-6 activates the phosphatase SHP-2 and Signal transducer and activator of transcription 3 (STAT3) causing increased expression of suppressor of cytokine signalling 3 (SOCS3) [105, 106]. IL-6 also activates several serine/threonine kinases such as JNK, p38 mitogen activated protein kinases and PKC-δ that contribute to reduced insulin sensitivity and glucose metabolism (Figure 4) [107, 108].

Information relating to the possible role of inflammation in the aetiology of myocardial insulin resistance is limited. A recent study however reported that high fat feeding caused increased myocardial macrophage infiltration and increased cytokine and SOCS levels in cardiomyocytes from these animals [109]. These changes were associated with reduced myocardial insulin sensitivity and glucose metabolism.

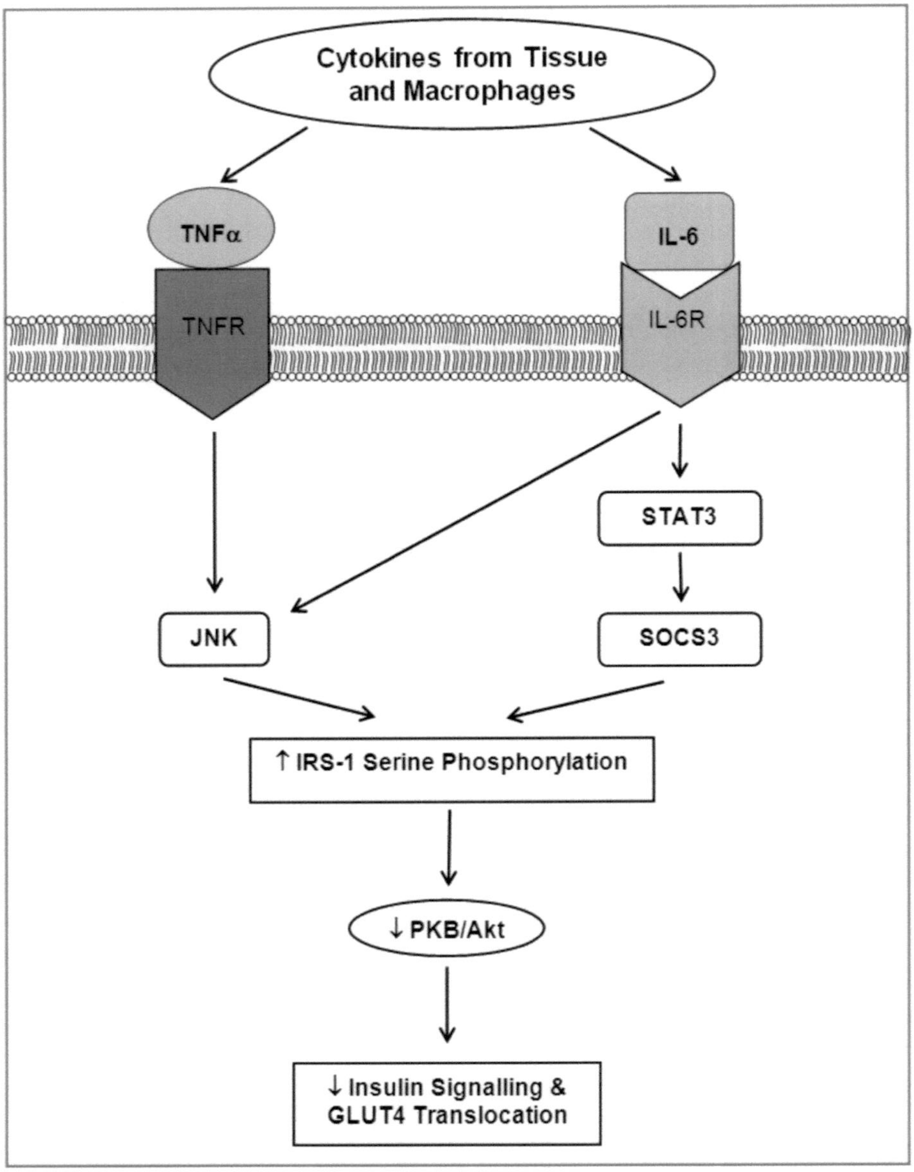

Figure 4. Proposed mechanism for inflammation induced insulin resistance in muscle. Cytokines from macrophages and myocytes activate their receptors and associated signalling pathways to increase serine (inhibitory) phosphorylation of IRS-1. IL-6 is known to activate the STAT3-SOCS3 pathways while TNFα activates JNK to phosphorylate IRS-1.

6. The role of the Renin-Angiotensin System (RAS) in insulin resistance

The authors [110] and others [111-115] have shown that the systemic and tissue renin-angiotensin systems (RAS) activity is increased in obesity. The role of increased RAS activity in metabolic and cardiovascular disease has been reviewed in detail [29, 116-118]. A key observation linking the RAS system to insulin resistance was made when it became apparent that hypertensive patients treated with angiotensin converting enzyme (ACE) inhibitors or angiotensin (AT) receptor blockers have a reduced risk of developing insulin resistance and type-2 diabetes when compared to patients on other conventional anti-hypertensive therapy [119, 120]. Subsequent studies have corroborated these observations with RAS inhibition improving blood glucose management [121] and lowering risk of type-2 diabetes [122]. These data provided indirect evidence to suggest that the RAS (and particularly over-activation) contributes to insulin resistance and type-2 diabetes.

Several human and animal studies support a role for RAS over-activity in insulin resistance. Genetic abnormalities leading to over-activation of the RAS provides strong evidence for the involvement of the RAS in insulin resistance. In infants [123] and adults [124, 125] the DD genotype of the ACE I/D polymorphism is associated with glucose intolerance and insulin insensitivity. Similarly, AGTT174M polymorphisms are associated with metabolic syndrome in aboriginal Canadians [126].

As mentioned previously, pharmacological blockade of the RAS in clinical trials has provided the most compelling evidence for a role for RAS over-activity in metabolic abnormalities such as insulin resistance. The use of ACE inhibitors for antihypertensive therapy reduces the risk of developing type-2 diabetes by 14% [119]. Studies on animals support these observations with RAS inhibition improving insulin sensitivity in rat [127] and mice [128]. Genetic deletion of renin [129] or ACE [130] or one of the two AT receptors also appears to be effective in preventing or reducing insulin resistance in mice [131, 132].

Besides the evidence showing that inhibition of RAS activity may improve insulin sensitivity, several studies also provide direct evidence implicating over-activation of the RAS in the aetiology of insulin resistance. Chronic angiotensin II infusion causes insulin resistance in rats [133, 134] while the TG(mREN2)27 rat which suffers from chronic systemic RAS over-activation develops muscle and systemic insulin resistance [135]. The RAS induced insulin resistance in these animals is improved by renin inhibition or angiotensin receptor blockade [135, 136].

The mechanism for angiotensin II (Ang II) induced insulin resistance has received significant attention. Ang II adversely affects glucose metabolism and decreases its uptake and utilisation by interfering with insulin signalling [137]. In L6 myocytes Ang II suppresses insulin induced phosphorylation of the tyrosine residue on IRS-1. This was associated with decreased activation of PKB/Akt and GLUT4 translocation to the sarcolemma. These changes were all AT_1 receptor, NADPH oxidase and NFκB dependent [138, 139]. Based on these observations it seems likely that Ang II activates NADPH oxidase and increases reactive oxygen species (ROS) generation through the angiotensin type 1 (AT_1) receptor. ROS activate the NFκB to increase transcription of cytokines that include TNFα and IL-6. These cytokines increase SOCS3 expression which inhibits insulin signalling (Figure 5) [140]. In rats Ang II also reduces skeletal muscle mitochondrial content (possibly through increased ROS generation) which would be expected to reduce muscle glucose utilisation [141].

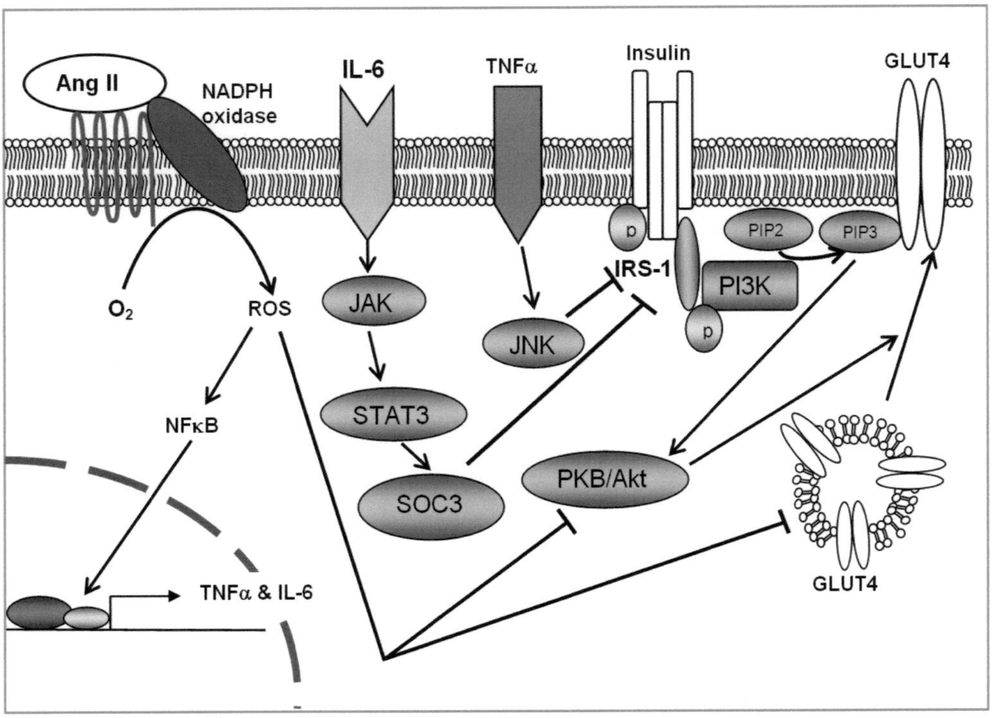

Figure 5. Proposed mechanism for renin-angiotensin system over-activation induced insulin resistance. Angiotensin II activates NADPH oxidase to generate reactive oxygen species (ROS) which activate the translocation of NFκB to the nucleus. Here it causes the transcription, synthesis and release of cytokines (TNFα and IL-6). The binding of these cytokines to their sarcolemmal receptors induce serine kinases and SOC3 which inhibits IRS-1 tyrosine phosphorylation, insulin signalling and GLUT4 translocation.

Adipose tissue RAS over-activity may also contribute to systemic insulin resistance since Ang II from adipose tissue contributes to circulating Ang II levels. This was well demonstrated by a study investigating the effect of adipose tissue angiotensinogen (Agt) over-expression on systemic glucose tolerance and insulin resistance [142]. The over-expression of Agt in adipose tissue caused cardiac and skeletal insulin resistance and reduced muscle glucose uptake.

7. The role of adipocytokines in the aetiology of insulin resistance

Adipocytokines released from adipose tissue perform regulatory functions in energy and fluid balance and satiety and have been implicated in conditions such as obesity, dyslipidaemia, insulin resistance/diabetes and cardiovascular disease. Besides the two pro-inflammatory cytokines discussed previously (TNFα and IL-6) adipocytes secrete several well characterised adipocytokines that include: leptin, adiponectin, and resistin. Dysregulation of the synthesis and secretion of these peptides has been associated with, and implicated in, the aetiology of metabolic diseases such as insulin resistance and type-2 diabetes. A possible role for adipokines in the regulation of myocardial metabolism only emerged recently [143-145].

Leptin is synthesised by white adipose tissue and is involved in appetite control and energy expenditure. Although the absence of leptin leads to obesity and insulin resistance, most obese patients have elevated leptin levels but do not respond to the appetite suppressing and other effects of the peptide [146, 147]. Mutations of the leptin receptor (Ob-R) are associated with obesity in the *db/db* mouse [148] and the Zucker (*fa/fa*) rat [149] and leptin deficiency occurs in obese (*ob/ob*) mice [150] while the treatment of patients [151, 152] and animals [150] with recombinant leptin reduces body weight and improves serum lipid levels.

Serum triglyceride levels and blood glucose handling also improved in women with lipodystrophy and leptin deficiency indicating that leptin may alter lipid metabolism and prevent lipotoxicity [153]. Animal studies demonstrate that leptin promotes lipid oxidation. In rat adipocytes leptin reduces insulin's' lipogenic effect by: 1) inhibiting insulin binding to its receptor [154], 2) increasing adipose and non-adipose tissue β-oxidation, and, 3) decreasing adipose tissue triglyceride content without elevating circulating free fatty acids (Figure 6) [74]. This reduction in serum fatty acid levels will also counter the effect of insulin on lipogenesis [74, 154].

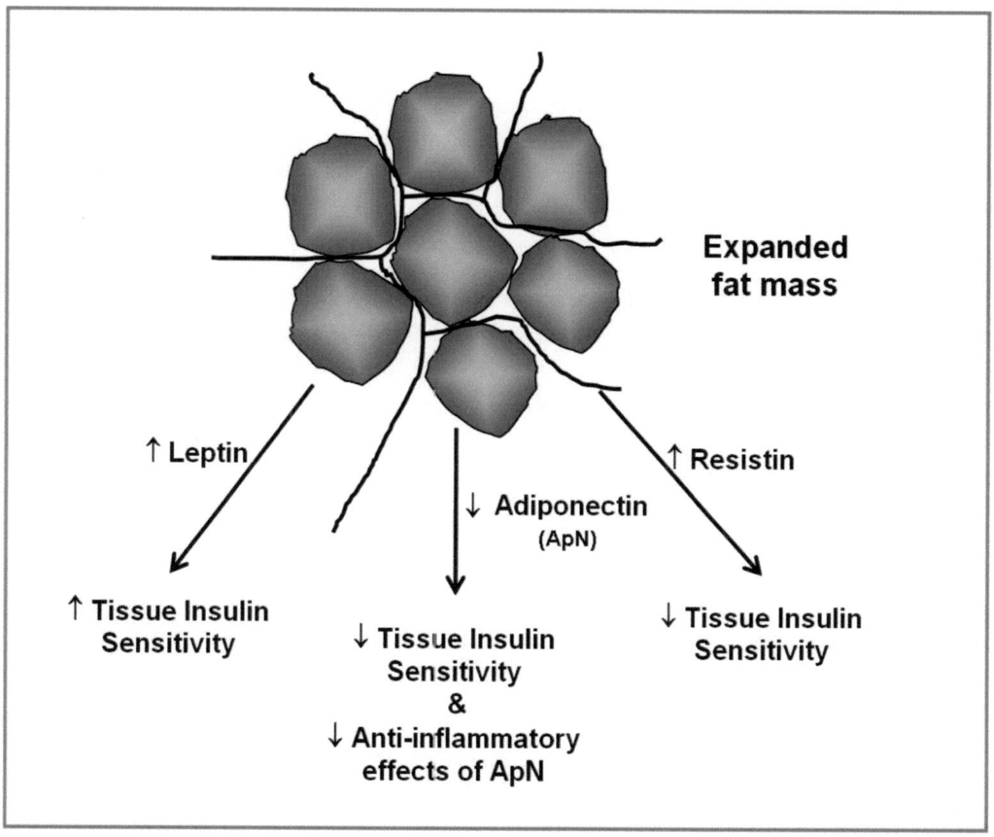

Figure 6. A simplified illustration to demonstrate the effects of adipocytokines on tissue insulin sensitivity and inflammation.

There is a strong association between leptin deficiency/resistance and lipotoxicity [155]. The lipid lowering effects of leptin in heart muscle was demonstrated in a study where 24 hour high fat feeding of mice was associated with cardiac lipid accumulation in animals with low leptin levels but not those with high plasma leptin levels [156]. Leptin administration decreases cardiac muscle lipotoxicity in a subsequent study by this group [157].

Leptin administration to the perfusate of isolated rat hearts perfused with palmitate and glucose significantly increased fatty acid oxidation and reduced intramyocardial triglyceride content without increasing cardiac work. This was accompanied by increased myocardial oxygen consumption and reduced cardiac efficiency [143]. The significance of leptin in metabolism is further highlighted in genetic models such as the leptin deficient *ob/ob* mouse and the leptin resistant *db/db* mouse that has a loss-of-function mutation on the leptin receptor. These animals are obese, insulin resistant and display excess intramyocardial lipid accumulation. They are also more prone to increased cardiomyocyte apoptosis and cardiac dysfunction than their control littermates [158-162].

Circulating adiponectin levels are reduced in obesity, insulin resistance and diabetes and correlate with the extent of insulin resistance and hyperinsulinaemia [163-165]. It is synthesised by adipocytes, skeletal muscle, heart muscle and endothelial cells [166] and is a key adipocytokine in the regulation of metabolism. It is considered to be an anti-diabetic, anti-inflammatory and anti-atherogenic agent with adiponectin deficient animals becoming glucose intolerant, insulin resistance and hyperleptinaemic [167, 168]. Studies utilising adiponectin replacement therapy have demonstrated its ability to decrease dyslipidaemia [169] and improve insulin sensitivity (Figure 6) [170-172].

Adiponectin acts via phosphorylation of 5'adenosine monophosphate-activated protein kinase (AMPK) to influence insulin sensitivity and fatty acid and glucose utilisation [172, 173]. Its action is mediated through the AdipoR1 and AdipoR2 receptors [170] that are both expressed in cardiac tissue [174]. Receptor activation is associated with modulation of AMPK, PI3K, p38 MAP kinase and extracellular signal-regulated kinase (Erk) 1/2 MAP kinase [175-177].

Resistin is secreted from white adipose tissue but is also expressed in other tissues [178]. It was given its name because it was originally shown to counter the effects of insulin by suppressing insulin signalling [179]. Over-expression of resistin is associated with dyslipidaemia and insulin resistance [180, 181] and inhibition of glucose uptake in cardiomyocytes [182]. In humans plasma resistin levels are closely correlated to insulin resistance irrespective of body weight [183]. However, these observations are not supported by two animal studies that found that resistin levels were not a good predictor of insulin resistance when corrected for body mass index (BMI) [184, 185]. In both high fat diet and genetic mutation induced obesity, resistin levels were closely associated with body weight with obese animals having significantly elevated resistin levels [179]. The exact role of resistin in insulin resistance is however poorly understood and unresolved.

8. Effects of myocardial insulin resistance on myocardial metabolism, mechanical function and tolerance to ischaemia and reperfusion

The heart utilises glucose, fatty acids and lactate as fuels for the production of ATP. Cardiac metabolism is under the control of several hormones with insulin being a key regulator of glucose, fatty acid and lactate metabolism. Changes in myocardial insulin sensitivity disrupt the hearts' normal substrate metabolism and potentially decrease mechanical function and myocardial tolerance to ischaemia/reperfusion.

8.1. Myocardial metabolism

The heart is a dynamic organ, constantly requiring energy in the form of ATP in order to meet its homeostatic and contractile demands. This is achieved through a constant supply of oxidizable substrates from the circulation. The most important substrates utilized by the heart are: fatty acids, glucose and lactate. Although the adult heart is capable of oxidizing a variety of substrates, the majority of ATP (60-70%) generated by the heart originates from the oxidation of fatty acids [186, 187]. However, in the presence of elevated glucose and insulin levels as occurs immediately following a meal, 60-70% of ATP may be derived from glucose metabolism [188].

Circulating fatty acids are taken up by the heart either in their free form (as free fatty acids (FFAs)) bound to albumin, or they can be released from the triglyceride component of chylomicrons or very-low-density-lipoproteins (VLDL) [189]. The concentration of fatty acids present in blood greatly dictates their uptake and metabolism by the heart [190]. Under normal physiological conditions, long chain fatty acids (LCFAs) are the principal fatty acids oxidized by the heart [191]. The entry of LCFAs across the sarcolemma into the cytoplasm of the cardiomyocyte occurs though passive diffusion or membrane protein mediated transport, the latter accounting for the majority of fatty acid translocation to the cytosol [192]. This membrane protein mediated transport is facilitated by fatty acid translocase (FAT)/CD36, plasma membrane fatty acid binding protein (FABPpm) and fatty acid transport protein (FATP) [192]. Once inside the cell, non-esterified LCFAs are transported via cytoplasmic heart-type FABPs through the cytoplasm to the location where they will be utilized [193-195]. LCFAs are then esterified by acyl-CoA synthetase to form long chain fatty acyl-CoA's (LCFA-CoA) [55]. LCFA-CoAs can be stored in intracellular lipid pools where they can be converted to additional lipid intermediates (triglycerides, diacylglycerol (DAG) or ceramide), or are transported to the mitochondria where they undergo β-oxidation.

Glucose enters the cardiomyocyte through either the basal uptake glucose transporter, GLUT1, or via the insulin dependent glucose transporter, GLUT4 [196]. GLUT4 is stored in cytoplasmic vesicles which are recruited to the sarcolemma in response to insulin stimulation or cardiac contraction. Glucose itself can also induce GLUT4 translocation with this and insulin stimulated translocation determining the glucose flux rate into the cardiomyocyte [197]. Inside the cell hexokinase converts glucose to glucose-6-phosphate which can be stored as glycogen (after conversion by glycogen synthase) or it can undergo glycolysis to yield pyruvate and ATP. During adequate myocardial oxygen availability pyruvate is transported into the mitochondria via a mitochondrial monocarboxylate transporter [198] and subsequently oxidized by pyruvate dehydrogenase (PDH) to produce acetyl-CoA (reviewed by Stanley *et al.* [199]). During anaerobic conditions as occurs during myocardial ischaemia, pyruvate may be converted to lactate.

The rate of glucose oxidation is also influenced by fatty acid β-oxidation rates since hexokinase, PFK and PDH activity are all inhibited by various products of fatty acid metabolism (for a review see Hue and Taegtmeyer [200]). There is a delicate interplay in the utilisation of these two myocardial substrates which is intricately related to their circulating levels. The common endpoint where glucose and fatty acid metabolism converge is the production of acetyl-CoA which enters the tricarboxylic acid/Krebs cycle where it is used to generate ATP during oxidative phosphorylation [187, 201]. Alternatively the acetyl-CoA can be utilised in non-oxidative pathways for the production of triglycerides, DAG and ceramide.

8.2. Impact of myocardial insulin resistance on myocardial metabolism

The early onset of insulin resistance in obesity may be a physiological response to increased lipid availability leading to increased lipid utilisation and a reciprocal reduction in glucose metabolism. Chronic dysregulation of glucose uptake and metabolism by dyslipidaemia and inflammation may however induce pathological changes in cardiac metabolism that compromise cardiac morphology and mechanical function.

High fat feeding of C57BL/6 mice induces myocardial insulin resistance within 10 days. This insulin resistance was associated with reduced myocardial glucose uptake, PKB/Akt activity and GLUT4 protein levels and preceded and occurred independently of systemic insulin resistance [202]. With myocardial insulin resistance, fatty acid oxidation rates are normal or elevated, while glucose oxidation rates are normally reduced both in the presence or absence of insulin stimulation [5, 44, 45, 203-205]. Although a limited number of studies have reported similar myocardial fatty acid and glucose oxidation rates in obese, insulin resistant animals when compared to lean controls, they have all found that insulin stimulated myocardial glycolytic flux rates remain suppressed with insulin resistance [89, 206]. In humans similar increases in myocardial fatty acid metabolism were reported in obese men and women. Gender however also played and important role in determining the impact of obesity of glucose and fatty acid uptake and utilization [207]. Women were less prone to obesity induced dysregulation of myocardial metabolism than their obese male counterparts. These gender based differences in myocardial metabolism in response to obesity may translate to differences in the development of obesity-related cardiovascular diseases.

8.3. Effect of insulin resistance on cardiac mechanical function

Increased lipid uptake and oxidation as seen with insulin resistance potentially leads to cellular lipid intermediate accumulation, excessive mitochondrial or peroxisomal ROS generation and functional derangement in the heart [71]. This is well demonstrated by a study showing that cardiac specific PPARα over-expression which increases cardiac lipid oxidation causes metabolic derangements and leads to adverse structural and function changes in the heart [208]

Pre-diabetic (insulin resistant) obese Zucker rats display cardiac dysfunction [47]. These observations were corroborated in obese insulin resistant mice (ob/ob and db/db) that had increased myocardial lipid oxidation rates, decreased glucose oxidation rates and decreased cardiac efficiency. These changes were also associated with systolic dysfunction when compared to lean insulin sensitive littermates [45].

Although genetic models of obesity do not accurately resemble the phenotype of human obesity, the recent development of a number of models of diet-induced obesity have contributed to a better understanding of the impact of obesity and insulin resistance on myocardial function. High fat feeding induced insulin resistance in C57BL/6 mice also causes cardiac remodelling and systolic dysfunction [202]. The authors and other research groups have however also shown that rodent models of diet-induced obesity with insulin resistance have either normal [90, 203, 205, 209, 210] or compromised [110, 203, 204, 211, 212] cardiac mechanical function. It is currently not possible to conclusively attribute the cardiac dysfunction reported in these studies to myocardial insulin resistance since there are several studies that have reported normal cardiac function in animal models with insulin resistance [90, 203, 205, 209, 210].

Reduced cardiac efficiency possibly contributes to cardiac dysfunction in obesity, insulin resistance and diabetes [44, 45, 213]. Animals [44, 45, 162, 213] and humans [95] that are obese and insulin resistant or diabetic have increased myocardial oxygen consumption which reflects a decreased cardiac efficiency as determined by the myocardial work to myocardial oxygen consumption ratio [214]. Mitochondria isolated from obese insulin resistant mice have reduced oxidative capacity, and display fatty acid induced uncoupling of mitochondrial oxygen consumption and ATP production which is evident from the reduced ATP-to-O ratios [162, 213]. This data from human and rodent studies also implicate impaired mitochondrial energetics in the cardiac dysfunction associated with obesity and insulin resistance. Recent epidemiological evidence points to an important mediatory role for insulin resistance in the development of obesity related congestive heart failure [215].

8.4. Effect of dyslipidaemia and insulin resistance on myocardial tolerance to ischaemia/reperfusion

A key feature of myocardial ischaemia is the reduced oxygen and substrate availability that results in lower mitochondrial oxidative phosphorylation rates. Ischaemia essentially disrupts the tightly coupled ATP breakdown and re-synthesis equilibrium that exists during normoxia and leads to an ATP deficit. Cellular ATP becomes depleted with the extent of this depletion being dependent on the duration and severity of ischaemia [216].

Although oxidative metabolism is reduced during ischaemia, reperfusion after ischaemia is associated with an initial increase in glycolytic flux rate which quickly declines to normal levels [217]. Despite glycolysis only accountings for a small amount of the total ATP production under aerobic conditions, glycolytically generated ATP becomes invaluable in the maintenance of cellular ion pump function and ion homeostasis and the reduction of myocardial damage during mild ischaemia [218]. While glycolytically produced ATP may aid in maintaining ion homeostasis during ischaemia, it is insufficient for the maintenance of myocardial contractile function [218]. Under conditions of severe ischaemia in the absence of a glucose and oxygen, myocardial glycogen stores undergoing glycolysis do not only contribute to the ATP synthesised, but greatly increase cytosolic proton accumulation and a decline in intracellular pH [219]. Despite its potential adverse effect on pH, elevated glycogen levels at the onset of myocardial ischaemia may be important in maintaining tissue ATP levels since it has been associated with improved functional recovery after ischaemia [220].

Despite myocardial ischaemia decreasing mitochondrial substrate oxidation, fatty acid oxidation predominates during ischaemia and subsequent early reperfusion [221]. During early ischaemia there is a transient increase in anaerobic glycolysis while glucose oxidation decreases [199, 221-224]. Under these conditions normal or increased glucose uptake (under the influence of insulin) may be important for the delivery of glycolytic ATP to maintain ion homeostasis. Hearts from animal models of obesity and insulin resistance [211], isolated insulin resistance [225] and diabetes [226] have a reduced tolerance to ischaemia and reperfusion and suffer more severe ischaemia/reperfusion injury. Myocardial insulin resistance potentially decreases myocardial tolerance to ischaemia by decreasing glucose uptake, glycogen synthesis and glycolysis which all play a critical role in the delivery of ATP for cellular homeostasis in the ischaemic/reperfused heart.

Although fatty acids are predominantly oxidized by the ischaemic heart, the preference for fatty acid oxidation as occurs under dyslipidaemic conditions also has adverse effects on the ischaemic and reperfused heart. The mitochondrion generates 12% less ATP per oxygen molecule through the oxidation of fatty acids compared to glucose oxidation during normoxia [187]. Increased fatty acid oxidation consequently reduces cardiac efficiency during ischaemia and subsequent reperfusion. During reperfusion the glycolytic flux rate exceeds glucose oxidation rates which remains suppressed due to increased fatty acid oxidation during reperfusion [224, 227]. This fatty acid induced uncoupling of glucose oxidation from glycolysis results in an accumulation of hydrogen ions which can damage the heart and affect post ischaemic function [199, 228-230]. These detrimental effects of increased fatty acid β-oxidation during both ischaemia and reperfusion would be expected to be pronounced in dyslipidaemia (as occurs in obesity and high fructose feeding) and insulin resistance and exacerbate ischaemic injury.

Pharmacological inhibition of myocardial fatty acid oxidation prior to the onset of, or during reperfusion results in increased glucose oxidation and improved cardiac functional recovery following the ischaemic episode [224, 227]. Hearts from prediabetic obese Zucker rats have reduced GLUT4 expression, reduced glucose uptake and larger reductions in tissue ATP levels during low-flow ischaemia. These changes are associated with poorer post-ischaemic functional recoveries when compared to their lean control littermates [231]. Treating these rats with rosiglitazone (the insulin sensitizer) normalized myocardial total GLUT4 protein expression, myocardial ischaemic substrate metabolism and improved reperfusion functional recovery.

8.5. The effect of insulin resistance on myocardial pro-survival signalling and ischaemic tolerance

The ability of the heart to withstand injury during ischaemia and reperfusion is not only dependent on myocardial metabolism but also upon the expression and functionality of its intrinsic pro-survival signalling pathways. Investigations into cardioprotection with preconditioning and postconditioning has revealed common signalling elements that transduce protective stimuli and converge on mitochondrial targets [232-234]. These stimuli recruit paths comprising cell surface G-protein coupled receptors (GPCRs), signalling kinase networks (*e.g.* PI3K-Akt-eNOS, Erk1/2, PKC, p38-MAPK, Glycogen synthase kinase 3 beta (GSK3β)) that have been dubbed the Reperfusion Injury Salvage Kinases (RISKs), and mitochondrial components that may represent end-effectors. These end-effectors include K_{ATP} channels and the mitochondrial permeability transition pore - mPTP (Figure. 7). Central to the RISK pathways is protein kinase B (PKB)/Akt which is not only key to myocardial insulin signalling [188] and physiological hypertrophy/remodelling [235] but is also considered a pro-survival/anti-apoptotic kinase in the context of myocardial ischaemia/reperfusion.

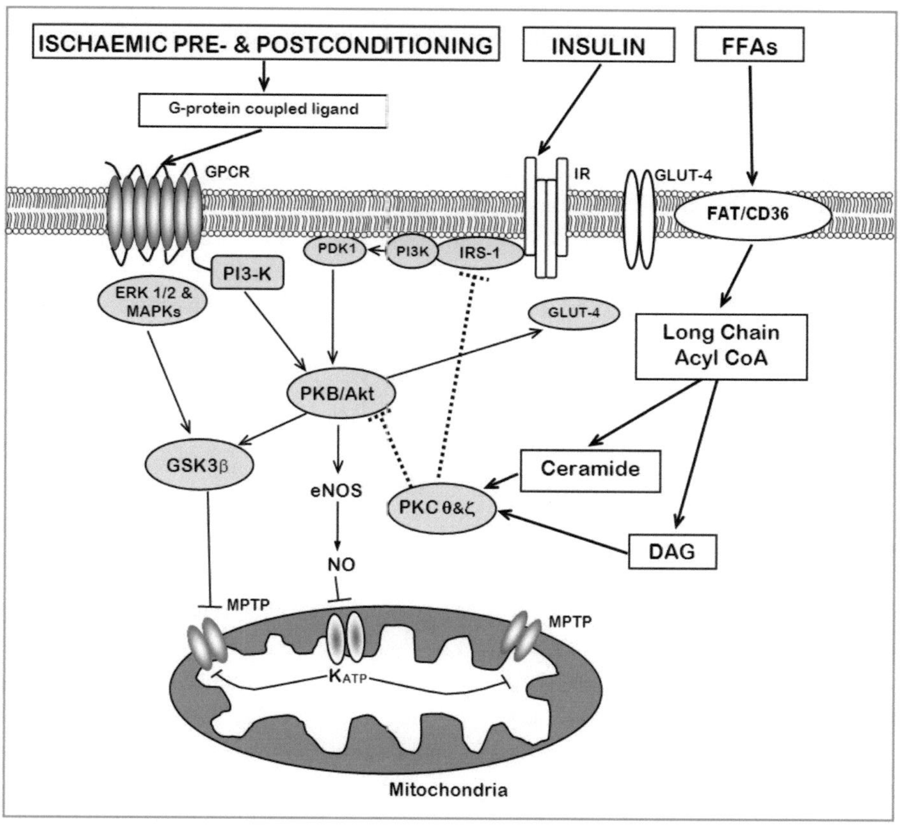

Figure 7. An illustration demonstrating the pivotal role of PKB/Akt in the RISK and insulin signalling pathways and the possible impact of dyslipidaemia and insulin resistance on these signalling pathways. Broken line represents the proposed mechanism linking insulin resistance with PKB/Akt inhibition/inactivation and Reperfusion Injury Salvage Kinase (RISK) pathway dysfunction.

Insulin regulates cardiac metabolism, growth and mitogen-activated protein kinase (MAPK) pathways through pivotal PKB/Akt. Dyslipidaemia induced insulin resistance which is characterized by PI3K/Akt dysregulation possibly also negatively influences the functionality of the RISK pathway in the heart during ischaemia/reperfusion.

Early experimental evidence has emerged to support a role for obesity with insulin resistance in RISK pathway dysfunction. Wagner and co-workers [236] have shown loss of preconditioning in a rat model of established metabolic syndrome. In the leptin-deficient (*ob/ob)* mouse cardiac benefit from postconditioning is impaired [237], while there is also evidence of failed preconditioning in obese insulin-resistant rats [238]. Failure of a variety of cardioprotective interventions involving multiple and varied triggers, implicates dysfunction of the signalling paths of the RISK pathway that are common to these interventions. This is also supported by the recent findings of Bouhidel and co-workers [237] who reported impaired phosphorylation of Akt, Erk1/2 and p70S6K1 in *ob/ob* mice while others [236] presented evidence of impaired Erk1/2 activation and failure to phosphorylate and inactivate GSK3β. Ineffective protection in obese insulin resistance rats is also associated with impaired activation of the mitochondrial K_{ATP} channel [238]. All early indications suggest that distinct changes in intrinsic cardioprotective signalling occur in myocardial insulin resistance.

9. Interventions and therapy for the treatment of insulin resistance

Compelling scientific evidence indicates that obesity and/or lipogenic diets that lead to dyslipidaemia promote insulin resistance. Besides the dyslipidaemia, abnormal RAS activity and perturbations in adipocytokine levels also contribute to tissue insulin insensitivity. The primary goal of therapy for the treatment of insulin resistance should therefore be to prevent or reduce obesity (adipose tissue expansion) and dyslipidaemia. In addition to normalising circulating lipid levels, weight loss would normalise adipose tissue content and its associated pro-inflammatory cytokine and adipocytokine levels and ultimately improve insulin resistance. Since there is a direct correlation between obesity and RAS over-activation, weight loss and/or RAS inhibition has the potential to attenuate the adverse effects of abnormal RAS activity on tissue insulin signalling.

9.1. Lifestyle changes: Physical activity and diet

Maintaining normal body weight or reducing body weight in overweight patients is the preferred approach for the prevention or treatment of the underlying causes of insulin resistance. Regular physical activity aimed at balancing caloric intake with caloric expenditure is recommended to maintain body weight. To reduce body weight caloric intake should be reduced and caloric expenditure increased until the desired body weight has been achieved. Current recommendations are to do 30 minutes moderate intensity exercise daily in order to maintain normal body weight and reduce the risk of developing medical conditions such as cancer, insulin resistance, diabetes and cardiovascular disease [239].

In addition to regular exercise to maintain normal body weight or promote weight loss, individuals with a genetic predisposition to obesity, insulin resistance and diabetes should carefully manage their diet and reduce their intake of refined sugars, trans- and saturated fats and cholesterol and increase their consumption of grains, and fruit and vegetables [240]. Based on recent evidence provided by studies investigating the potential role of fructose in dyslipidaemia and metabolic diseases [24, 27, 41], it would also be prudent to avoid the overconsumption of fructose rich foods and beverages.

The larger the BMI loss achieved through exercise and/or dietary restriction, the larger the metabolic improvements that are achieved. Weight loss improves lipid profiles and blood glucose levels in metabolic syndrome patients [241] with a weight loss of more than 10% reversing metabolic disorders in two-thirds of metabolic syndrome patients studied [242]. These patients no longer met the criteria for metabolic syndrome. Lifestyle interventions also decreases the progression from insulin resistance to type-2 diabetes. In the US Diabetes Prevention Program, interventions aimed at reducing body weight by 7% succeeded in preventing progression from insulin resistance to type- 2 diabetes by 58% [243]. In this study 38% of the patients with metabolic syndrome at entry into the study had a reversal of metabolic syndrome with body weight loss.

9.2. Drug therapy that improves insulin sensitivity

Although lifestyle changes should remain the therapy of choice for the reduction of body weight and normalisation of metabolic disorders, not all patients respond to lifestyle changes to the same extent. In many cases lifestyle changes fail to achieve the intended objective of adequate weight loss. Under these circumstances pharmacological interventions have to be considered. Several drugs have been developed to improve lipid profiles and insulin sensitivity/action but have been disappointing and have in some cases had adverse side effects.

9.2.1. Lipid lowering drugs

Dyslipidaemia which presents as elevated circulating triglycerides and LDL-cholesterol and low HDL-cholesterol can be treated with statins (3-hydroxy-3-methylglutaryl-coenzyme A (HMG-CoA) reductase inhibitors) that reduce levels of all forms of Apo B containing lipoproteins [244-247]. These drugs reduce the conversion of acetyl-CoA to mevalonate and the eventual synthesis of cholesterol in the liver by blocking HMG-CoA reductase. There are several studies that have demonstrated that statins (simvastatin and atorvastatin) improve plasma triglyceride and glycosylated haemoglobin in non insulin dependent diabetics [246]. Fluvastatin also improved lipid profiles and insulin resistance in nondiabetic dyslipidaemic patients. These researchers however concluded that the insulin sensitising effects of fluvastatin were not related to its triglyceride lowering effects [247].

Another class of lipid lowering drug that has achieved satisfactory results is the fibrates that activate peroxisome proliferator-activated receptor (PPARs) and facilitate lipid metabolism. In humans, fibrates lower circulating triglyceride and LDL-C levels [248, 249] and elevate HDL-C levels [249]. PPARα agonists possibly improve lipid profiles by increasing the synthesis of both apolipoprotein A-I [248] and A-II [250] which would assist in increasing HDL-cholesterol while reducing apolipoprotein B which is a major lipoprotein constituent of LDL-cholesterol. PPARα agonists also increase hepatic mitochondrial β-oxidation which reduces hepatic free fatty acids that are an essential component of VLDL and LDL-cholesterol.

Since PPARα agonists have repeatedly been demonstrated to have both systemic and tissue specific insulin sensitizing effects [251-254] their potential for the treatment of insulin resistance and diabetes is encouraging. The insulin sensitising effects of the fibrates probably relate to their lipid lowering effects since a PPARα agonist significantly increases hepatic and skeletal muscle insulin receptor and IRS-1 tyrosine phosphorylation, while increasing IRS-associated PI3K activity in obese (*ob/ob*) mice [252]. These insulin sensitising effects were accompanied by reduced hepatic, skeletal muscle [252] and heart muscle [255] lipid accumulation.

Combination therapy using statins and fibrates has been an attractive possibility but the results have been disappointing. The fibrate gemfibrozil in combination with statins has been associated with increased risk of myopathy [256]. It has however been proposed that the adverse effects of gemfibrozil and statin combination therapy may be due to a pharmacological interaction between these two drugs and that other fenofibrates may be more suitable for combination therapy with statins [257].

9.2.2. Insulin sensitizers

The two most promising insulin sensitizers are metformin and the glitazones. Metformin decreases hepatic gluconeogenesis and triglyceride production which in turn enhances insulin sensitivity [258]. Metformin reduced the progression of insulin resistance (pre-diabetic) to type-2 diabetes in the Diabetes Prevention Program [243].

Thiazolidinediones (TZDs) are PPARγ agonists that regulate insulin sensitivity in the liver, muscle and adipose tissue by increasing fatty acid oxidation and decreasing fatty acid synthesis [258]. TZDs are also believed to have anti-inflammatory effects. Pioglitazone was used in the ACT-NOW study in which it improved HDL-cholesterol and triglyceride levels and reduced the incidence of type-2 diabetes by 78% in prediabetic patients followed up over 2 years [259]. The Pioglitazone In Prevention Of Diabetes (PIPOD) study demonstrated that pioglitazone reduced the incidence of diabetes in premenopausal women [260]. It similarly improves insulin sensitivity and reduces both blood FFA and triglycerides levels in obese non-diabetic patients [261]. The usefulness of pioglitazone for the management of insulin sensitivity is however limited since it promotes fluid retention which increases risk of heart failure in certain patient populations with cardiovascular disease. In the diabetes reduction assessment with ramipril and rosiglitazone medication (DREAM) trial, rosiglitazone showed potential in preventing diabetes but appeared to increase the risk of heart failure [262].

9.2.3. RAS inhibitors or AT receptor blockers

Obesity and high fat feeding increases both systemic and adipose tissue RAS activity [110, 112-115]. As discussed previously in this chapter, the most compelling evidence for a role for the RAS in the aetiology of insulin resistance comes from studies using ACE inhibitors and AT receptor antagonists to control blood pressure. Both these therapies are associated with reduced risk of developing insulin resistance and type-2 diabetes in patients [119, 122, 263-266] and in rodent models of obesity and insulin resistance [127, 128]. Although these antihypertensives are not prescribed for the treatment of abnormal RAS activity, they potentially improve insulin sensitivity in a patient population that is at high risk of cardiovascular disease due to their hypertension.

9.2.4. Anti-inflammatory therapy

Several lines of evidence implicate chronic inflammation in the aetiology of insulin resistance. Obesity is associated with elevated circulating cytokines and C-reactive protein which can be normalised by weight loss [267]. Although no drugs are currently available to treat chronic systemic inflammation, the use of lipid lowering drugs have been associated with reduced C-reactive protein levels in patients [267-269]. These drugs are not prescribed to specifically reduce inflammation but may contribute to improved insulin sensitivity by improving dyslipidaemia and decreasing its stimulation of β-oxidation and ROS generation. Increase ROS generation potentially increase cytokine synthesis and release in certain organs (Figure 2).

Author details

Eugene F. du Toit and Daniel G. Donner
Heart Foundation Research Center, Griffith Health Institute, School of Medical Science, Griffith University, Gold Coast, Queensland, Australia

10. References

[1] Stefan, N., K. Kantartzis, and H.U. Haring, *Causes and metabolic consequences of Fatty liver.* Endocr Rev, 2008. 29(7): p. 939-60.
[2] Najjar, S.M., et al., *Insulin acutely decreases hepatic fatty acid synthase activity.* Cell Metab, 2005. 2(1): p. 43-53.
[3] Reaven, G.M., *Banting lecture 1988. Role of insulin resistance in human disease.* Diabetes, 1988. 37(12): p. 1595-607.
[4] Reaven, G.M., *Pathophysiology of insulin resistance in human disease.* Physiol Rev, 1995. 75(3): p. 473-86.
[5] Zhang, L., et al., *Role of fatty acid uptake and fatty acid beta-oxidation in mediating insulin resistance in heart and skeletal muscle.* Biochim Biophys Acta, 2010. 1801(1): p. 1-22.
[6] White, M.F. and C.R. Kahn, *The insulin signaling system.* J Biol Chem, 1994. 269(1): p. 1-4.
[7] Myers, M.G., Jr., et al., *IRS-1 activates phosphatidylinositol 3'-kinase by associating with src homology 2 domains of p85.* Proc Natl Acad Sci U S A, 1992. 89(21): p. 10350-4.

[8] Yonezawa, K., et al., *Insulin-dependent formation of a complex containing an 85-kDa subunit of phosphatidylinositol 3-kinase and tyrosine-phosphorylated insulin receptor substrate 1.* J Biol Chem, 1992. 267(36): p. 25958-65.

[9] Shepherd, P.R., D.J. Withers, and K. Siddle, *Phosphoinositide 3-kinase: the key switch mechanism in insulin signalling.* Biochem J, 1998. 333 (Pt 3): p. 471-90.

[10] Chang, L., S.H. Chiang, and A.R. Saltiel, *Insulin signaling and the regulation of glucose transport.* Mol Med, 2004. 10(7-12): p. 65-71.

[11] Alessi, D.R., et al., *Mechanism of activation of protein kinase B by insulin and IGF-1.* EMBO J, 1996. 15(23): p. 6541-51.

[12] Alessi, D.R. and P. Cohen, *Mechanism of activation and function of protein kinase B.* Curr Opin Genet Dev, 1998. 8(1): p. 55-62.

[13] Foran, P.G., et al., *Protein kinase B stimulates the translocation of GLUT4 but not GLUT1 or transferrin receptors in 3T3-L1 adipocytes by a pathway involving SNAP-23, synaptobrevin-2, and/or cellubrevin.* J Biol Chem, 1999. 274(40): p. 28087-95.

[14] Clarke, J.F., et al., *Inhibition of the translocation of GLUT1 and GLUT4 in 3T3-L1 cells by the phosphatidylinositol 3-kinase inhibitor, wortmannin.* Biochem J, 1994. 300 (Pt 3): p. 631-5.

[15] Summers, S.A., et al., *Regulation of insulin-stimulated glucose transporter GLUT4 translocation and Akt kinase activity by ceramide.* Mol Cell Biol, 1998. 18(9): p. 5457-64.

[16] Rider, M.H. and L. Hue, *Activation of rat heart phosphofructokinase-2 by insulin in vivo.* FEBS Lett, 1984. 176(2): p. 484-8.

[17] Hue, L. and M.H. Rider, *Role of fructose 2,6-bisphosphate in the control of glycolysis in mammalian tissues.* Biochem J, 1987. 245(2): p. 313-24.

[18] Hue, L., et al., *Insulin and ischemia stimulate glycolysis by acting on the same targets through different and opposing signaling pathways.* J Mol Cell Cardiol, 2002. 34(9): p. 1091-7.

[19] Luiken, J.J., et al., *Insulin stimulates long-chain fatty acid utilization by rat cardiac myocytes through cellular redistribution of FAT/CD36.* Diabetes, 2002. 51(10): p. 3113-9.

[20] Saddik, M., et al., *Acetyl-CoA carboxylase regulation of fatty acid oxidation in the heart.* J Biol Chem, 1993. 268(34): p. 25836-45.

[21] Kahn, S.E., R.L. Hull, and K.M. Utzschneider, *Mechanisms linking obesity to insulin resistance and type 2 diabetes.* Nature, 2006. 444(7121): p. 840-6.

[22] Rutledge, A.C. and K. Adeli, *Fructose and the metabolic syndrome: pathophysiology and molecular mechanisms.* Nutr Rev, 2007. 65(6 Pt 2): p. S13-23.

[23] Tappy, L. and K.A. Le, *Metabolic effects of fructose and the worldwide increase in obesity.* Physiol Rev, 2010. 90(1): p. 23-46.

[24] Tappy, L., et al., *Fructose and metabolic diseases: new findings, new questions.* Nutrition, 2010. 26(11-12): p. 1044-9.

[25] Boden, G., *Obesity, insulin resistance and free fatty acids.* Curr Opin Endocrinol Diabetes Obes, 2011. 18(2): p. 139-43.

[26] Kershaw, E.E. and J.S. Flier, *Adipose tissue as an endocrine organ.* J Clin Endocrinol Metab, 2004. 89(6): p. 2548-56.

[27] Dekker, M.J., et al., *Fructose: a highly lipogenic nutrient implicated in insulin resistance, hepatic steatosis, and the metabolic syndrome.* Am J Physiol Endocrinol Metab, 2010. 299(5): p. E685-94.

[28] Kannel, W.B., T. Gordon, and W.P. Castelli, *Obesity, lipids, and glucose intolerance. The Framingham Study.* Am J Clin Nutr, 1979. 32(6): p. 1238-45.

[29] Folli, F., et al., *Crosstalk between insulin and angiotensin II signalling systems.* Exp Clin Endocrinol Diabetes, 1999. 107(2): p. 133-9.

[30] Kalupahana, N.S. and N. Moustaid-Moussa, *The renin-angiotensin system: a link between obesity, inflammation and insulin resistance.* Obes Rev, 2012. 13(2): p. 136-49.

[31] Ryden, M. and P. Arner, *Tumour necrosis factor-alpha in human adipose tissue -- from signalling mechanisms to clinical implications.* J Intern Med, 2007. 262(4): p. 431-8.

[32] Bizeau, M.E. and M.J. Pagliassotti, *Hepatic adaptations to sucrose and fructose.* Metabolism, 2005. 54(9): p. 1189-201.

[33] Stanhope, K.L. and P.J. Havel, *Fructose consumption: potential mechanisms for its effects to increase visceral adiposity and induce dyslipidemia and insulin resistance.* Curr Opin Lipidol, 2008. 19(1): p. 16-24.

[34] Faeh, D., et al., *Effect of fructose overfeeding and fish oil administration on hepatic de novo lipogenesis and insulin sensitivity in healthy men.* Diabetes, 2005. 54(7): p. 1907-13.

[35] Chong, M.F., B.A. Fielding, and K.N. Frayn, *Mechanisms for the acute effect of fructose on postprandial lipemia.* Am J Clin Nutr, 2007. 85(6): p. 1511-20.

[36] Matsuzaka, T., et al., *Insulin-independent induction of sterol regulatory element-binding protein-1c expression in the livers of streptozotocin-treated mice.* Diabetes, 2004. 53(3): p. 560-9.

[37] Nagai, Y., et al., *Amelioration of high fructose-induced metabolic derangements by activation of PPARalpha.* Am J Physiol Endocrinol Metab, 2002. 282(5): p. E1180-90.

[38] Adiels, M., et al., *Overproduction of large VLDL particles is driven by increased liver fat content in man.* Diabetologia, 2006. 49(4): p. 755-65.

[39] Stanhope, K.L., et al., *Twenty-four-hour endocrine and metabolic profiles following consumption of high-fructose corn syrup-, sucrose-, fructose-, and glucose-sweetened beverages with meals.* Am J Clin Nutr, 2008. 87(5): p. 1194-203.

[40] Taghibiglou, C., et al., *Mechanisms of hepatic very low density lipoprotein overproduction in insulin resistance. Evidence for enhanced lipoprotein assembly, reduced intracellular ApoB degradation, and increased microsomal triglyceride transfer protein in a fructose-fed hamster model.* J Biol Chem, 2000. 275(12): p. 8416-25.

[41] Le, K.A., et al., *Fructose overconsumption causes dyslipidemia and ectopic lipid deposition in healthy subjects with and without a family history of type 2 diabetes.* Am J Clin Nutr, 2009. 89(6): p. 1760-5.

[42] Wildman, R.P., *Healthy obesity.* Curr Opin Clin Nutr Metab Care, 2009. 12(4): p. 438-43.

[43] Fabbrini, E., Magkos, F.,Mohammed, B.S., Pietka, T., Abumrad, N.A., Patterson, B.W., Okunade, A., Klein, S., *Intrahepatic fat, not visceral fat, is linked with metabolic complications of obesity.* Proceedings of the National Academy of Sciences of the United States of America, 2009. 106 (36): p. 15430-15435.

[44] Mazumder, P.K., et al., *Impaired cardiac efficiency and increased fatty acid oxidation in insulin-resistant ob/ob mouse hearts.* Diabetes, 2004. 53(9): p. 2366-74.

[45] Buchanan, J., et al., *Reduced cardiac efficiency and altered substrate metabolism precedes the onset of hyperglycemia and contractile dysfunction in two mouse models of insulin resistance and obesity.* Endocrinology, 2005. 146(12): p. 5341-9.

[46] Luiken, J.J., et al., *Increased rates of fatty acid uptake and plasmalemmal fatty acid transporters in obese Zucker rats.* J Biol Chem, 2001. 276(44): p. 40567-73.

[47] Young, M.E., et al., *Impaired long-chain fatty acid oxidation and contractile dysfunction in the obese Zucker rat heart.* Diabetes, 2002. 51(8): p. 2587-95.

[48] Coort, S.L., et al., *Increased FAT (fatty acid translocase)/CD36-mediated long-chain fatty acid uptake in cardiac myocytes from obese Zucker rats.* Biochem Soc Trans, 2004. 32(Pt 1): p. 83-5.

[49] Thakker, G.D., et al., *Effects of diet-induced obesity on inflammation and remodeling after myocardial infarction.* Am J Physiol Heart Circ Physiol, 2006. 291(5): p. H2504-14.

[50] Unger, R.H., *Lipotoxic diseases.* Annu Rev Med, 2002. 53: p. 319-36.

[51] Chess, D.J. and W.C. Stanley, *Role of diet and fuel overabundance in the development and progression of heart failure.* Cardiovasc Res, 2008. 79(2): p. 269-78.

[52] Chiu, H.C., et al., *A novel mouse model of lipotoxic cardiomyopathy.* J Clin Invest, 2001. 107(7): p. 813-22.

[53] Carley, A.N., et al., *Mechanisms responsible for enhanced fatty acid utilization by perfused hearts from type 2 diabetic db/db mice.* Arch Physiol Biochem, 2007. 113(2): p. 65-75.

[54] Koonen, D.P., et al., *Long-chain fatty acid uptake and FAT/CD36 translocation in heart and skeletal muscle.* Biochim Biophys Acta, 2005. 1736(3): p. 163-80.

[55] Luiken, J.J., et al., *Regulation of cardiac long-chain fatty acid and glucose uptake by translocation of substrate transporters.* Pflugers Arch, 2004. 448(1): p. 1-15.

[56] Chabowski, A., et al., *The subcellular compartmentation of fatty acid transporters is regulated differently by insulin and by AICAR.* FEBS Lett, 2005. 579(11): p. 2428-32.

[57] van Herpen, N.A. and V.B. Schrauwen-Hinderling, *Lipid accumulation in non-adipose tissue and lipotoxicity.* Physiol Behav, 2008. 94(2): p. 231-41.

[58] Turinsky, J., D.M. O'Sullivan, and B.P. Bayly, *1,2-Diacylglycerol and ceramide levels in insulin-resistant tissues of the rat in vivo.* J Biol Chem, 1990. 265(28): p. 16880-5.

[59] Ussher, J.R., et al., *Inhibition of de novo ceramide synthesis reverses diet-induced insulin resistance and enhances whole-body oxygen consumption.* Diabetes, 2010. 59(10): p. 2453-64.

[60] Yu, C., et al., *Mechanism by which fatty acids inhibit insulin activation of insulin receptor substrate-1 (IRS-1)-associated phosphatidylinositol 3-kinase activity in muscle.* J Biol Chem, 2002. 277(52): p. 50230-6.

[61] Jean-Baptiste, G., et al., *Lysophosphatidic acid mediates pleiotropic responses in skeletal muscle cells.* Biochem Biophys Res Commun, 2005. 335(4): p. 1155-62.

[62] Wang, X., et al., *Insulin resistance accelerates muscle protein degradation: Activation of the ubiquitin-proteasome pathway by defects in muscle cell signaling.* Endocrinology, 2006. 147(9): p. 4160-8.

[63] Schenk, S., M. Saberi, and J.M. Olefsky, *Insulin sensitivity: modulation by nutrients and inflammation.* J Clin Invest, 2008. 118(9): p. 2992-3002.

[64] Hannun, Y.A. and L.M. Obeid, *The Ceramide-centric universe of lipid-mediated cell regulation: stress encounters of the lipid kind.* J Biol Chem, 2002. 277(29): p. 25847-50.

[65] Merrill, A.H., Jr. and D.D. Jones, *An update of the enzymology and regulation of sphingomyelin metabolism.* Biochim Biophys Acta, 1990. 1044(1): p. 1-12.

[66] Kim, J.K., et al., *PKC-theta knockout mice are protected from fat-induced insulin resistance.* J Clin Invest, 2004. 114(6): p. 823-7.

[67] Hajduch, E., et al., *Ceramide impairs the insulin-dependent membrane recruitment of protein kinase B leading to a loss in downstream signalling in L6 skeletal muscle cells.* Diabetologia, 2001. 44(2): p. 173-83.

[68] Adams, J.M., 2nd, et al., *Ceramide content is increased in skeletal muscle from obese insulin-resistant humans.* Diabetes, 2004. 53(1): p. 25-31.

[69] Summers, S.A., *Ceramides in insulin resistance and lipotoxicity.* Prog Lipid Res, 2006. 45(1): p. 42-72.

[70] Holland, W.L., et al., *Inhibition of ceramide synthesis ameliorates glucocorticoid-, saturated-fat-, and obesity-induced insulin resistance.* Cell Metab, 2007. 5(3): p. 167-79.

[71] Zhou, Y.T., et al., *Lipotoxic heart disease in obese rats: implications for human obesity.* Proc Natl Acad Sci U S A, 2000. 97(4): p. 1784-9.

[72] Hickson-Bick, D.L., L.M. Buja, and J.B. McMillin, *Palmitate-mediated alterations in the fatty acid metabolism of rat neonatal cardiac myocytes.* J Mol Cell Cardiol, 2000. 32(3): p. 511-9.

[73] Katsuyama, K., et al., *Role of nuclear factor-kappaB activation in cytokine- and sphingomyelinase-stimulated inducible nitric oxide synthase gene expression in vascular smooth muscle cells.* Endocrinology, 1998. 139(11): p. 4506-12.

[74] Shimabukuro, M., et al., *Direct antidiabetic effect of leptin through triglyceride depletion of tissues.* Proc Natl Acad Sci U S A, 1997. 94(9): p. 4637-41.

[75] Ghafourifar, P., et al., *Mitochondrial nitric-oxide synthase stimulation causes cytochrome c release from isolated mitochondria. Evidence for intramitochondrial peroxynitrite formation.* J Biol Chem, 1999. 274(44): p. 31185-8.

[76] Garcia-Ruiz, C., et al., *Direct effect of ceramide on the mitochondrial electron transport chain leads to generation of reactive oxygen species. Role of mitochondrial glutathione.* J Biol Chem, 1997. 272(17): p. 11369-77.

[77] Heydrick, S.J., et al., *Enhanced stimulation of diacylglycerol and lipid synthesis by insulin in denervated muscle. Altered protein kinase C activity and possible link to insulin resistance.* Diabetes, 1991. 40(12): p. 1707-11.

[78] Avignon, A., et al., *Chronic activation of protein kinase C in soleus muscles and other tissues of insulin-resistant type II diabetic Goto-Kakizaki (GK), obese/aged, and obese/Zucker rats. A mechanism for inhibiting glycogen synthesis.* Diabetes, 1996. 45(10): p. 1396-404.

[79] Itani, S.I., et al., *Lipid-induced insulin resistance in human muscle is associated with changes in diacylglycerol, protein kinase C, and IkappaB-alpha.* Diabetes, 2002. 51(7): p. 2005-11.

[80] Itani, S.I., et al., *Involvement of protein kinase C in human skeletal muscle insulin resistance and obesity.* Diabetes, 2000. 49(8): p. 1353-8.

[81] Itani, S.I., et al., *Increased protein kinase C theta in skeletal muscle of diabetic patients.* Metabolism, 2001. 50(5): p. 553-7.

[82] Sebastian, D., et al., *CPT I overexpression protects L6E9 muscle cells from fatty acid-induced insulin resistance.* Am J Physiol Endocrinol Metab, 2007. 292(3): p. E677-86.

[83] Virkamaki, A., et al., *Intramyocellular lipid is associated with resistance to in vivo insulin actions on glucose uptake, antilipolysis, and early insulin signaling pathways in human skeletal muscle.* Diabetes, 2001. 50(10): p. 2337-43.

[84] Manco, M., et al., *Insulin resistance directly correlates with increased saturated fatty acids in skeletal muscle triglycerides.* Metabolism, 2000. 49(2): p. 220-4.

[85] Sinha, R., et al., *Assessment of skeletal muscle triglyceride content by (1)H nuclear magnetic resonance spectroscopy in lean and obese adolescents: relationships to insulin sensitivity, total body fat, and central adiposity.* Diabetes, 2002. 51(4): p. 1022-7.

[86] Boden, G., et al., *Effects of acute changes of plasma free fatty acids on intramyocellular fat content and insulin resistance in healthy subjects.* Diabetes, 2001. 50(7): p. 1612-7.

[87] Kelley, D.E., et al., *Interaction between glucose and free fatty acid metabolism in human skeletal muscle.* J Clin Invest, 1993. 92(1): p. 91-8.

[88] Griffin, M.E., et al., *Free fatty acid-induced insulin resistance is associated with activation of protein kinase C theta and alterations in the insulin signaling cascade.* Diabetes, 1999. 48(6): p. 1270-4.

[89] Atkinson, L.L., et al., *Potential mechanisms and consequences of cardiac triacylglycerol accumulation in insulin-resistant rats.* Am J Physiol Endocrinol Metab, 2003. 284(5): p. E923-30.

[90] Yan, J., et al., *Increased glucose uptake and oxidation in mouse hearts prevent high fatty acid oxidation but cause cardiac dysfunction in diet-induced obesity.* Circulation, 2009. 119(21): p. 2818-28.

[91] Kankaanpaa, M., et al., *Myocardial triglyceride content and epicardial fat mass in human obesity: relationship to left ventricular function and serum free fatty acid levels.* J Clin Endocrinol Metab, 2006. 91(11): p. 4689-95.

[92] Szczepaniak, L.S., et al., *Myocardial triglycerides and systolic function in humans: in vivo evaluation by localized proton spectroscopy and cardiac imaging.* Magn Reson Med, 2003. 49(3): p. 417-23.

[93] McGavock, J.M., et al., *Cardiac steatosis in diabetes mellitus: a 1H-magnetic resonance spectroscopy study.* Circulation, 2007. 116(10): p. 1170-5.

[94] Rijzewijk, L.J., et al., *Myocardial steatosis is an independent predictor of diastolic dysfunction in type 2 diabetes mellitus.* J Am Coll Cardiol, 2008. 52(22): p. 1793-9.

[95] Peterson, L.R., et al., *Effect of obesity and insulin resistance on myocardial substrate metabolism and efficiency in young women.* Circulation, 2004. 109(18): p. 2191-6.

[96] Lazar, M.A., *The humoral side of insulin resistance.* Nat Med, 2006. 12(1): p. 43-4.

[97] Weisberg, S.P., et al., *Obesity is associated with macrophage accumulation in adipose tissue.* J Clin Invest, 2003. 112(12): p. 1796-808.

[98] Li, Z. and A.M. Diehl, *Innate immunity in the liver.* Curr Opin Gastroenterol, 2003. 19(6): p. 565-71.

[99] Kewalramani, G., P.J. Bilan, and A. Klip, *Muscle insulin resistance: assault by lipids, cytokines and local macrophages.* Curr Opin Clin Nutr Metab Care, 2010. 13(4): p. 382-90.

[100] Boden, G., et al., *Free fatty acids produce insulin resistance and activate the proinflammatory nuclear factor-kappaB pathway in rat liver.* Diabetes, 2005. 54(12): p. 3458-65.

[101] Boden, G., *Fatty acid-induced inflammation and insulin resistance in skeletal muscle and liver.* Curr Diab Rep, 2006. 6(3): p. 177-81.

[102] Gao, Z., et al., *Inactivation of PKCtheta leads to increased susceptibility to obesity and dietary insulin resistance in mice.* Am J Physiol Endocrinol Metab, 2007. 292(1): p. E84-91.

[103] Shi, H., et al., *TLR4 links innate immunity and fatty acid-induced insulin resistance.* J Clin Invest, 2006. 116(11): p. 3015-25.

[104] Kosteli, A., et al., *Weight loss and lipolysis promote a dynamic immune response in murine adipose tissue.* J Clin Invest, 2010. 120(10): p. 3466-79.

[105] Hotamisligil, G.S., N.S. Shargill, and B.M. Spiegelman, *Adipose expression of tumor necrosis factor-alpha: direct role in obesity-linked insulin resistance.* Science, 1993. 259(5091): p. 87-91.

[106] Lebrun, P. and E. Van Obberghen, *SOCS proteins causing trouble in insulin action.* Acta Physiol (Oxf), 2008. 192(1): p. 29-36.

[107] Hirosumi, J., et al., *A central role for JNK in obesity and insulin resistance.* Nature, 2002. 420(6913): p. 333-6.

[108] Kim, H.J., et al., *Differential effects of interleukin-6 and -10 on skeletal muscle and liver insulin action in vivo.* Diabetes, 2004. 53(4): p. 1060-7.

[109] Ko, H.J., et al., *Nutrient stress activates inflammation and reduces glucose metabolism by suppressing AMP-activated protein kinase in the heart.* Diabetes, 2009. 58(11): p. 2536-46.

[110] du Toit, E.F., M. Nabben, and A. Lochner, *A potential role for angiotensin II in obesity induced cardiac hypertrophy and ischaemic/reperfusion injury.* Basic Res Cardiol, 2005. 100(4): p. 346-54.

[111] Dobrian, A.D., et al., *Development of hypertension in a rat model of diet-induced obesity.* Hypertension, 2000. 35(4): p. 1009-15.

[112] Engeli, S., et al., *Weight loss and the renin-angiotensin-aldosterone system.* Hypertension, 2005. 45(3): p. 356-62.

[113] Uckaya, G., et al., *Plasma leptin levels strongly correlate with plasma renin activity in patients with essential hypertension.* Horm Metab Res, 1999. 31(7): p. 435-8.

[114] Goossens, G.H., et al., *Endocrine role of the renin-angiotensin system in human adipose tissue and muscle: effect of beta-adrenergic stimulation.* Hypertension, 2007. 49(3): p. 542-7.

[115] Boustany, C.M., et al., *Activation of the systemic and adipose renin-angiotensin system in rats with diet-induced obesity and hypertension.* Am J Physiol Regul Integr Comp Physiol, 2004. 287(4): p. R943-9.

[116] Steckelings, U.M., et al., *The evolving story of the RAAS in hypertension, diabetes and CV disease: moving from macrovascular to microvascular targets.* Fundam Clin Pharmacol, 2009. 23(6): p. 693-703.

[117] Thatcher, S., et al., *The adipose renin-angiotensin system: role in cardiovascular disease.* Mol Cell Endocrinol, 2009. 302(2): p. 111-7.

[118] Yvan-Charvet, L. and A. Quignard-Boulange, *Role of adipose tissue renin-angiotensin system in metabolic and inflammatory diseases associated with obesity.* Kidney Int, 2011. 79(2): p. 162-8.

[119] Yusuf, S., et al., *Ramipril and the development of diabetes.* JAMA, 2001. 286(15): p. 1882-5.

[120] Vermes, E., et al., *Enalapril reduces the incidence of diabetes in patients with chronic heart failure: insight from the Studies Of Left Ventricular Dysfunction (SOLVD).* Circulation, 2003. 107(9): p. 1291-6.

[121] Bosch, J., et al., *Effect of ramipril on the incidence of diabetes.* N Engl J Med, 2006. 355(15): p. 1551-62.

[122] Hansson, L., et al., *Effect of angiotensin-converting-enzyme inhibition compared with conventional therapy on cardiovascular morbidity and mortality in hypertension: the Captopril Prevention Project (CAPPP) randomised trial.* Lancet, 1999. 353(9153): p. 611-6.

[123] Han, T., et al., *Relationship between angiotensin-converting enzyme gene insertion or deletion polymorphism and insulin sensitivity in healthy newborns.* Pediatrics, 2007. 119(6): p. 1089-94.

[124] Cong, N.D., et al., *The I/D polymorphism of angiotensin-converting enzyme gene but not the angiotensinogen gene is associated with insulin response to oral glucose in Japanese.* Proc Soc Exp Biol Med, 1999. 220(1): p. 46-51.

[125] Bonnet, F., et al., *Influence of the ACE gene insertion/deletion polymorphism on insulin sensitivity and impaired glucose tolerance in healthy subjects.* Diabetes Care, 2008. 31(4): p. 789-94.

[126] Pollex, R.L., et al., *Metabolic syndrome in aboriginal Canadians: prevalence and genetic associations.* Atherosclerosis, 2006. 184(1): p. 121-9.

[127] Henriksen, E.J., et al., *Selective angiotensin II receptor receptor antagonism reduces insulin resistance in obese Zucker rats.* Hypertension, 2001. 38(4): p. 884-90.

[128] Iwai, M., et al., *Direct renin inhibition improved insulin resistance and adipose tissue dysfunction in type 2 diabetic KK-A(y) mice.* J Hypertens, 2010. 28(7): p. 1471-81.

[129] Takahashi, N., et al., *Increased energy expenditure, dietary fat wasting, and resistance to diet-induced obesity in mice lacking renin.* Cell Metab, 2007. 6(6): p. 506-12.

[130] Jayasooriya, A.P., et al., *Mice lacking angiotensin-converting enzyme have increased energy expenditure, with reduced fat mass and improved glucose clearance.* Proc Natl Acad Sci U S A, 2008. 105(18): p. 6531-6.

[131] Kouyama, R., et al., *Attenuation of diet-induced weight gain and adiposity through increased energy expenditure in mice lacking angiotensin II type 1a receptor.* Endocrinology, 2005. 146(8): p. 3481-9.

[132] Yvan-Charvet, L., et al., *Deletion of the angiotensin type 2 receptor (AT2R) reduces adipose cell size and protects from diet-induced obesity and insulin resistance.* Diabetes, 2005. 54(4): p. 991-9.

[133] Ogihara, T., et al., *Angiotensin II-induced insulin resistance is associated with enhanced insulin signaling.* Hypertension, 2002. 40(6): p. 872-9.

[134] Ran, J., T. Hirano, and M. Adachi, *Chronic ANG II infusion increases plasma triglyceride level by stimulating hepatic triglyceride production in rats.* Am J Physiol Endocrinol Metab, 2004. 287(5): p. E955-61.

[135] Sloniger, J.A., et al., *Selective angiotensin II receptor antagonism enhances whole-body insulin sensitivity and muscle glucose transport in hypertensive TG(mREN2)27 rats.* Metabolism, 2005. 54(12): p. 1659-68.

[136] Lastra, G., et al., *Direct renin inhibition improves systemic insulin resistance and skeletal muscle glucose transport in a transgenic rodent model of tissue renin overexpression.* Endocrinology, 2009. 150(6): p. 2561-8.

[137] Richey, J.M., et al., *Angiotensin II induces insulin resistance independent of changes in interstitial insulin.* Am J Physiol, 1999. 277(5 Pt 1): p. E920-6.

[138] Wei, Y., et al., *Angiotensin II-induced NADPH oxidase activation impairs insulin signaling in skeletal muscle cells.* J Biol Chem, 2006. 281(46): p. 35137-46.

[139] Wei, Y., et al., *Angiotensin II-induced skeletal muscle insulin resistance mediated by NF-kappaB activation via NADPH oxidase.* Am J Physiol Endocrinol Metab, 2008. 294(2): p. E345-51.

[140] Calegari, V.C., et al., *Suppressor of cytokine signaling-3 Provides a novel interface in the cross-talk between angiotensin II and insulin signaling systems.* Endocrinology, 2005. 146(2): p. 579-88.

[141] Mitsuishi, M., et al., *Angiotensin II reduces mitochondrial content in skeletal muscle and affects glycemic control.* Diabetes, 2009. 58(3): p. 710-7.

[142] Kalupahana, N.S., et al., *Overproduction of angiotensinogen from adipose tissue induces adipose inflammation, glucose intolerance, and insulin resistance.* Obesity (Silver Spring), 2012. 20(1): p. 48-56.

[143] Atkinson, L.L., M.A. Fischer, and G.D. Lopaschuk, *Leptin activates cardiac fatty acid oxidation independent of changes in the AMP-activated protein kinase-acetyl-CoA carboxylase-malonyl-CoA axis.* J Biol Chem, 2002. 277(33): p. 29424-30.

[144] Ding, G., et al., *Adiponectin and its receptors are expressed in adult ventricular cardiomyocytes and upregulated by activation of peroxisome proliferator-activated receptor gamma.* J Mol Cell Cardiol, 2007. 43(1): p. 73-84.

[145] Palanivel, R., et al., *Globular and full-length forms of adiponectin mediate specific changes in glucose and fatty acid uptake and metabolism in cardiomyocytes.* Cardiovasc Res, 2007. 75(1): p. 148-57.

[146] Buettner, C., et al., *Leptin controls adipose tissue lipogenesis via central, STAT3-independent mechanisms.* Nat Med, 2008. 14(6): p. 667-75.

[147] Ren, J., *Leptin and hyperleptinemia - from friend to foe for cardiovascular function.* J Endocrinol, 2004. 181(1): p. 1-10.

[148] Chua, S.C., Jr., et al., *Phenotypes of mouse diabetes and rat fatty due to mutations in the OB (leptin) receptor.* Science, 1996. 271(5251): p. 994-6.

[149] Takaya, K., et al., *Molecular cloning of rat leptin receptor isoform complementary DNAs--identification of a missense mutation in Zucker fatty (fa/fa) rats.* Biochem Biophys Res Commun, 1996. 225(1): p. 75-83.

[150] Zhang, Y., et al., *Positional cloning of the mouse obese gene and its human homologue.* Nature, 1994. 372(6505): p. 425-32.

[151] Montague, C.T., et al., *Congenital leptin deficiency is associated with severe early-onset obesity in humans.* Nature, 1997. 387(6636): p. 903-8.

[152] Farooqi, I.S., et al., *Effects of recombinant leptin therapy in a child with congenital leptin deficiency.* N Engl J Med, 1999. 341(12): p. 879-84.

[153] Oral, E.A., et al., *Leptin-replacement therapy for lipodystrophy.* N Engl J Med, 2002. 346(8): p. 570-8.

[154] Lago, F., et al., *Adipokines as novel modulators of lipid metabolism.* Trends Biochem Sci, 2009. 34(10): p. 500-10.

[155] Unger, R.H., *Hyperleptinemia: protecting the heart from lipid overload.* Hypertension, 2005. 45(6): p. 1031-4.

[156] Lee, Y., et al., *Liporegulation in diet-induced obesity. The antisteatotic role of hyperleptinemia.* J Biol Chem, 2001. 276(8): p. 5629-35.

[157] Lee, Y., et al., *Hyperleptinemia prevents lipotoxic cardiomyopathy in acyl CoA synthase transgenic mice.* Proc Natl Acad Sci U S A, 2004. 101(37): p. 13624-9.

[158] Christoffersen, C., et al., *Cardiac lipid accumulation associated with diastolic dysfunction in obese mice.* Endocrinology, 2003. 144(8): p. 3483-90.

[159] Barouch, L.A., et al., *Cardiac myocyte apoptosis is associated with increased DNA damage and decreased survival in murine models of obesity.* Circ Res, 2006. 98(1): p. 119-24.

[160] Dong, F., et al., *Impaired cardiac contractile function in ventricular myocytes from leptin-deficient ob/ob obese mice.* J Endocrinol, 2006. 188(1): p. 25-36.

[161] Li, S.Y., et al., *Cardiac contractile dysfunction in Lep/Lep obesity is accompanied by NADPH oxidase activation, oxidative modification of sarco(endo)plasmic reticulum Ca2+-ATPase and myosin heavy chain isozyme switch.* Diabetologia, 2006. 49(6): p. 1434-46.

[162] Boudina, S. and E.D. Abel, *Diabetic cardiomyopathy revisited.* Circulation, 2007. 115(25): p. 3213-23.

[163] Arita, Y., et al., *Paradoxical decrease of an adipose-specific protein, adiponectin, in obesity.* Biochem Biophys Res Commun, 1999. 257(1): p. 79-83.

[164] Weyer, C., et al., *Hypoadiponectinemia in obesity and type 2 diabetes: close association with insulin resistance and hyperinsulinemia.* J Clin Endocrinol Metab, 2001. 86(5): p. 1930-5.

[165] Matsubara, M., S. Maruoka, and S. Katayose, *Inverse relationship between plasma adiponectin and leptin concentrations in normal-weight and obese women.* Eur J Endocrinol, 2002. 147(2): p. 173-80.

[166] Kadowaki, T. and T. Yamauchi, *Adiponectin and adiponectin receptors.* Endocr Rev, 2005. 26(3): p. 439-51.

[167] Kubota, N., et al., *Disruption of adiponectin causes insulin resistance and neointimal formation.* J Biol Chem, 2002. 277(29): p. 25863-6.

[168] Matsuda, M., et al., *Role of adiponectin in preventing vascular stenosis. The missing link of adipo-vascular axis.* J Biol Chem, 2002. 277(40): p. 37487-91.

[169] Xu, A., et al., *Adiponectin ameliorates dyslipidemia induced by the human immunodeficiency virus protease inhibitor ritonavir in mice.* Endocrinology, 2004. 145(2): p. 487-94.

[170] Yamauchi, T., et al., *Globular adiponectin protected ob/ob mice from diabetes and ApoE-deficient mice from atherosclerosis.* J Biol Chem, 2003. 278(4): p. 2461-8.

[171] Yamauchi, T., et al., *The fat-derived hormone adiponectin reverses insulin resistance associated with both lipoatrophy and obesity.* Nat Med, 2001. 7(8): p. 941-6.

[172] Yamauchi, T., et al., *Adiponectin stimulates glucose utilization and fatty-acid oxidation by activating AMP-activated protein kinase.* Nat Med, 2002. 8(11): p. 1288-95.

[173] Tomas, E., et al., *Enhanced muscle fat oxidation and glucose transport by ACRP30 globular domain: acetyl-CoA carboxylase inhibition and AMP-activated protein kinase activation.* Proc Natl Acad Sci U S A, 2002. 99(25): p. 16309-13.

[174] Fujioka, D., et al., *Role of adiponectin receptors in endothelin-induced cellular hypertrophy in cultured cardiomyocytes and their expression in infarcted heart.* Am J Physiol Heart Circ Physiol, 2006. 290(6): p. H2409-16.

[175] Shibata, R., et al., *Adiponectin-mediated modulation of hypertrophic signals in the heart.* Nat Med, 2004. 10(12): p. 1384-9.

[176] Shibata, R., et al., *Adiponectin protects against myocardial ischemia-reperfusion injury through AMPK- and COX-2-dependent mechanisms.* Nat Med, 2005. 11(10): p. 1096-103.

[177] Karmazyn, M., et al., *Signalling mechanisms underlying the metabolic and other effects of adipokines on the heart.* Cardiovasc Res, 2008. 79(2): p. 279-86.

[178] Adeghate, E., *An update on the biology and physiology of resistin.* Cell Mol Life Sci, 2004. 61(19-20): p. 2485-96.

[179] Kusminski, C.M., P.G. McTernan, and S. Kumar, *Role of resistin in obesity, insulin resistance and Type II diabetes.* Clin Sci (Lond), 2005. 109(3): p. 243-56.

[180] Rajala, M.W., et al., *Regulation of resistin expression and circulating levels in obesity, diabetes, and fasting.* Diabetes, 2004. 53(7): p. 1671-9.

[181] Sato, N., et al., *Adenovirus-mediated high expression of resistin causes dyslipidemia in mice.* Endocrinology, 2005. 146(1): p. 273-9.

[182] Graveleau, C., et al., *Mouse and human resistins impair glucose transport in primary mouse cardiomyocytes, and oligomerization is required for this biological action.* J Biol Chem, 2005. 280(36): p. 31679-85.

[183] Silha, J.V., et al., *Plasma resistin, adiponectin and leptin levels in lean and obese subjects: correlations with insulin resistance.* Eur J Endocrinol, 2003. 149(4): p. 331-5.

[184] Youn, B.S., et al., *Plasma resistin concentrations measured by enzyme-linked immunosorbent assay using a newly developed monoclonal antibody are elevated in individuals with type 2 diabetes mellitus.* J Clin Endocrinol Metab, 2004. 89(1): p. 150-6.

[185] Rea, R. and R. Donnelly, *Resistin: an adipocyte-derived hormone. Has it a role in diabetes and obesity?* Diabetes Obes Metab, 2004. 6(3): p. 163-70.

[186] Zierler, K.L., *Fatty acids as substrates for heart and skeletal muscle.* Circ Res, 1976. 38(6): p. 459-63.

[187] Opie, L.H., *The Heart; Physiology, from Cell to Circulation. 3rd Edition*, 1998, Raven Press: Philadelphia, NY. p. Chapter 11, pp295-342.

[188] Bertrand, L., et al., *Insulin signalling in the heart.* Cardiovasc Res, 2008. 79(2): p. 238-48.

[189] van der Vusse, G.J., M. van Bilsen, and J.F. Glatz, *Cardiac fatty acid uptake and transport in health and disease.* Cardiovasc Res, 2000. 45(2): p. 279-93.

[190] Scott, J.C., L.J. Finkelstein, and J.J. Spitzer, *Myocardial removal of free fatty acids under normal pathological conditions.* Am J Physiol, 1962. 203: p. 482-6.

[191] Coort, S.L., et al., *Cardiac substrate uptake and metabolism in obesity and type-2 diabetes: role of sarcolemmal substrate transporters.* Mol Cell Biochem, 2007. 299(1-2): p. 5-18.

[192] Luiken, J.J., et al., *Uptake and metabolism of palmitate by isolated cardiac myocytes from adult rats: involvement of sarcolemmal proteins.* J Lipid Res, 1997. 38(4): p. 745-58.

[193] Fournier, N., M. Geoffroy, and J. Deshusses, *Purification and characterization of a long chain, fatty-acid-binding protein supplying the mitochondrial beta-oxidative system in the heart.* Biochim Biophys Acta, 1978. 533(2): p. 457-64.

[194] Vork, M.M., J.F. Glatz, and G.J. Van Der Vusse, *On the mechanism of long chain fatty acid transport in cardiomyocytes as facilitated by cytoplasmic fatty acid-binding protein.* J Theor Biol, 1993. 160(2): p. 207-22.

[195] Schaap, F.G., et al., *Impaired long-chain fatty acid utilization by cardiac myocytes isolated from mice lacking the heart-type fatty acid binding protein gene.* Circ Res, 1999. 85(4): p. 329-37.

[196] Kraegen, E.W., et al., *Glucose transporters and in vivo glucose uptake in skeletal and cardiac muscle: fasting, insulin stimulation and immunoisolation studies of GLUT1 and GLUT4.* Biochem J, 1993. 295 (Pt 1): p. 287-93.

[197] Zaninetti, D., R. Greco-Perotto, and B. Jeanrenaud, *Heart glucose transport and transporters in rat heart: regulation by insulin, workload and glucose.* Diabetologia, 1988. 31(2): p. 108-13.

[198] Halestrap, A.P. and N.T. Price, *The proton-linked monocarboxylate transporter (MCT) family: structure, function and regulation.* Biochem J, 1999. 343 Pt 2: p. 281-99.

[199] Stanley, W.C., et al., *Regulation of myocardial carbohydrate metabolism under normal and ischaemic conditions. Potential for pharmacological interventions.* Cardiovasc Res, 1997. 33(2): p. 243-57.

[200] Hue, L. and H. Taegtmeyer, *The Randle cycle revisited: a new head for an old hat.* Am J Physiol Endocrinol Metab, 2009. 297(3): p. E578-91.

[201] Depre, C., J.L. Vanoverschelde, and H. Taegtmeyer, *Glucose for the heart.* Circulation, 1999. 99(4): p. 578-88.

[202] Park, S.Y., et al., *Cardiac-specific overexpression of peroxisome proliferator-activated receptor-alpha causes insulin resistance in heart and liver.* Diabetes, 2005. 54(9): p. 2514-24.

[203] Wilson, C.R., et al., *Western diet, but not high fat diet, causes derangements of fatty acid metabolism and contractile dysfunction in the heart of Wistar rats.* Biochem J, 2007. 406(3): p. 457-67.

[204] Aasum, E., et al., *Fenofibrate modulates cardiac and hepatic metabolism and increases ischemic tolerance in diet-induced obese mice.* J Mol Cell Cardiol, 2008. 44(1): p. 201-9.

[205] Wright, J.J., et al., *Mechanisms for increased myocardial fatty acid utilization following short-term high-fat feeding.* Cardiovasc Res, 2009. 82(2): p. 351-60.

[206] Lopaschuk, G.D. and J.C. Russell, *Myocardial function and energy substrate metabolism in the insulin-resistant JCR:LA corpulent rat.* J Appl Physiol, 1991. 71(4): p. 1302-8.

[207] Peterson, L.R., et al., *Impact of gender on the myocardial metabolic response to obesity.* JACC Cardiovasc Imaging, 2008. 1(4): p. 424-33.

[208] Finck, B.N., et al., *The cardiac phenotype induced by PPARalpha overexpression mimics that caused by diabetes mellitus.* J Clin Invest, 2002. 109(1): p. 121-30.

[209] Carroll, J.F., W.J. Zenebe, and T.B. Strange, *Cardiovascular function in a rat model of diet-induced obesity.* Hypertension, 2006. 48(1): p. 65-72.

[210] Maarman, G., et al., *Effect of Chronic CPT-1 Inhibition on Myocardial Ischemia-Reperfusion Injury (I/R) in a Model of Diet-Induced Obesity.* Cardiovasc Drugs Ther, 2012.

[211] du Toit, E.F., et al., *Myocardial susceptibility to ischemic-reperfusion injury in a prediabetic model of dietary-induced obesity.* Am J Physiol Heart Circ Physiol, 2008. 294(5): p. H2336-43.

[212] Ouwens, D.M., et al., *Cardiac contractile dysfunction in insulin-resistant rats fed a high-fat diet is associated with elevated CD36-mediated fatty acid uptake and esterification.* Diabetologia, 2007. 50(9): p. 1938-48.

[213] Boudina, S., et al., *Reduced mitochondrial oxidative capacity and increased mitochondrial uncoupling impair myocardial energetics in obesity.* Circulation, 2005. 112(17): p. 2686-95.

[214] How, O.J., et al., *Increased myocardial oxygen consumption reduces cardiac efficiency in diabetic mice.* Diabetes, 2006. 55(2): p. 466-73.

[215] Ingelsson, E., et al., *Insulin resistance and risk of congestive heart failure.* JAMA, 2005. 294(3): p. 334-41.

[216] Puri, P.S., et al., *Alterations in energy metabolism and ultrastructure upon reperfusion of the ischemic myocardium after coronary occlusion.* Am J Cardiol, 1975. 36(2): p. 234-43.

[217] Opie, L.H., *Effects of regional ischemia on metabolism of glucose and fatty acids. Relative rates of aerobic and anaerobic energy production during myocardial infarction and comparison with effects of anoxia.* Circ Res, 1976. 38(5 Suppl 1): p. I52-74.

[218] Opie, L.H., *The Heart; Physiology, from Cell to Circulation. 4th Edition*, 2004, Lippincott Williams & Wilkins: Philadelphia, PA. p. Chapter 11, pp330-333; Chapter 17, p533.

[219] Garlick, P.B., G.K. Radda, and P.J. Seeley, *Studies of acidosis in the ischaemic heart by phosphorus nuclear magnetic resonance.* Biochem J, 1979. 184(3): p. 547-54.

[220] Van Rooyen, J., J. McCarthy, and L.H. Opie, *Increased glycolysis during ischaemia mediates the protective effect of glucose and insulin in the isolated rat heart despite the presence of cardiodepressant exogenous substrates.* Cardiovasc J S Afr, 2002. 13(3): p. 103-9.

[221] Stanley, W.C., *Changes in cardiac metabolism: a critical step from stable angina to ischaemic cardiomyopathy.* Eur Heart J, 2001. 3((Supplement O)): p. O2-O7.

[222] Liedtke, A.J., *Alterations of carbohydrate and lipid metabolism in the acutely ischemic heart.* Prog Cardiovasc Dis, 1981. 23(5): p. 321-36.

[223] Liedtke, A.J., et al., *Changes in substrate metabolism and effects of excess fatty acids in reperfused myocardium.* Circ Res, 1988. 62(3): p. 535-42.

[224] Lopaschuk, G.D., et al., *Glucose and palmitate oxidation in isolated working rat hearts reperfused after a period of transient global ischemia.* Circ Res, 1990. 66(2): p. 546-53.

[225] Morel, S., et al., *Insulin resistance modifies plasma fatty acid distribution and decreases cardiac tolerance to in vivo ischaemia/reperfusion in rats.* Clin Exp Pharmacol Physiol, 2003. 30(7): p. 446-51.

[226] Aasum, E., et al., *Age-dependent changes in metabolism, contractile function, and ischemic sensitivity in hearts from db/db mice.* Diabetes, 2003. 52(2): p. 434-41.

[227] Lopaschuk, G.D., R.B. Wambolt, and R.L. Barr, *An imbalance between glycolysis and glucose oxidation is a possible explanation for the detrimental effects of high levels of fatty acids during aerobic reperfusion of ischemic hearts.* J Pharmacol Exp Ther, 1993. 264(1): p. 135-44.

[228] Liu, Q., et al., *High levels of fatty acids delay the recovery of intracellular pH and cardiac efficiency in post-ischemic hearts by inhibiting glucose oxidation.* J Am Coll Cardiol, 2002. 39(4): p. 718-25.

[229] Liu, B., et al., *Cardiac efficiency is improved after ischemia by altering both the source and fate of protons.* Circ Res, 1996. 79(5): p. 940-8.

[230] Orchard, C.H. and J.C. Kentish, *Effects of changes of pH on the contractile function of cardiac muscle.* Am J Physiol, 1990. 258(6 Pt 1): p. C967-81.

[231] Sidell, R.J., et al., *Thiazolidinedione treatment normalizes insulin resistance and ischemic injury in the zucker Fatty rat heart.* Diabetes, 2002. 51(4): p. 1110-7.

[232] Downey, J.M., A.M. Davis, and M.V. Cohen, *Signaling pathways in ischemic preconditioning.* Heart Fail Rev, 2007. 12(3-4): p. 181-8.

[233] Halestrap, A.P., S.J. Clarke, and I. Khaliulin, *The role of mitochondria in protection of the heart by preconditioning.* Biochim Biophys Acta, 2007. 1767(8): p. 1007-31.

[234] Hausenloy, D.J. and D.M. Yellon, *Preconditioning and postconditioning: underlying mechanisms and clinical application.* Atherosclerosis, 2009. 204(2): p. 334-41.

[235] Bernardo, B.C., et al., *Molecular distinction between physiological and pathological cardiac hypertrophy: experimental findings and therapeutic strategies.* Pharmacol Ther, 2010. 128(1): p. 191-227.

[236] Wagner, C., et al., *Cardioprotection by postconditioning is lost in WOKW rats with metabolic syndrome: role of glycogen synthase kinase 3beta.* J Cardiovasc Pharmacol, 2008. 52(5): p. 430-7.

[237] Bouhidel, O., et al., *Myocardial ischemic postconditioning against ischemia-reperfusion is impaired in ob/ob mice.* Am J Physiol Heart Circ Physiol, 2008. 295(4): p. H1580-6.

[238] Katakam, P.V., et al., *Myocardial preconditioning against ischemia-reperfusion injury is abolished in Zucker obese rats with insulin resistance.* Am J Physiol Regul Integr Comp Physiol, 2007. 292(2): p. R920-6.

[239] Thompson, P.D., et al., *Exercise and physical activity in the prevention and treatment of atherosclerotic cardiovascular disease: a statement from the Council on Clinical Cardiology (Subcommittee on Exercise, Rehabilitation, and Prevention) and the Council on Nutrition, Physical Activity, and Metabolism (Subcommittee on Physical Activity).* Circulation, 2003. 107(24): p. 3109-16.

[240] *Third Report of the National Cholesterol Education Program (NCEP) Ecpert Panel on Detection, Evaluation and Treatment of High Blood Cholesterol in Adults (Adult Treatment Panel III) final report.* Circulation, 2002. 106: p. 3143-21.

[241] Phelan, S., et al., *Impact of weight loss on the metabolic syndrome.* Int J Obes (Lond), 2007. 31(9): p. 1442-8.

[242] Muzio, F., et al., *Long-term effects of low-calorie diet on the metabolic syndrome in obese nondiabetic patients.* Diabetes Care, 2005. 28(6): p. 1485-6.

[243] Orchard, T.J., et al., *The effect of metformin and intensive lifestyle intervention on the metabolic syndrome: the Diabetes Prevention Program randomized trial.* Ann Intern Med, 2005. 142(8): p. 611-9.

[244] Ballantyne, C.M., et al., *Influence of low high-density lipoprotein cholesterol and elevated triglyceride on coronary heart disease events and response to simvastatin therapy in 4S.* Circulation, 2001. 104(25): p. 3046-51.

[245] Pyorala, K., et al., *Reduction of cardiovascular events by simvastatin in nondiabetic coronary heart disease patients with and without the metabolic syndrome: subgroup analyses of the Scandinavian Simvastatin Survival Study (4S).* Diabetes Care, 2004. 27(7): p. 1735-40.

[246] Paolisso, G., et al., *Effects of simvastatin and atorvastatin administration on insulin resistance and respiratory quotient in aged dyslipidemic non-insulin dependent diabetic patients.* Atherosclerosis, 2000. 150(1): p. 121-7.

[247] Sonmez A, B.Y., Kilic M, Saglam K, Buluku F and Kocar IH., *Fluvastatin improves insulin resistance in nondiabetic dyslipidemic patients.* Endocrine, 2003. 22(2): p. 151-154.

[248] Malmendier, C.L. and C. Delcroix, *Effects of fenofibrate on high and low density lipoprotein metabolism in heterozygous familial hypercholesterolemia.* Atherosclerosis, 1985. 55(2): p. 161-9.

[249] Robins, S.J., et al., *Relation of gemfibrozil treatment and lipid levels with major coronary events: VA-HIT: a randomized controlled trial.* JAMA, 2001. 285(12): p. 1585-91.

[250] Vu-Dac, N., et al., *Fibrates increase human apolipoprotein A-II expression through activation of the peroxisome proliferator-activated receptor.* J Clin Invest, 1995. 96(2): p. 741-50.

[251] Guerre-Millo, M., et al., *Peroxisome proliferator-activated receptor alpha activators improve insulin sensitivity and reduce adiposity.* J Biol Chem, 2000. 275(22): p. 16638-42.

[252] Ide, T., et al., *Enhancement of insulin signaling through inhibition of tissue lipid accumulation by activation of peroxisome proliferator-activated receptor (PPAR) alpha in obese mice.* Med Sci Monit, 2004. 10(10): p. BR388-95.

[253] Bergeron, R., et al., *Peroxisome proliferator-activated receptor (PPAR)-alpha agonism prevents the onset of type 2 diabetes in Zucker diabetic fatty rats: A comparison with PPAR gamma agonism.* Endocrinology, 2006. 147(9): p. 4252-62.

[254] Tsunoda, M., et al., *A novel PPARalpha agonist ameliorates insulin resistance in dogs fed a high-fat diet.* Am J Physiol Endocrinol Metab, 2008. 294(5): p. E833-40.

[255] Forcheron, F., et al., *Diabetic cardiomyopathy: effects of fenofibrate and metformin in an experimental model--the Zucker diabetic rat.* Cardiovasc Diabetol, 2009. 8: p. 16.

[256] Chang, J.T., et al., *Rhabdomyolysis with HMG-CoA reductase inhibitors and gemfibrozil combination therapy.* Pharmacoepidemiol Drug Saf, 2004. 13(7): p. 417-26.

[257] van Puijenbroek, E.P., et al., *Possible increased risk of rhabdomyolysis during concomitant use of simvastatin and gemfibrozil.* J Intern Med, 1996. 240(6): p. 403-4.

[258] Moscatiello, S., et al., *Managing the combination of nonalcoholic fatty liver disease and metabolic syndrome.* Expert Opin Pharmacother, 2011. 12(17): p. 2657-72.

[259] DeFronzo, R.A., et al., *Pioglitazone for diabetes prevention in impaired glucose tolerance.* N Engl J Med, 2011. 364(12): p. 1104-15.

[260] Xiang, A.H., et al., *Effect of pioglitazone on pancreatic beta-cell function and diabetes risk in Hispanic women with prior gestational diabetes.* Diabetes, 2006. 55(2): p. 517-22.

[261] Campia, U., L.A. Matuskey, and J.A. Panza, *Peroxisome proliferator-activated receptor-gamma activation with pioglitazone improves endothelium-dependent dilation in nondiabetic patients with major cardiovascular risk factors.* Circulation, 2006. 113(6): p. 867-75.

[262] Dagenais, G.R., et al., *Effects of ramipril and rosiglitazone on cardiovascular and renal outcomes in people with impaired glucose tolerance or impaired fasting glucose: results of the*

Diabetes REduction Assessment with ramipril and rosiglitazone Medication (DREAM) trial. Diabetes Care, 2008. 31(5): p. 1007-14.

[263] Fogari, R., et al., *Comparative effects of lisinopril and losartan on insulin sensitivity in the treatment of non diabetic hypertensive patients.* Br J Clin Pharmacol, 1998. 46(5): p. 467-71.

[264] Yavuz, D., et al., *Effects of ACE inhibition and AT1-receptor antagonism on endothelial function and insulin sensitivity in essential hypertensive patients.* J Renin Angiotensin Aldosterone Syst, 2003. 4(3): p. 197-203.

[265] Aksnes, T.A., et al., *Improved insulin sensitivity with the angiotensin II-receptor blocker losartan in patients with hypertension and other cardiovascular risk factors.* J Hum Hypertens, 2006. 20(11): p. 860-6.

[266] Jin, H.M. and Y. Pan, *Angiotensin type-1 receptor blockade with losartan increases insulin sensitivity and improves glucose homeostasis in subjects with type 2 diabetes and nephropathy.* Nephrol Dial Transplant, 2007. 22(7): p. 1943-9.

[267] van Dielen, F.M., et al., *Macrophage inhibitory factor, plasminogen activator inhibitor-1, other acute phase proteins, and inflammatory mediators normalize as a result of weight loss in morbidly obese subjects treated with gastric restrictive surgery.* J Clin Endocrinol Metab, 2004. 89(8): p. 4062-8.

[268] Jialal, I., et al., *Effect of hydroxymethyl glutaryl coenzyme a reductase inhibitor therapy on high sensitive C-reactive protein levels.* Circulation, 2001. 103(15): p. 1933-5.

[269] Nesto, R., *C-reactive protein, its role in inflammation, Type 2 diabetes and cardiovascular disease, and the effects of insulin-sensitizing treatment with thiazolidinediones.* Diabet Med, 2004. 21(8): p. 810-7.

Section 5

Diagnostic and Therapeutic Aspects in Insulin Resistance

Chapter 9

Ultrasonographic Measurement of Visceral Fat

Tamara Alempijevic, Aleksandra Pavlovic Markovic
and Aleksandra Sokic Milutinovic

Additional information is available at the end of the chapter

http://dx.doi.org/10.5772/54812

1. Introduction

Metabolic syndrome (MS), that has received increased attention in the past few years, consists of multiple, interrelated risk factors of metabolic origin that appear to directly promote the development of atherosclerotic cardiovascular disease (ASCVD). Most important of these underlying risk factors are abdominal obesity and insulin resistance. Other associated conditions include physical inactivity, aging, hormonal imbalance, and genetic or ethnic predisposition [1].

The measurement of abdominal obesity through waist circumference (WC) has been established as a simple, inexpensive and useful method for the diagnosis of abdominal obesity. Thus, WC has been proposed as a key element for the diagnosis of MS and its use suggested as a part of the routine general physical examination in clinical practice[2].

Moreover, WC correlates with visceral obesity, and in clinical studies, it has been associated with increased cardiovascular risk[3]. It has been proposed as a part of the routine general physical examination in clinical practice.

It is shown that mesenteric fat thickness is an independent determinant of metabolic syndrome, with an odds ratio of 1.35 for every 1 mm increase, at least within the observed range of mesenteric fat thickness. The discriminating cut-off point of 10 mm indicates the presence of metabolic syndrome and identifies subjects with increased intima-media thickness[4].

Hypotheses relating central adiposity to the metabolic syndrome focus on the newly emerging understanding that adipose tissue (particularly visceral adipose tissue) is a source of factors [including free fatty acids, tumour necrosis factor-alpha (TNF-α)] that impair insulin action in skeletal muscle. In addition, the adipose specific collagen-like molecule, adiponectin, has been found to have antidiabetic, anti-atherosclerotic and anti-inflammatory functions. Excessive adipose tissue is associated with a decreased production of adiponectin which may impair insulin sensitivity.

Measurement of mesenteric fat thickness may potentially be developed into an alternative tool to identify subjects at risk for cardiovascular diseases[5].

Newer clinical studies showed that WC not always correlates with visceral obesity and associated risk for cardiovascular diseases in clinical studies[6]. Therefor, several imaging methods have been proposed for estimation of visceral adipose tissue. Recent advances in imaging techniques and an understanding of differences in the molecular biology of the different adipose tissue depots have been reported. Computed tomography (CT) and especially Magnetic Resonance Imaging (MRI), the gold standard technique, provide non invasive estimation of VAT (visceral adipose tissue) amount safely and accurately. Unfortunately, both MRI and CT are high-cost technologies, and CT requires radiation exposure. In addition, a great variability in the precise definition of adipose tissue compartments by CT and MRI measurements is found in clinical studies. The measurement of visceral fat volume using ultrasonography (US) could calculate as effective as using CT. This method should be practiced in clinics due to its low cost, no side effects and technical suitability[7,8].

2. Computed tomography

In 1999, Yoshizumi et al. presented the standard technique for fat visceral fat measurement at CT which is used in all further published studies[9]. CT (TCT-900S Helix; Toshiba, Tokyo, Japan) was performed with all subjects supine (120 kV, 200 mA, section thickness of 5 mm, scanning time of 2 seconds, field of view of 400 mm). In subjects, subcutaneous and visceral fat areas were measured on one cross-sectional scan obtained at the umbilicus. A region of interest of the subcutaneous fat layer was defined by tracing its contour on each scan, and the attenuation range of CT numbers (in Hounsfield units) for fat tissue was calculated. A histogram for fat tissue was computed on the basis of mean attenuation plus or minus 2 SD. Intraperitoneal tissue was defined by tracing its contour on the scan; within that region of interest, tissue with attenuation within the mean plus or minus 2 SD was considered to be the visceral fat area. The pixels with attenuation values in the selected attenuation range were depicted as white. From those white regions, the total fat area was calculated by counting the number of pixels in each; the visceral fat area was subtracted, and the remainder was defined as the subcutaneous fat area. Results with this method were compared to those with a computerized planimetric method (KL 4300 Digitizer; Graphtec, Tokyo) and with a fixed attenuation range from 2190 to 230 HU as the standard of reference.

3. Magnetic Resonance Imaging

The basic method of visceral fat measurement by MR is as described by Demerath et al[10]. Images were obtained with a Magnetom Vision 1.5 Tesla whole-body scanner (Siemens, Mississauga, Canada) using a T1-weighted fast-spin echo pulse sequence (TR 322 ms, TE

12 ms). The subjects were instructed to lie in the magnet in a supine position with arms extended above the head. A breath-hold sequence (≈22 s per acquisition) was used to minimize the effects of respiratory motion on the images. All images were acquired on a 256 × 256 mm matrix and a 480-mm field of view. Slice thickness was 10 mm, and images were obtained every 10 mm from the 9th thoracic vertebra (T9) to the first sacral vertebra (S1). Depending on the height of the person, this resulted in a total of 21–40 axial images per person. The images were retrieved from the scanner according to a DICOM (Digital Imaging and Communications in Medicine) protocol (National Electrical Manufacturer's Association, Rosslyn, VA). Segmentation of the axial images into VAT and subcutaneous adipose tissue (SAT) areas was performed by 2 trained observers using image analysis software (Slice-O-Matic, version 4.2; Tomovision Inc, Montreal, Canada). Tagging of adipose tissue began at the first image, containing the upper margin of the liver and continued down to the L5-S1 image, which increased the likelihood that all intraabdominal adipose tissue was included in the estimate. To calculate VAT and SAT volumes, the VAT and SAT areas for each image were summed across all images. A significant advantage of the contiguous image approach is that no geometrical assumptions have to be made regarding how to interpolate between consecutive slices for the calculation of total volumes.

4. Ultrasonography

Ultrasonography (US) is a simple and reliable method for measuring both subcutaneous and visceral fat showing a strong correlation with both adiposities measured with computed tomography scan[11].

Different techniques are presented by different authors, and no standard method of measurement is still proposed.

In 1990. Armellini et al.[12] proposed the use of ultrasonography for the first time for the quantification of visceral adiposity as an alternative technique to CT.

There are several proposed techniques, but the most reliable technique of ultrasonographic measurement of fat tissue thickness was presented by Meriño-Ibarra et al.[13]. Sonography measurements were performed using a linear-array probe (Aloka SSD-900, Tokyo, Japan) (7.5 MHz and 42 mm) in supine position. It was kept perpendicular to the skin on the upper median abdomen, and longitudinal scan was done in the midpoint between the xiphoid appendix and the navel along the alba line with regard to the surface of the liver, to be almost parallel to the skin. Subcutaneous fat thickness (STh) and area (SA) were measured on the xiphoumbilical line in both longitudinal and transverse views. Measurements were taken 3 times directly from the screen using the electronic calipers at the inner edge of the skin and at the outer edge of the alba line and the fat-muscle interfaces for area. Preperitoneal fat thickness or visceral-fat thickness (VTh) and area (VA) were measured in the same sites and views (Fig. 1). In this case, measurements were taken at the inner edge of the alba line and at the peritoneal line for thickness and area. Then mean values were calculated. Preperitoneal circumference (PC) was calculated as:

$$PC = WC - (2\pi - STh)$$

This measurement assumes that WC is a circumference, hence after measuring WC and STh, the intra-abdominal radius and PC can be easily calculated with the formula cited previously. All the subjects were asked to hold their breath during the examination. Special care was taken to keep the probe just touching the skin to prevent compression of the fat layers.

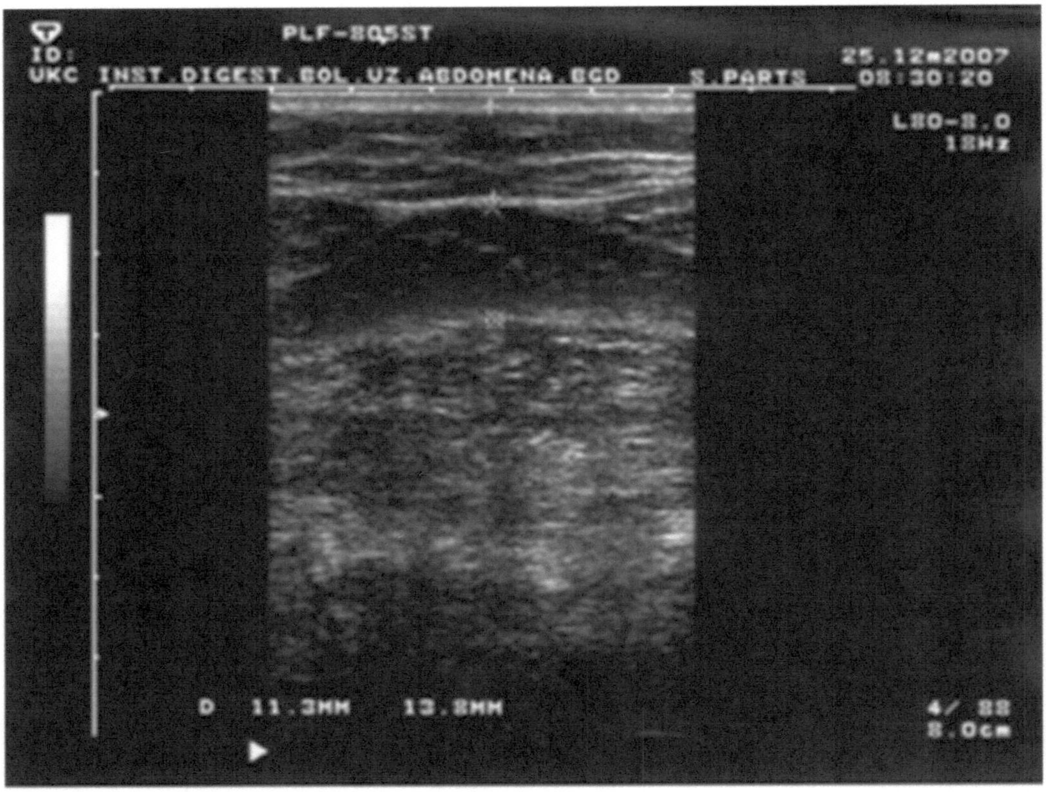

Figure 1. Subcutaneous and visceral fat thickness measurement

Other authors, as well contributed to this topic, Suzuki et al.[14] proposed a new index as a good non/invasive indicator of viscerl fat deposition. They calculated the abdominal wall fat index as preperitoneal fat/subcutaneous fat ratio. The thickness of subcutaneous as preperitoneal fat layers was measured directly on the screen using electronic callipers. The maximum thickness of preperitoneal fat and the minimum thickness of subcutaneous fat were used as representative markers.

Hirooka et al.[15] proposed an another technique. This group measured the distance between the internal surface of the abdominal muscle and splenic vein, the distance between the internal surface of the abdominal muscle and the posterior wall of the aorta of the aorta on the umbilicus and the thickness of the posterior right renal wall in the right posterior perinephritic space. A 3.5MHz convex-array probe was used to measure each parameter,other than the thickness of both the subcutaneous and the preperitoneal fat layers at the xyphoid process by performing a longitudinal scan, which was measured using 7.5MHz linear-array probe. The transducer was placed vertically against the skin as lightly as possible to prevent compression of the fat layers. The distance between the internal surface of the abdominal muscle and the splenic vein was scanned transversely in the midline. When the splenic vein could not be visualized clearly, this vein was detected by using color Doppler flow. The equation was calculated as follows:

$$\left[\textit{visceral fat volume}\right] = -9.008 + 1.191 \times \begin{bmatrix} \textit{distance} \\ \textit{between the internal surface of} \\ \textit{the abdominal muscle and the} \\ \textit{splenic vein } (mm) \end{bmatrix} + \\ + 0.987 \times \begin{bmatrix} \textit{distance between the internal} \\ \textit{surface of the abdominal muscle and} \\ \textit{the posterior wall of the aorta on the} \\ \textit{umbilicus } (mm) \end{bmatrix} + \\ + 3.644 \times \begin{bmatrix} \textit{thickness of the fat layer of the} \\ \textit{posterior right renal wall } (mm) \end{bmatrix}$$

There was a good correlation between the visceral fat volume calculated by the above equation and the volume by CT described.

Visceral fat amount can be estimated by measurement of perirenal fat, as presented by Kawasaki et al.[16]. This group performed sonography using a Power Vision 8000 scanner (Toshiba, Tokyo, Japan) equipped with a 3.75-MHz convex probe. On sonography, the thickness of combined para- and perirenal fat was measured between the kidney and the inner aspect of the abdominal musculature. Measurements on both sides were averaged. The results correlated with CT measurement, as well as with laboratory values.

5. Conclusion

Since 1990, CT has been proposed as the gold standard method to quantify abdominal adiposity[17]. Despre´s and Lamarche[18] observed that a visceral fat area of 130 cm^2 was associated with a high risk of cardiovascular events, although prospective studies are still lacking to confirm such an association. In the meantime, other techniques have been used to predict cardiovascular risk. Undoubtedly, BMI is the most common method for estimating body fat, and several epidemiological studies have reinforced its role in the prediction of morbidity and mortality[19,20]. However, an increased BMI does not show which body compartment (fat or lean mass) is inadequate and cannot differentiate subcutaneous from visceral fat accumulation. The use of US in the assessment of intra-abdominal fat, initially proposed by Armellini et al.[12], was further confirmed by strong correlations with the CT-determined visceral fat area[14,21]. US is expected to be the most specific method because it allows the individual visualization of subcutaneous and intra-abdominal (visceral) fat. In addition, US is a noninvasive and quick method with good reproducibility rates (intra-examination variation <1%) and lower costs than CT scans. However, specific equipment and a welltrained examiner are required. Despite the fact that body composition might be attributable to ethnic differences, changes in the US-determined visceral-to-subcutaneous fat ratio can potentially be monitored for the risk associated with visceral fat accumulation. Also, US may represent a useful method for monitoring weight loss, variations in visceral fat, and associated risks[22].

Whatever technique is used, ultrasonography is a reliable method for measurement visceral fat amount and assessment of metabolic syndrome presence and risk for cardiovascular diseases development.

Author details

Tamara Alempijevic, Aleksandra Pavlovic Markovic and Aleksandra Sokic Milutinovic
School of Medicine, University of Belgrade, Serbia
Clinic for Gastroenterology and Hepatology, Clinical Center of Serbia, Belgrade, Serbia

6. References

[1] Grundy SM, Cleeman JI, MD, Daniels SR, Donato KA, Eckel RH, Franklin BA, et al. Diagnosis and Management of the Metabolic Syndrome. An American Heart Association/National Heart, Lung, and Blood Institute. Scientific Statement. Circulation 2005; 112(17): e285–90.

[2] Wang J. Waist circumference: a simple, inexpensive, and reliable tool that should be included as part of physical examinations in the doctor's office. Am J Clin Nutr 2003; 78(5): 902–3.

[3] Zhu S, Wang Z, Heshka S, Heo M, Faith MS, Heymsfield SB. Waist circumference and obesity-associated risk factors among whites in the third National Health and Nutrition Examination Survey: clinical action thresholds. Am J Clin Nutr 2002; 76(4): 743–9.

[4] Liu KH, Chan YL, Chan WB, Ngor Chan JC, Winnie Chu CW. Mesenteric fat thickness is an independent determinant of metabolic syndrome and identifies subjects with increased carotid intima-media thickness. Diabetes Care 2006; 29(2): 379– 84.

[5] Mangge H, Almer G, Truschnig-Wilders M, Schmidt A, Gasser R, Fuchs D. Inflammation, adiponectin, obesity and cardiovascular risk. Curr Med Chem. 2010;17(36):4511-20.

[6] Ness-Abramof R, Apovian CM. Waist circumference measurement in clinical practice. Nutr Clin Pract 2008;23(4):397-404.

[7] Schlett CL, Hoffmann U. [Identification and quantification of fat compartments with CT and MRI and their importance]. Radiologe 2011; 51(5):372-8.

[8] Meng K, Lee CH, Saremi F. Metabolic syndrome and ectopic fat deposition: what can CT and MR provide? Acad Radiol 2010; 17(10):1302-12.

[9] Yoshizumi T, Nakamura T, Yamane M, Islam AHMW, Menju M, Yamasaki K, et al. Abdominal fat: Standardized technique for measurement at CT. Radiology 1999; 211: 283 – 286.

[10] Demerath EW, Shen W, Lee M, Choh AC, Czerwinski SA, Siervogel RM, Towne B. Approximation of total visceral adipose tissue with a single magnetic resonance image. Am J Clin Nutr 2007; 85(2): 362-8.

[11] Ribeiro-Filho FF, Faria AN, Kohlmann O Jr, Ajzen S, Ribeiro AB, Zanella MT, et al. Ultrasonography for the evaluation of visceral fat and cardiovascular risk. Hypertension 2001; 38(3 Pt 2): 713–7.

[12] Armellini F, Zamboni M, Rigo L, Todesco T, Bergamo-Andreis IA, Procacci C, et al. The contribution of sonography to the measurement of intra- abdominal fat. J Clin Ultrasound 1990 ;18(7):563-7.

[13] Meriño-Ibarra E, Artieda M, Cenarro A, Goicoechea J, Calvo L, Guallar A, et al. Ultrasonography for the evaluation of visceralfat and the metabolic syndrome. Metabolism 2005; 54(9): 1230–5.

[14] Suzuki R, Watanabe S, Hirai Y, Akiyama K, Nishide T, Matsushima Y, rt al. Abdominal wall fat index, estimated by ultrasonography, for assessment of the ratio of visceral fat to subcutaneous fat in the abdomen. Am J Med 1993 Sep;95(3):309-14.

[15] Hirooka M, Kumagi T, Kurose K, Nakanishi S, Michitaka K, Matsuura B, et al. A technique for the measurement of visceral fat by ultrasonography: comparison of measurements by ultrasonography and computed tomography. Intern Med 2005; 44(8):794-9.

[16] Kawasaki S, Hasegawa O, Satoh S, Numata K, Terauchi Y. Sonographic assessment of fatty liver infiltration using the measurement of para- and perirenal fat thickness. J Clin Ultrasound 2010; 38(9):470-4.

[17] Rossner S, Bo WJ, Hiltbrandt E, et al. Adipose tissue determinations in cadavers—a comparison between cross-sectional planimetry and computed tomography. Int J Obes Relat Metab Disord. 1990;14:893–902.

[18] Despre´s JP, Lamarche B. Effects of diet and physical activity on adiposity and body fat distribution: implications for the prevention of cardiovascular disease. Nutr Res Rev. 1993;6: 137–59.

[19] World Health Organization. Obesity: Preventing and Managing the Global Epidemic. Report of a WHO Consulation on Obesity. Geneva, Switzerland; World Health Organization; 1997.

[20] Calle EE, Thun MJ, Petrelli JM, Rodriguez C, Heath CW Jr. Body mass index and mortality in a prospective cohort of US adults. N Engl J Med 1999;341:1097–105.

[21] Tornaghi G, Raiteri R, Pozzato C, et al. Anthropometric or ultrasonic measurements in assessment of visceral fat? A comparative study. Int J Obes Relat Metab Disord 1994;18: 771–5.

[22] Wirth A, Steinmetz B. Gender differences in changes in subcutaneous and intra-abdominal fat during weight reduction: an ultrasound study. Obes Res 1998;6:393–9.

Chapter 10

The Effects of Antihypertensive Agents in Metabolic Syndrome – Benefits Beyond Blood Pressure Control

Nadya Merchant and Bobby V. Khan

Additional information is available at the end of the chapter

http://dx.doi.org/10.5772/54292

1. Introduction

Vascular dysfunction is a highly complex biological process, and cardiovascular diseases are a leading cause of morbidity and mortality in the United States [1]. It is estimated that approximately 80 million US adults (>1 in 3) have one or more types of cardiovascular (CV) disease, including hypertension, atherosclerosis, and congestive heart failure. CV disease has been estimated to account for 34.3% of all deaths in the United States in 2006 [1]. Vascular or endothelial dysfunction is caused by many interrelated factors including oxidative stress, hypertension, diabetes mellitus, renal disease, smoking, inflammation and atherosclerosis.

In this chapter we will review results from large-scale clinical trials to determine if inhibitors of the renin–angiotensin system (RAS), including angiotensin-converting enzyme inhibitors (ACEIs) and angiotensin type II receptor blockers (ARBs) and calcium channel blockers (CCBs), may have beneficial effects on central aortic pressure (CAP) and the biomarkers high-sensitivity C-reactive protein (hsCRP), adiponectin, cystatin C, homeostasis model assessment of insulin resistance (HOMA-IR), procollagen, tumor necrosis factor-α (TNF-α), and interleukin-6 (IL-6).

Biomarkers are playing an increasing role in the study of CV disease and we attempt to define their function in improving clinical management and outcomes [2, 3]. By definition, biomarkers are objectively measured indicators of biological processes, and to be of use, they must be relevant, predictable, accurate, and reproducible [3]. They provide readily quantifiable surrogate endpoints and allow accurate assessment of the effects of therapy on particular pathological processes, thereby allowing for prompt diagnosis and more timely initiation of appropriate treatment, improved monitoring, and treatment augmentation [4].

Some of the benefits of inhibiting RAS with ARBs and ACEIs have been shown to be independent of blood pressure (BP) reduction [5] [6]. Surrogate biomarkers are diverse, and they may provide a viable means of measuring the response to treatment. This chapter will focus on the following eight biomarkers, which have been used as predictors of vascular outcome in patients with hypertension and those with metabolic syndrome: CAP, hsCRP, adiponectin, cystatin C, HOMA-IR, procollagen, TNF-α, and IL-6.

Anti-inflammatory, anti-atherogenic, and/or improved metabolic homeostasis, independent of BP lowering, which is seen with some antihypertensives, may benefit high-risk patient populations or those who do not achieve adequate BP control. These include ethnic groups such as African Americans, obese patients, and patients with renal disease, metabolic syndrome, diabetes mellitus, and/or existing vascular disease. Improvements in inflammatory and other biomarkers has been reported with ARBs and ACEIs in obese patients with metabolic syndrome [7, 8] and in hypertensive patients with and without type 2 diabetes mellitus (T2DM) [9, 10]. Similarly, CCBs have been shown to improve markers of inflammation in patients with hypertension [11, 12], while β-blockers such as nebivolol were shown to modify markers of inflammation and obesity in obese African Americans with hypertension [13]. As a class, ARBs are known to have anti-inflammatory properties, which may contribute to their pharmacologic effects. Biomarker studies in hypertensive patients have demonstrated the effects of ARBs on inflammatory and other biomarkers [7, 14], including CAP [15, 16], hsCRP [14, 17-19], adiponectin [20], cystatin [21, 22], HOMA-IR [23-25], procollagen [26-28], TNF-α [29-31], and IL-6 [32-34].

This chapter summarizes the role of biomarkers as surrogate endpoints in the treatment of hypertensive patients and discusses the evidence for the effects of ARBs and other antihypertensive drugs on biomarkers and their correlation with clinical efficacy. The source material for this review was derived from a MEDLINE literature search, performed from 1999 to 2011, to identify published studies investigating the use of selective antihypertensive agents using at least one of the eight previously mentioned biomarkers. The agents specified in the search were amlodipine, olmesartan medoxomil, combination amlodipine plus olmesartan medoxomil, losartan, hydrochlorothiazide (HCTZ), and combination losartan plus HCTZ.

2. A review of anti-hypertensive drugs

Hypertension is a strong contributor to cardiovascular disease in patients with the cardiometabolic syndrome. It has been shown to not only be an independent risk factor, but it also contributes to the development of other risk factors for cardiovascular disease. Over the last few decades, a number of classes of anti-hypertensive drugs have been used to treat hypertension, with the ultimate goal of reducing the incidence of endpoints such as heart attacks and stroke. Some of the broad categories of antihypertensives include thiazide diuretics, ARBs, ACEIs, CCBs and β-blockers.

The first step in atherosclerosis is endothelial dysfunction. It has been shown that the RAS is involved in the development of atherosclerosis through many different mechanisms including increasing oxidative stress, vasoconstriction, inflammation and reduced ability of the endothelium to regenerate itself (reviewed in [35]). The blockage of the RAS through ACEIs and ARBs, aids in slowing down the processes of endothelial dysfunction and subsequent atherosclerosis. ACEIs reduce angiotensin II production and suppress the degradation of bradykinin. This results in reduced oxidative stress, improved vasodilation and improved endothelial function [36, 37]. Some common ACEIs include ramipril, enalapril, lisinopril, perindopril and fosinopril. The Heart Outcomes Prevention Evaluation (HOPE) study evaluated the benefits of ramipril as compared to placebo [38]. Ramipril (10mg/day) resulted in a reduction of cardiovascular death (26% RR), nonfatal myocardial infarction (MI) (20% RR) and stroke (32% RR). Ramipril was shown to be beneficial in all subgroups of patients in the HOPE Study. The Efficacy of Perindopril in Reduction of Cardiovascular Events Among Patients with Stable Coronary Artery Disease (EUROPA) study, Perindopril Protection Against Recurrent Stroke (PROGRESS) study and the Anglo-Scandinavian Cardiac Outcomes Trial-Blood Pressure Lowering Arm (ASCOT-BPLA) study are some other large, outcome trials which also showed a positive effect of ACEIs on cardiovascular events and mortality [39-41].

ARBs also block the RAS. This is accomplished through blocking of the angiotensin I receptor which leads to an upregulation of the angiotensin II receptor and the conversion of of angiotensin II to angiotensin $_{(1-7)}$ which has vasodilatory, antioxidant and pro-apoptotic properties [42, 43]. Some common ARBs include losartan, telmisartan, valsartan, olmesartan, candesartan and irbesartan. Large outcome trials such as the Renal Outcomes with Telmisartan, Ramipril, or Both, in People at High Vascular Risk (ONTARGET) study, and the Valsartan in Acute Myocardial Infarction (VALIANT) study have shown that ARBs are comparable to ACEIs in reducing cardiovascular risk, without the side effect of excess coughing that is frequently experienced by patients who are taking ACEIs [44] [45]. Combination of ARBs with β-blockers or statins have also shown positive results [46, 47].

CCBs are another class of antihypertensives which provide similar blood pressure lowering effects of ACEIs and ARBs, but they provide better protection against stroke and heart failure [48]. CCBs inhibit the flow of extracellular calcium through ion-specific channels that span the cell wall. This causes vascular smooth muscle cells to relax and thereby results in vasodilation, blood pressure lowering and reduced peripheral arterial resistance. Commonly prescribed CCBs include amlodipine, benidipine, azelnidipine and manidipine.

β-blockers are another group of antihypertensives which are divided into two main categories. Traditional (non-vasodilatory) β-blockers such as atenolol, metropolol and propanolol reduce blood pressure by reducing cardiac output [49]. These β-blockers are effective at lowering brachial blood pressure, however data from studies including the Conduit Artery Function Evaluation (CAFÉ) study suggests that these compounds do not adequately control central aortic pressure [50]. This can then lead to an increase in vascular events including stroke [51]. Additionally, these agents have been shown to increase plasma triglyceride levels [52] and the risk of new-onset diabetes by about 20-30% [53, 54]. The other group of β-blockers are the vasodilatory β-blockers which includes labetalol, carvediol and nebivolol. These drugs reduce systemic vascular resistance while maintaining cardiac output. Additionally, these agents do not negatively affect glycemic control and may even provide beneficial metabolic effects [55-57].

Diuretics include HCTZ , chlorthalidone and the loop diuretics such as furosemide. According to the Joint National Committee on Prevention, Detection, Evaluation , and Treatment of High Blood Pressure (JNC 7) guidelines, diuretics are recommended as the first line of therapy for hypertension [58]. Chlorothalidone is more potent at 25mg dosing than 50mg of HCTZ. Also, chlorothalidone has been shown to improve cardiovascular outcomes [59]. Certain subpopulations, including diabetics, the elderly and blacks have lower renin levels and they respond favorably to diuretic therapy [60]. Diuretics, particularly HCTZ, are often combined with antihypertensives from another class, such as ARBs and ACEIs, to provide enhanced therapeutic benefits [61].

The newest category of anytihypertensives include direct renin inhibitors (DRIs). Aliskiren is the most common DRI. This class of drugs works by inhibiting the first rate-limiting step in the RAS, resulting in a more complete inhibition of the RAS cascade as compared to ACEIs and ARBs [62]. Additionally, DRIs reduce the production of aldosterone, which in addition to its sodium retension effects, also is a mediator in oxidative stress and inflammation [63] [64]. The Aliskiren in the Evaluation of Proteinuria in Diabetes (AVOID) study and the Aliskiren Observation of Heart Failure Treatment (ALOFT) trial show that aliskiren has renal and cardio protective effects in addition to blood pressure regulation [65, 66].

3. Role of biomarkers and mechanisms in specific patient groups

3.1. CAP

While brachial BP is easily measured and has been shown to be predictive of CV morbidity and mortality, it is an imperfect surrogate measure of CAP. Peripheral systolic BP (SBP) measured at the brachial artery does not accurately reflect CAP, particularly in youths, as a result of peripheral amplification of the pulse pressure wave [67-69]. This amplification difference decreases with age and arterial stiffness. Central aortic systolic pressure or pulse pressure has been shown to be a powerful and more robust predictor of end organ damage and CV mortality than brachial BP, irrespective of whether the central pressures were derived from noninvasive pulse wave analysis or measured directly during routine catheterization [68]. Although techniques have been developed to a stage where direct noninvasive measurement of CAP could be readily applied to routine clinical practice, the studies conducted to-date, assessing the predictive value of CAP, have been relatively small. Thus, additional data from large interventional studies of clinical outcomes and larger-scale longitudinal epidemiological studies of clinical outcomes are required to confirm the utility of CAP as a predictor of vascular risk before it becomes part of routine clinical practice [67-69].

Noninvasive assessment of the central pulse pressure waveform is performed by applanation tonometry, which involves applying a pressure sensor (tonometer) with mild pressure over the radial or carotid artery. The recorded waveform is then used to algorithmically derive central pressure indices from a peripheral brachial BP measurement [69]. In addition, aortic pulse wave velocity (PWV), which is usually recorded between the carotid and femoral arteries, is used to determine vessel distensibility; the velocity of the pulse wave increases with decreasing vessel distensibility (increased arterial stiffness) [67]. Increased PWV, an indication of arterial stiffness, appears to be associated with endothelial dysfunction, inflammation, and atherosclerosis, and has been shown to be an independent predictor of coronary events and CV mortality [67]. Hence, arterial stiffness is an emerging biomarker for therapeutic interventions.

3.2. hsCRP

C-reactive protein (CRP), an acute phase reactant predominantly produced in the liver in response to IL-6, interleukin-1β, and TNF-α, is a marker of the general inflammatory response. Current technology permits the quantification of CRP through a high-sensitivity assay, therefore this marker is referred to as hsCRP. Epidemiological studies have established that individuals with higher levels of hsCRP have increased CV risk [70]. The nature of the relationship between hsCRP and CV disease is unclear, but hsCRP provides a useful measure of risk and the effects of interventions [70, 71].

Studies have shown a continuous independent association between serum CRP levels and elevated BP [72]. In elderly, normotensive individuals, higher baseline CRP levels were associated with a higher incidence of new-onset hypertension after 2 years [73]. Moreover, in apparently healthy adults representative of the US population, a 10-mmHg increase in pulse pressure was associated with significant increases of 12%–15% in the odds of having an elevated CRP level, independent of SBP or diastolic BP (DBP), or demographic factors [74]. There are even suggestions that hsCRP may be a better marker of coronary artery disease (CAD) than low-density lipoprotein cholesterol (LDL-C) [2, 75]. Evidence suggests that inhibition of the RAS with certain agents, particularly ARBs and ACEIs, may improve CV outcomes by reducing vascular inflammation and remodeling independently of BP reductions [76].

3.3. Adiponectin

Adiponectin is one of the adipocyte-derived hormones that has profound anti-inflammatory and anti-atherogenic properties. It is also thought to play an important role in the modulation of glucose and lipid metabolism [2, 77]. Reduced adiponectin levels have been noted in males, obese subjects, and patients with hypertension, CAD, or T2DM [78]. Reduced adiponectin levels are predictive of CAD and MI [79]. Animal studies have shown that increased adiponectin levels are protective against atherosclerosis, while clinical studies with antihypertensive drugs, including ARBs, ACEIs, and CCBs, have associated improvements in BP and insulin resistance with increased adiponectin levels [78, 80]. In obese subjects, serum adiponectin levels were inversely associated with intima-media thickness, a surrogate measure of subclinical atherosclerosis, and positively associated with arterial compliance [79]. The mechanism behind the beneficial effects of adiponectin is uncertain; one hypothesis suggests that adiponectin increases nitric oxide activity, thereby inhibiting platelet activation, while another hypothesis suggests it suppresses monocyte activation [78].

3.4. Cystatin C

The serum cystatin C level directly correlates with the glomerular filtration rate (GFR) and is produced constantly, independent of muscle mass, age, or sex. It is therefore an easily obtained biomarker for renal dysfunction that may be more reliable than measurement of creatinine levels in certain patient populations, particularly in children [81-83]. However, there are concerns over the cost of the immunoassay, intraindividual variability, and its sensitivity in transplant patients or its suitability in patients with cancer, where cystatin C production may vary [82]. Notably, a study in patients after heart transplantation found that cystatin C was superior to creatinine as a prognostic indicator of early renal dysfunction during 4 years of follow-up [84].

Cystatin C is a predictor of CV morbidity and mortality, and it has been suggested that this association may be independent of renal function [85, 86]. In one study, cystatin C, but not creatinine or GFR, was closely associated with left ventricular (LV) mass in patients with hypertension, suggesting utility as a marker for cardiac hypertrophy [86].

3.5. HOMA-IR

HOMA-IR is a mathematical model prediction that provides an accurate quantitative assessment of insulin resistance [87], which is associated with hypertension, obesity, and diabetes, and an increased risk of CAD [88].

Many CV drugs adversely affect glucose and lipid homeostasis, and insulin resistance is an important mediator of these adverse effects on glucose metabolism [88]. Direct RAS inhibitors (ARBs and ACEIs) and some other antihypertensives provide beneficial effects in terms of glucose homeostasis [88].

3.6. Procollagen

Collagen fractions in the extracellular matrix are intimately involved in the atherosclerotic process and the vascular remodeling that occurs in CV disease [89]. There is evidence that altered collagen metabolism (eg, elevated serum levels of tissue inhibitor of metalloproteinase-1) is associated with hypertension [89], and that plasma markers of collagen metabolism are positively correlated with arterial stiffness measured by PWV in hypertensive patients with LV hypertrophy [90].

Therefore, measurement of serum procollagen fractions as indicators of myocardial fibrosis may be useful in the clinical assessment of CV risk [91].

3.7. TNF-α

TNF-α is a marker of inflammation and is believed to promote the development of insulin resistance and hyperinsulinemia, and thereby affect BP [29]. TNF-α is released from mast cells and macrophages in the myocardial endothelium during acute MI, and from cardiomyocytes during persistent ischemia. The released TNF-α contributes to ischemic and/or reperfusion injury and is believed to contribute to cardiac contractile dysfunction after MI via a local inflammatory reaction [31]. Surprisingly, low levels of TNF-α may be beneficial and display a cardioprotective effect, reducing infarct size [31]. TNF-α is also believed to play a role in the development of atherosclerosis by up-regulating cell surface receptors for advanced glycation end products that promote the release of inflammatory mediators in the endothelium [30]. The differential effects are possibly related to which of the two tumor necrosis receptor types (TNF-R1 or TNF-R2) the TNF-α molecule interacts.

3.8. IL-6

IL-6 is an inflammatory cytokine that, along with TNF-α, is one of the main inducers of acute phase reactants, such as CRP. It has been positively correlated with CV risk. For instance, in elderly subjects without known CV disease, serum levels of IL-6 were significantly associated with CAD, stroke, and congestive heart failure events, and to a greater extent than CRP or TNF-α levels [92]. Similarly, in older men without CAD, IL-6 was found to be more discriminating than CRP and fibrinogen in predicting a first coronary artery ischemic event, being associated with MI/coronary death but not CAD endpoints (angina) [33]. However, not all studies have found strong correlations between IL-6 and CAD [34].

4. Antihypertensive drugs: benefits beyond just blood pressure lowering

Clinical evidence that many current antihypertensive agents have a beneficial effect on putative biomarkers of CV pathology or risk continues to accumulate and indicates that not all drugs or patient subpopulations are equal.

4.1. CAP

Of the various antihypertensive drug classes, RAS inhibitors (ARBs and ACEIs) and CCBs generally appear to have greater effects on CAP than β-blockers and thiazide diuretics. Despite similar brachial BP reductions, the combination of amlodipine plus perindopril was associated with greater reductions in CAP than atenolol plus a thiazide diuretic [93]. Lisinopril also significantly reduced central SBP, central pulse pressure, and the augmentation index, while bisoprolol only significantly lowered central DBP and actually increased the augmentation index [94]. The combination of olmesartan and azelnidipine was compared to olmesartan and amlodipine [95]. While both combinations had similar brachial BP lowering effects, there was a greater reduction in CAP with the olmesartan/azelnidipine combination. Another study showed significant reductions in both brachial and central BP reductions with different drug classes in the following order: CCBs > diuretics (HCTZ) > ACEIs [96]. β-blockers did not significantly lower peripheral or central BP.

Similar brachial BP and CAP reductions were achieved with valsartan plus HCTZ versus amlodipine; however, valsartan plus HCTZ provided a greater reduction in arterial stiffness (estimated by aortic PWV) [97]. Reductions in central SBP were greater with fosinopril plus HCTZ than with indapamide or amlodipine; this correlated with 24-hour and nighttime SBP reductions, but not with seated cuff SBP [98].

Recent studies have shown that PWV is significantly reduced with candesartan or benidipine treatment, as compared to amlodipine [99, 100]. Arterial stiffness, measured through cardioankle vascular index was significantly decreased with combination of olmesartan and azelnidipine, but not with olmesartan monotheraphy [101]. However, arterial index decreased significantly with monotheraphy and combination therapy in this study. On the other hand, another recent study showed that monotheraphy with olmesartan does significantly decrease arterial stiffness [102].

The effects of antihypertensives on flow mediated dilation (FMD) has also been measured. Olmesartan has been shown to positively impact FMD and while amlodipine treatment has no effect on FMD [103], the combination of amlodipine and atorvastatin has significant improvements on this marker, even more than atorvastatin alone [104]. Another study found the same effects of amlodipine and atorvastatin combination on patients with hypertension and hyperglycemia [105]. The combination of amlodipine and valsartan was also found to improve FMD in diabetics with early hypertension, even more than the effects of the individual drugs [106].

4.2. hsCRP

Several antihypertensive drug classes, such as ARBs, ACEIs, and CCBs, lower serum hsCRP in addition to BP, indicating a reduction in the inflammatory processes involved in the progression of atherosclerosis. ARBs, in particular, seem to have a strong depressor effect on this marker of inflammation. Patients with chronic kidney disease (CKD), who have higher baseline levels of inflammation than control subjects with normal renal function, displayed significant reductions in hsCRP and brachial BP with olmesartan medoxomil treatment [107]. In a small study of 10 patients with mild-to-moderate hypertension, olmesartan medoxomil did not reduce BP significantly, but did produce significant reductions in hsCRP and appeared to improve myocardial function independent of BP lowering [19]. In another study, hsCRP levels significantly dropped in hypertensive patients who were treated with olmesartan for 6 month [102]. In non-diabetic patients with hypertension and the metabolic syndrome, both olmesartan medoxomil plus amlodipine and olmesartan medoxomil plus HCTZ effectively reduced BP and CRP with no differences between groups. However, olmesartan plus amlodipine produced greater reductions in all other inflammatory markers [108]. Olmesartan treatment was compared to candesartan treatment in hypertensive patients with T2DM [109]. BP and hsCRP reductions were similar in both treatment groups. In a separate study, these researchers also found that monotherapy with either losartan or ramapril is equally beneficial in lowering hsCRP [109].

In a study comparing the CCB azelnidipine or the thiazide diuretic trichlormethiazide added to an ARB, the ARB plus azelnidipine combination produced significantly greater reductions in hsCRP than the ARB plus thiazide combination; this reduction mirrored the BP-lowering effects [110]. Similar data were shown in a 4-month crossover study comparing olmesartan medoxomil plus azelnidipine or trichlormethiazide [111]. Azelnidipine was shown to be superior to amlodipine with regards to hsCRP lowering in nondiabetic hypertensive patients and the beneficial effects of azelnidipine also included improved glucose tolerance and insulin sensitivity [112]. When combined with atorvastatin, amlodipine therapy reduces plasma hsCRP significantly [104]. In the recent Effects of Manidipine and its Combination with an ACE Inhibitor on Insulin Sensitivity and Metabolic, Inflammatory and Prothrombotic Markers in Hypertensive Patients with Metabolic Syndrome: the MARCADO Study, a number of monotherapies (manidipine, amlodipine, teimisartan) and combination therapy (manidipine/lisionpril) were compared for treatment of non-diabetic, hypertensive patients with the metabolic syndrome. Levels of hsCRP reduced with all of these treatments, but the most significant reduction was with the manidipine/lisinopril combination therapy [113]. Comparison of 12 weeks of combination therapy with enalapril plus add-on losartan with higher dose enalapril monotherapy showed a significant reduction in hsCRP with combination therapy, but not with high-dose enalapril alone; BP reductions were significant and similar in both groups [114]. In another study, patients who were on olmesartan therapy received additional HCTZ or azelnidipine therapy for 24 weeks. HsCRP levels dropped significantly with the azelnidipine add-on therapy but there was no change with HCTZ therapy [115].

Evidence suggests that ARBs may differ in their anti-inflammatory effects. For instance, in patients with CAD, olmesartan medoxomil and valsartan both produced significant reductions in BP, but only olmesartan medoxomil induced a significant reduction in hsCRP [116]. Losartan has also been shown to reduce hsCRP in newly diagnosed hypertensive patients who are at CV disease risk [117]. Studies comparing the hsCRP-lowering effects of ARBs and CCBs have shown variable results. One study found no difference in hsCRP reductions after 8 weeks of therapy with losartan or amlodipine regimens [118]. The effects on hsCRP and other inflammatory markers did not explain the greater improvements in insulin sensitivity seen with ARBs over CCBs. However, in patients with hypertension and other CV risk factors, therapy with valsartan plus HCTZ was significantly more effective than amlodipine in reducing hsCRP. These biomarker results correlated with BP reductions [119]. HsCRP improvement did not correlate with endothelial function in a study comparing candesartan with amlodipine; both treatments significantly improved endothelial function (assessed by changes in forearm blood flow in reactive hyperemia), whereas significant reductions in hsCRP levels were seen only with candesartan and not amlodipine therapy [120]. The study investigators concluded that the anti-inflammatory effects observed with candesartan may be related to observed improvement in insulin sensitivity. In a study of patients with CAD, treatment with irbesartan did not lower hsCRP levels. [121] The lack of effect of irbesartan may have been due to low levels of hsCRP at study baseline. Patients were also receiving statin and aspirin therapy, which also lower levels of this marker. In a recent study, olmesartan reduced hsCRP levels in patients with essential hypertension while amlodipine had no effects on hsCRP [103].

As with ARBs, CCBs seem to differ in their ability to reduce inflammatory markers. In hypertensive patients with the metabolic syndrome, similar significant reductions in hsCRP and BP were seen with manidipine and amlodipine, but these data did not correlate with changes in other biomarkers, such as adiponectin, HOMA-IR, and TNF-α, which showed greater improvements with manidipine than with amlodipine [122]. In a different study in patients with arterial hypertension and insulin resistance who were already receiving at least two antihypertensive agents, neither moxonidine nor amlodipine showed significant changes in hsCRP, whereas both treatments resulted in significant BP lowering [123].

Adding a 3-hydroxy-3-methylglutaryl-coenzyme A (HMG-CoA) reductase inhibitor (atorvastatin) to amlodipine therapy produced significantly greater reductions in BP and hsCRP than was seen with amlodipine alone [124], but losartan plus simvastatin achieved similar reductions in hsCRP compared with losartan or simvastatin alone [47]. BP reductions were significantly greater with losartan or losartan plus simvastatin than with simvastatin alone. The combination of rosuvastatin and a number of ARBs was studied as treatment in adults with the metabolic syndrome [125]. While rosuvastatin and telmisartan reduced hsCRP by 44% after 24 weeks of therapy, there was less reduction in hsCRP with the combination of rosuvastatin and irbesartan or rosuvastatin and olmesartan.

These observations suggest that RAS antagonists such as ARBs and ACEIs have a significant anti-inflammatory effect, and there may be variations within these classes. As diseases such as diabetes mellitus and atherosclerosis are inflammatory processes, the clinical benefits seen with these classes of antihypertensives may be a combination of the suppression of inflammation and the reduction of BP.

4.3. Adiponectin

Studies assessing the effect of the selected antihypertensive drugs on the serum levels of adiponectin are discussed here. Antihypertensive agents do not uniformly influence metabolic parameters in patients with hypertension. In a comparison of telmisartan and irbesartan in obese, insulin-resistant, hypertensive patients, increases were significantly greater with telmisartan, although both treatments resulted in significant increases in adiponectin levels [126]. Adiponectin changes correlated inversely with changes in BP for telmisartan, but not for irbesartan. The investigators speculate that the differences between the two agents may be partly due to partial peroxisome proliferator-activated receptor-γ (PPAR-γ) agonist activity exhibited by telmisartan, although a study by Kintscher et al in 14,200 patients confirmed that irbesartan also activates PPAR-γ [127]. Despite similar reductions in BP, olmesartan medoxomil plus amlodipine produced significant increases in adiponectin levels in patients with hypertension and the metabolic syndrome, whereas olmesartan medoxomil plus HCTZ did not [108]. The increase in adiponectin correlated with a lower risk for developing T2DM and paralleled reductions (improvements) in HOMA-IR index and fasting plasma insulin levels.

In nondiabetic, proteinuric patients, treatment with losartan plus HCTZ reduced BP, proteinuria, and LDL-C, and increased adiponectin, but the change in adiponectin correlated with adverse reductions in high-density lipoprotein cholesterol (HDL-C) levels [128]. In a crossover study that investigated possible factors to explain improvements in insulin sensitivity with ARB therapy compared with CCB therapy in patients with hypertension, between group differences were not noted for increases in adiponectin levels or reductions in BP after 8 weeks of therapy with losartan or amlodipine [118]. In contrast, although both telmisartan and amlodipine increased adiponectin levels in patients with hypertension and T2DM, the increases were higher with telmisartan than with amlodipine [129]. Both groups showed a similar significant decrease in BP. Similarly, in patients with prediabetes, losartan produced greater increases in adiponectin than a CCB, whereas BP reduction was similar and significant in both groups [130]. Within CCBs, candesartan, but not olmesartan therapy, over the period of a year resulted in increased adiponectin and insulin sensitivity in T2DM hypertensive patients, even though BP lowering was similar in both treatment groups [109]. When compared to the ACEI ramipril, losartan treatment significantly improved adiponectin levels and overall metabolic parameters while ramipril had no effect on adiponectin or any other metabolic markers [131]. In obese hypertensive patients, telmisartan, but not losartan raised serum adiponectin levels [132].

ARBs and statins have additive effects on adiponectin. Losartan plus simvastatin or losartan alone resulted in significantly greater increases in adiponectin levels from baseline than with simvastatin alone [47]. This correlated with BP reductions, which were greater with losartan or losartan plus simvastatin than with simvastatin alone. A correlation was also observed with LDL reductions, which were greater with simvastatin or simvastatin with losartan relative to losartan alone.

There were no changes in adiponectin levels with the aldosterone blocker spironolactone or the CCB amlodipine in patients with diabetic nephropathy or in controls. However, spironolactone, but not amlodipine, increased adiponectin in a subgroup of patients with poor baseline glycemic control, i.e. glycosylated hemoglobin (HbA_{1c}) ≥8%. A significant decrease in SBP, but not DBP, was observed in both treatment groups [133]. This link between the renin-angiotensin cascade and aldosterone suggests a possible mechanism by which spironolactone provides an increased level of adiponectin in hyperglycemia.

In a comparison of enalapril, metoprolol, amlodipine, and indapamide, no changes in adiponectin level were seen with enalapril, amlodipine, or metoprolol, whereas a reduction in adiponectin was seen with indapamide. This reduction in adiponectin with the thiazide-like diuretic correlated with increased insulin resistance [134]. In a comparison of metoprolol, amlodipine, ramipril, doxazosin, and valsartan in hypertensive patients with the metabolic syndrome, both ramipril and valsartan resulted in significantly higher increases in adiponectin than the other regimens; adiponectin levels inversely correlated with SBP [135]. In a study comparing manidipine, amlodipine, telmisartan, and the combination therapy of manidipine and lisinopril, adiponectin levels increased with all of the treatments except amlodipine. The greatest increase in adiponectin was seen with manidipine [113]. The combination of amlodipine and atorvastatin resulted in a greater increase in adiponectin than treatment with amlodipine alone [104]. Similar results were seen in patients with hypertension and hyperglycemia that were treated with amlodipine and atorvastatin [105].

In a small study in patients with hypertension, ramipril, candesartan, and amlodipine were associated with greater increases in adiponectin levels while thiazide and atenolol were associated with a decrease in adiponectin. There were no correlations with BP lowering, which was greatest with atenolol, amlodipine, and candesartan therapies than with ramipril [136].

Unlike the situation with hypertensive, obese, or diabetic patients, where adiponectin levels are reportedly reduced, the levels of adiponectin are raised in patients with renal disease when compared with healthy controls. Thus, in patients with renal disease, a positive correlation between adiponectin and insulin resistance is seen, and increased adiponectin levels are associated with increased all-cause and CV mortality (the opposite of that seen in obese patients or those with T2DM without renal disease). Paradoxically, short-term losartan therapy in patients with T2DM nephropathy was associated with a significant decrease in adiponectin levels compared with amlodipine therapy [137].

Adiponectin, secreted by fat cells, regulates the insulin response and has a favorable effect on glucose and lipid metabolism. Insulin resistance is a hallmark for the progression of vascular disease. The quantitative changes in adiponectin provide insight into how antihypertensive agents such as ARBs may be effective in attenuating or reversing the pathogenesis of atherosclerosis and diabetes mellitus.

4.4. Cystatin C

Only three studies have assessed the effect of the selected antihypertensive drugs on serum cystatin C levels. In one study, a significant decrease in cystatin C with olmesartan medoxomil therapy correlated with improvements in BP, LV mass index, and LV hypertrophy at 6 months [138]. Another study found that cystatin C levels decreased in patients who were on olmesartan or olmesartan with HCTZ, but in this study, there was no correlation between cyctatin C and BP levels [139]. However, the third study found no significant decrease in cystatin C with enalapril/losartan combination therapy or with high-dose enalapril, despite significant reductions in BP [114].

The use of cystatin C as an early marker for CKD may be helpful in longitudinal follow-up analyses. The findings in the above studies are preliminary but suggest that BP reduction may be associated with lower cystatin C levels. It is too early to determine whether inhibition of the RAS (in the form of ACEIs or ARBs) may have an effect on cystatin C that is superior to other antihypertensive drugs.

4.5. HOMA-IR

HOMA-IR is a model and calculation to determine quantification of insulin resistance. Antihypertensive drugs appear to have differing effects on insulin resistance, with ARBs foremost among those improving insulin sensitivity, although considerable variability has been observed and not all ARBs may be equal in this regard. RAS inhibitors generally have greater effects on glucose homeostasis than CCBs, which are usually considered to have neutral effects.

In hypertensive patients, a significantly greater reduction in HOMA-IR was seen with losartan/amlodipine therapy than with high-dose amlodipine [118]. The addition of losartan therapy to chronic heart failure patients who were on ACEIs resulted in a reduction of HOMA-IR as well as inflammatory cytokines after 24 weeks of therapy [140]. The MARCADOR Study compared the effects of manidipine, amlodipine, telmisartan, and manidipine combined with lisinopril. While BP lowering was similar with all of these treatments, HOMA-IR levels improved in all of the treatments except for amlodipine, and the greatest change in HOMA-IR was seen with manidipine treatment [113]. In contrast to previous results, both losartan and telmisartan had neutral effects on insulin resistance in 42 hypertensive patients with the metabolic syndrome, with no significant reductions in HOMA-IR in either group; BP reductions were similar for both ARBs [141]. In a more recent study, obese hypertensive patients were treated with telmisartan or olmesartan. While olmesartan improved BP levels, only telmisartan improved insulin glucose and HOMA-IR levels in addition to improving BP levels [25]. Others have also shown that telmisartan therapy helps to reduce HOMA-IR levels as compared to other ARBs and CCBs [132, 142]. Researchers studied the effects of irbesartan as compared to olmesartan in obese hypertensive females and found that while both treatments improved BP and lipid levels, only olmesartan resulted in HOMA-IR changes [143]. Olmesartan was also found to reduce HOMA-IR in hypertensive patients with sleep disordered breathing. Positive changes in BP level and left ventricular ejection fraction were also seen in these patients with olmesartan treatment [144].

Non-diabetic CKD patients have a high prevalence of insulin resistance, metabolic syndrome, and chronic inflammation. Treatment with olmesartan medoxomil for 16 weeks was associated with a significant reduction in HOMA-IR, along with reductions in markers of inflammation [107]. Losartan therapy was associated with improvements in fasting plasma insulin and HOMA-IR in patients with T2DM nephropathy, in parallel with reductions in adiponectin levels [137]. Both olmesartan medoxomil and telmisartan were shown to improve HOMA-IR in patients with nonalcoholic fatty liver disease and chronic hepatitis C, conditions with a greater incidence of insulin resistance than other liver diseases [145].

In a study investigating the effect of combination therapy with amlodipine plus olmesartan medoxomil on HOMA-IR in hypertensive patients with the metabolic syndrome, HOMA-IR was significantly reduced with olmesartan medoxomil/amlodipine, whereas no significant changes were seen with olmesartan medoxomil/HCTZ. The reductions in the HOMA-IR index strongly correlated with the increases in adiponectin level in the group treated with olmesartan medoxomil/amlodipine [108].

In a crossover study of amlodipine with or without atorvastatin therapy in obese patients with hypertension and normal lipid profiles, combination amlodipine/atorvastatin therapy produced a significantly greater reduction in HOMA-IR than amlodipine monotherapy; there was no correlation with BP reduction with either treatment [29]. The combination of rosuvastatin with telmisartan significantly lowered HOMA-IR and fasting serum insulin levels in metabolic syndrome patients, but when irbesartan or olmesartan was combined with rosuvastatin, HOMA-IR and fasting insulin levels increased [125]. In non-diabetic patients with the metabolic syndrome, manidipine, but not amlodipine, significantly reduced HOMA-IR [122].

In patients with hypertension and insulin resistance, neither moxonidine nor amlodipine produced changes in HOMA-IR. Both treatments significantly lowered BP and increased HDL-C, but only moxonidine reduced serum triglycerides. Neither drug affected serum CRP levels [123].

In patients with T2DM nephropathy, losartan, but not amlodipine, reduced HOMA-IR from baseline, but the between-group difference was not significant. However, other parameters of glucose metabolism (eg, fasting blood glucose, HbA_{1c}, and insulin sensitivity) were improved to a greater extent with losartan than with amlodipine [146]. In patients with hypertension and T2DM, telmisartan resulted in greater improvements in HOMA-IR than amlodipine [129].

Similar results with losartan and amlodipine were seen in patients with prediabetes, with greater improvements in HOMA-IR with losartan than with amlodipine; the two agents resulted in similar BP reductions [130].

In a study in hypertensive patients, both candesartan and amlodipine significantly improved endothelial function, but significant decreases in HOMA-IR and CRP were only observed with candesartan [120].

In a comparison of losartan and amlodipine in Japanese patients with hypertension, with or without diabetes, losartan provided greater increases in adiponectin than amlodipine. These increases correlated with HOMA-IR changes [147].

In agreement with the adiponectin results discussed earlier, indapamide treatment increased HOMA-IR in patients with hypertension, whereas no changes in HOMA-IR were seen with enalapril, metoprolol, or amlodipine [134]. In patients with hypertension and the metabolic syndrome, doxazosin, amlodipine, ramipril, and valsartan produced significant reductions in HOMA-IR, whereas no changes were seen with metoprolol [135].

Insulin resistance is a central force in the pathogenesis of vascular diseases, and HOMA-IR provides a reasonable assessment of the quantification of insulin resistance. Several long-term clinical studies have demonstrated the clinical benefit of ARBs in diabetic kidney disease, both in late stage [the Reduction of Endpoints in NIDDM with Angiotensin II

Antagonist Losartan (RENAAL) study and the Irbesartan Diabetic Nephropathy Trial (IDNT) study] and early stage [The Effect of Irbesartan on the Development of Diabetic Nephropathy in Patients with Type 2 Diabetes (IRMA-2) study]. The role of HOMA-IR may be beneficial in clinical practice, and quantitative and longitudinal analysis could provide long-term follow-up of disease management.

4.6. Procollagen

Several studies have assessed the effect of antihypertensive agents on procollagen fractions as a marker of atherogenesis and vascular remodeling. Valsartan and ramipril, but not amlodipine, were associated with reductions in procollagen. Despite similar BP lowering, valsartan and ramipril were more effective than amlodipine in preventing new episodes of atrial fibrillation [148].

Another study showed a significant difference in procollagen type I carboxy-terminal peptide (PICP) lowering between candesartan and amlodipine. Although BP control was similar, 24-hour SBP was significantly lower and LV mass index significantly decreased with amlodipine, while the effect of ARBs on procollagen indicate that they protect against CV fibrosis and renal injury [149].

There were no differences in procollagen markers with losartan- or atenolol-based regimens after the first year of treatment; changes in PICP during the first year of treatment were related to subsequent changes in LV mass index after 2 and 3 years of treatment in patients randomized to losartan, but not atenolol [26]. Losartan-related reduction in procollagen was shown to be greater in patients with higher baseline levels (those with hypertension and severe myocardial fibrosis) [150] and was significantly associated with symptom improvement [151].

4.7. TNF-α and IL-6

The effects of antihypertensive drugs on the inflammatory biomarker TNF-α have been somewhat variable. In patients with hypertension, olmesartan medoxomil reduced TNF-α levels in one study [152], but in another study in Japanese patients, neither losartan nor the CCB amlodipine significantly affected TNF-α levels [147]. In obese hypertensive patients, telmisartan, but not losartan treatment, was shown to reduce serum TNF-α levels [132]. Conversely, another study showed that in newly diagnosed hypertension patients, losartan lowers TNF-α levels [117]. In chronic heart failure patients, the addition of losartan to ACEI therapy resulted in a significant reduction of TNF-α levels [140]. Amlodipine was effective in reducing TNF-α, but was significantly more effective when combined with atorvastatin [153]. Another study found no difference between losartan and amlodipine in TNF-α levels after treatment, but the investigators did not appear to perform baseline assessments in order to determine if either drug reduced TNF-α from baseline levels [118]. Manidipine and lisinopril combination therapy was shown to have a highly significant effect on TNF-α levels in non-diabetic, hypertensive patients with the metabolic syndrome [113].

Losartan therapy significantly reduced TNF-α in patients with hypertension and T2DM [154]. However, olmesartan medoxomil combined with HCTZ had no effect on TNF-α in patients with hypertension and the metabolic syndrome (without diabetes), but when olmesartan medoxomil was combined with amlodipine, the combination did significantly reduce TNF-α levels [108]. Amlodipine was shown to reduce serum TNF-α levels, as well as mRNA expression of TNF-α in hypertensives with and without diabetes [155]. Interestingly, amlodipine alone was shown in another study to have no effect on TNF-α levels in patients with hypertension and the metabolic syndrome, whereas manidipine monotherapy was effective in lowering TNF-α [122]. Olmesartan medoxomil had no effect on TNF-α levels in patients with stage 3 or 4 CKD [107], and TNF-α was unaffected by amlodipine or spironolactone in patients with diabetic nephropathy [133].

Studies investigating the effect of antihypertensive drugs on IL-6 levels are summarized here. In an open-labeled study, losartan therapy reduced IL-6 levels in recently diagnosed hypertension without other CV disease risk factors [117]. Olmesartan medoxomil reduced IL-6 levels in one study in patients with hypertension [152], but had no effect in patients with stage 3 or 4 CKD [107]. Olmesartan medoxomil was ineffective when combined with HCTZ in patients with hypertension and the metabolic syndrome, but was effective in these patients when combined with amlodipine [108]. Valsartan combined with HCTZ was more effective than amlodipine alone in reducing IL-6 [156]. Another study showed that diabetics with hypertension have higher IL-6 levels than non-diabetics with hypertension, and amlodipine reduced serum IL-6 as well as mRNA expression of IL-6 in diabetics and non-diabtetics [155]. In a crossover study with non-diabetic hypertensive patients, IL-6 levels were reduced with azelnidipine therapy, but not with amlodipine [112]. In the MARCADOR study, the greatest reduction in IL-6 was achieved with a combination of manidipine and lisinopril, while there was no change in IL-6 with amlodipine [113]. Another study found a greater reduction in IL-6 with benidipine treatment as compared to amlodipine treatment [100]. Losartan, as add-on therapy has also been shown to reduce IL-6 levels [140].

These cytokines are rather non-specific for quantification of inflammation; however, these studies do reflect the general state of inflammation in the vasculature. Clinical studies that measure the level of the cytokines demonstrate variable results. Multiple studies with antihypertensives indicate a general reduction in the levels of cytokines, suggesting a decrease in vascular inflammation. In context with the clinical situation and other risk factors, the measurement of these biomarkers may be useful.

5. Conclusions

It can be expected that biomarkers will continue to play an increasing role in the management of CV disease. Their importance or significance is likely to increase in direct proportion to the growth in our knowledge of disease pathophysiology and the mechanisms of drug action. The use of biomarkers does, however, depend upon the markers being accurate, relevant to the purpose, easy to measure, and consistently reproducible.

There is a wealth of evidence for improvement of validated biomarkers of vascular disease with most classes of antihypertensive treatment in a range of high-risk patient populations. These include obese patients, patients with diabetes, patients with renal disease and/or metabolic syndrome, existing vascular disease, and African American patients. Benefits have also been observed in those with normal BP, but with other CV risk factors. There is some evidence to suggest that at least part of the effect seen with some antihypertensives on these biomarkers may be independent of BP reduction. Different drugs may have quite different effects on biomarkers, despite very similar or equivalent effects on BP. However, with other drugs, the changes in certain biomarkers appear to parallel changes in BP. In addition, there appear to be clear associations between certain biomarkers, such as HOMA-IR and adiponectin, and the manner in which they are affected by certain antihypertensive drugs.

There is particularly compelling evidence that RAS inhibitors (ACEIs and ARBs) and CCBs may have beneficial effects beyond BP control, making them particularly attractive for either monotherapy or combination therapy. In contrast, other drugs, such as the thiazide diuretic HCTZ, appear to counter the beneficial effects on biomarkers normally observed with ARBs when they are used in combination.

Of the biomarkers selected for review in this chapter, the benefits of antihypertensive therapy on hsCRP, adiponectin, and HOMA-IR reflect a potential for quantifiable long-term vascular benefits. However, more evidence is required to elucidate the mechanisms involved and understand the variability and apparent anomalies observed. In addition, more information about any differences between specific antihypertensive agents within the same class is needed. Additional evidence is required to determine the relevance of improvements observed with antihypertensive therapy on CAP, cystatin C, procollagen, TNF-α, and IL-6 to a reduction in the risk of subsequent vascular events.

Further research is required to determine the extent to which these antihypertensive-related improvements in biomarkers contribute to the overall clinical outcome achieved in tandem with other CV risk reduction strategies and interventions. In addition, long-term studies with biomarkers are also required to show whether biomarkers correlate with long-term clinical outcomes.

Author details

Nadya Merchant and Bobby V. Khan
Atlanta Vascular Research Foundation, Atlanta, GA, USA

6. References

[1] Writing Group, M., et al., Heart disease and stroke statistics--2010 update: a report from the American Heart Association. Circulation, 2010. 121(7): p. e46-e215.

[2] Packard, R.R. and P. Libby, Inflammation in atherosclerosis: from vascular biology to biomarker discovery and risk prediction. Clin Chem, 2008. 54(1): p. 24-38.

[3] Maisel, A.S., Cardiovascular and renal surrogate markers in the clinical management of hypertension. Cardiovasc Drugs Ther, 2009. 23(4): p. 317-26.

[4] Vasan, R.S., Biomarkers of cardiovascular disease: molecular basis and practical considerations. Circulation, 2006. 113(19): p. 2335-62.

[5] Lambers Heerspink, H.J., V. Perkovic, and D. de Zeeuw, Renal and cardio-protective effects of direct renin inhibition: a systematic literature review. J Hypertens, 2009. 27(12): p. 2321-31.

[6] Novo, S., et al., Role of ARBs in the blood hypertension therapy and prevention of cardiovascular events. Curr Drug Targets, 2009. 10(1): p. 20-5.

[7] Sola, S., et al., Irbesartan and lipoic acid improve endothelial function and reduce markers of inflammation in the metabolic syndrome: results of the Irbesartan and Lipoic Acid in Endothelial Dysfunction (ISLAND) study. Circulation, 2005. 111(3): p. 343-8.

[8] Nagamia, S., et al., The role of quinapril in the presence of a weight loss regimen: endothelial function and markers of obesity in patients with the metabolic syndrome. Prev Cardiol, 2007. 10(4): p. 204-9.

[9] Persson, F., et al., Irbesartan treatment reduces biomarkers of inflammatory activity in patients with type 2 diabetes and microalbuminuria: an IRMA 2 substudy. Diabetes, 2006. 55(12): p. 3550-5.

[10] Derosa, G., et al., Candesartan effect on inflammation in hypertension. Hypertens Res, 2010. 33(3): p. 209-13.

[11] Shurtz-Swirski, R., et al., [The effect of calcium channel blocker lercanidipine on lowgrade inflammation parameters in essential hypertension patients]. Harefuah, 2006. 145(12): p. 895-9, 942.

[12] Komoda, H., T. Inoue, and K. Node, Anti-inflammatory properties of azelnidipine, a dihydropyridine-based calcium channel blocker. Clin Exp Hypertens, 2010. 32(2): p. 121-8.

[13] Merchant, N., et al., Effects of nebivolol in obese African Americans with hypertension (NOAAH): markers of inflammation and obesity in response to exercise-induced stress. J Hum Hypertens, 2011. 25(3): p. 196-202.

[14] Del Fiorentino, A., et al., The effect of angiotensin receptor blockers on C-reactive protein and other circulating inflammatory indices in man. Vasc Health Risk Manag, 2009. 5(1): p. 233-42.

[15] Polonia, J., et al., Different influences on central and peripheral pulse pressure, aortic wave reflections and pulse wave velocity of three different types of antihypertensive drugs. Rev Port Cardiol, 2003. 22(12): p. 1485-92.

[16] Karalliedde, J., et al., Valsartan improves arterial stiffness in type 2 diabetes independently of blood pressure lowering. Hypertension, 2008. 51(6): p. 1617-23.

[17] Ridker, P.M., et al., Valsartan, blood pressure reduction, and C-reactive protein: primary report of the Val-MARC trial. Hypertension, 2006. 48(1): p. 73-9.

[18] Bloch, M.J., Do angiotensin receptor antagonists decrease hsCRP independent of blood pressure - and does it matter? J Clin Hypertens (Greenwich), 2007. 9(1): p. 57-9.
[19] Futai, R., et al., Olmesartan ameliorates myocardial function independent of blood pressure control in patients with mild-to-moderate hypertension. Heart Vessels, 2009. 24(4): p. 294-300.
[20] Moriuchi, A., et al., Induction of human adiponectin gene transcription by telmisartan, angiotensin receptor blocker, independently on PPAR-gamma activation. Biochem Biophys Res Commun, 2007. 356(4): p. 1024-30.
[21] Schepke, M., et al., Hemodynamic effects of the angiotensin II receptor antagonist irbesartan in patients with cirrhosis and portal hypertension. Gastroenterology, 2001. 121(2): p. 389-95.
[22] Watanabe, S., et al., Valsartan reduces serum cystatin C and the renal vascular resistance in patients with essential hypertension. Clin Exp Hypertens, 2006. 28(5): p. 451-61.
[23] Derosa, G., et al., Metabolic effects of telmisartan and irbesartan in type 2 diabetic patients with metabolic syndrome treated with rosiglitazone. J Clin Pharm Ther, 2007. 32(3): p. 261-8.
[24] Usui, I., et al., Telmisartan reduced blood pressure and HOMA-IR with increasing plasma leptin level in hypertensive and type 2 diabetic patients. Diabetes Res Clin Pract, 2007. 77(2): p. 210-4.
[25] de Luis, D.A., et al., Effects of telmisartan vs olmesartan on metabolic parameters, insulin resistance and adipocytokines in hypertensive obese patients. Nutr Hosp, 2010. 25(2): p. 275-9.
[26] Christensen, M.K., et al., Does long-term losartan- vs atenolol-based antihypertensive treatment influence collagen markers differently in hypertensive patients? A LIFE substudy. Blood Press, 2006. 15(4): p. 198-206.
[27] Muller-Brunotte, R., et al., Myocardial fibrosis and diastolic dysfunction in patients with hypertension: results from the Swedish Irbesartan Left Ventricular Hypertrophy Investigation versus Atenolol (SILVHIA). J Hypertens, 2007. 25(9): p. 1958-66.
[28] Kawamura, M., et al., Candesartan decreases type III procollagen-N-peptide levels and inflammatory marker levels and maintains sinus rhythm in patients with atrial fibrillation. J Cardiovasc Pharmacol, 2010. 55(5): p. 511-7.
[29] Fogari, R., et al., Effects of amlodipine-atorvastatin combination on inflammation markers and insulin sensitivity in normocholesterolemic obese hypertensive patients. Eur J Clin Pharmacol, 2006. 62(10): p. 817-22.
[30] Fujita, M., et al., Blockade of angiotensin II receptors reduces the expression of receptors for advanced glycation end products in human endothelial cells. Arterioscler Thromb Vasc Biol, 2006. 26(10): p. e138-42.
[31] Schulz, R. and G. Heusch, Tumor necrosis factor-alpha and its receptors 1 and 2: Yin and Yang in myocardial infarction? Circulation, 2009. 119(10): p. 1355-7.
[32] Cesari, M., et al., Inflammatory markers and onset of cardiovascular events: results from the Health ABC study. Circulation, 2003. 108(19): p. 2317-22.

[33] Luc, G., et al., C-reactive protein, interleukin-6, and fibrinogen as predictors of coronary heart disease: the PRIME Study. Arterioscler Thromb Vasc Biol, 2003. 23(7): p. 1255-61.
[34] Pai, J.K., et al., Inflammatory markers and the risk of coronary heart disease in men and women. N Engl J Med, 2004. 351(25): p. 2599-610.
[35] Patarroyo Aponte, M.M. and G.S. Francis, Effect of Angiotensin-Converting Enzyme Inhibitors and Angiotensin Receptor Antagonists in Atherosclerosis Prevention. Curr Cardiol Rep, 2012.
[36] Lonn, E., Angiotensin-converting enzyme inhibitors and angiotensin receptor blockers in atherosclerosis. Curr Atheroscler Rep, 2002. 4(5): p. 363-72.
[37] Shahin, Y., et al., Angiotensin converting enzyme inhibitors effect on endothelial dysfunction: a meta-analysis of randomised controlled trials. Atherosclerosis, 2011. 216(1): p. 7-16.
[38] Yusuf, S., [After the HOPE Study. ACE inhibitor now for every diabetic patient?. Interview by Dr. Dirk Einecke]. MMW Fortschr Med, 2000. 142(44): p. 10.
[39] Fox, K.M. and E.U.t.O.r.o.c.e.w.P.i.s.c.A.d. Investigators, Efficacy of perindopril in reduction of cardiovascular events among patients with stable coronary artery disease: randomised, double-blind, placebo-controlled, multicentre trial (the EUROPA study). Lancet, 2003. 362(9386): p. 782-8.
[40] PROGRESS will change the way we view stroke treatment. Cardiovasc J S Afr, 2001. 12(5): p. 288.
[41] Dahlof, B., et al., Prevention of cardiovascular events with an antihypertensive regimen of amlodipine adding perindopril as required versus atenolol adding bendroflumethiazide as required, in the Anglo-Scandinavian Cardiac Outcomes Trial-Blood Pressure Lowering Arm (ASCOT-BPLA): a multicentre randomised controlled trial. Lancet, 2005. 366(9489): p. 895-906.
[42] Dzau, V.J., Theodore Cooper Lecture: Tissue angiotensin and pathobiology of vascular disease: a unifying hypothesis. Hypertension, 2001. 37(4): p. 1047-52.
[43] Dzau, V.J., et al., The relevance of tissue angiotensin-converting enzyme: manifestations in mechanistic and endpoint data. Am J Cardiol, 2001. 88(9A): p. 1L-20L.
[44] Investigators, O., et al., Telmisartan, ramipril, or both in patients at high risk for vascular events. N Engl J Med, 2008. 358(15): p. 1547-59.
[45] Velazquez, E.J., et al., VALsartan In Acute myocardial iNfarcTion (VALIANT) trial: baseline characteristics in context. Eur J Heart Fail, 2003. 5(4): p. 537-44.
[46] Dahlof, B., et al., Effects of losartan and atenolol on left ventricular mass and neurohormonal profile in patients with essential hypertension and left ventricular hypertrophy. J Hypertens, 2002. 20(9): p. 1855-64.
[47] Koh, K.K., et al., Additive beneficial effects of losartan combined with simvastatin in the treatment of hypercholesterolemic, hypertensive patients. Circulation, 2004. 110(24): p. 3687-92.
[48] Turnbull, F. and C. Blood Pressure Lowering Treatment Trialists, Effects of different blood-pressure-lowering regimens on major cardiovascular events: results of prospectively-designed overviews of randomised trials. Lancet, 2003. 362(9395): p. 1527-35.

[49] Messerli, F.H., Calcium antagonists and beta-blockers: impact on cardiovascular and cerebrovascular events. Clin Cornerstone, 2004. 6(4): p. 18-27.

[50] Williams, B., et al., Differential impact of blood pressure-lowering drugs on central aortic pressure and clinical outcomes: principal results of the Conduit Artery Function Evaluation (CAFE) study. Circulation, 2006. 113(9): p. 1213-25.

[51] Terai, M., et al., Comparison of arterial functional evaluations as a predictor of cardiovascular events in hypertensive patients: the Non-Invasive Atherosclerotic Evaluation in Hypertension (NOAH) study. Hypertens Res, 2008. 31(6): p. 1135-45.

[52] Luna, B. and M.N. Feinglos, Drug-induced hyperglycemia. JAMA, 2001. 286(16): p. 1945-8.

[53] Bangalore, S., et al., A meta-analysis of 94,492 patients with hypertension treated with beta blockers to determine the risk of new-onset diabetes mellitus. Am J Cardiol, 2007. 100(8): p. 1254-62.

[54] Dahlof, B., et al., Cardiovascular morbidity and mortality in the Losartan Intervention For Endpoint reduction in hypertension study (LIFE): a randomised trial against atenolol. Lancet, 2002. 359(9311): p. 995-1003.

[55] Wright, J.T., Jr., et al., Lowering blood pressure with beta-blockers in combination with other renin-angiotensin system blockers in patients with hypertension and type 2 diabetes: results from the GEMINI Trial. J Clin Hypertens (Greenwich), 2007. 9(11): p. 842-9.

[56] Bakris, G.L., et al., Metabolic effects of carvedilol vs metoprolol in patients with type 2 diabetes mellitus and hypertension: a randomized controlled trial. JAMA, 2004. 292(18): p. 2227-36.

[57] Agabiti Rosei, E. and D. Rizzoni, Metabolic profile of nebivolol, a beta-adrenoceptor antagonist with unique characteristics. Drugs, 2007. 67(8): p. 1097-107.

[58] Chobanian, A.V., et al., The Seventh Report of the Joint National Committee on Prevention, Detection, Evaluation, and Treatment of High Blood Pressure: the JNC 7 report. JAMA, 2003. 289(19): p. 2560-72.

[59] Prevention of stroke by antihypertensive drug treatment in older persons with isolated systolic hypertension. Final results of the Systolic Hypertension in the Elderly Program (SHEP). SHEP Cooperative Research Group. JAMA, 1991. 265(24): p. 3255-64.

[60] Sica, D.A., et al., Thiazide and loop diuretics. J Clin Hypertens (Greenwich), 2011. 13(9): p. 639-43.

[61] Materson, B.J., et al., Results of combination anti-hypertensive therapy after failure of each of the components. Department of Veterans Affairs Cooperative Study Group on Anti-hypertensive Agents. J Hum Hypertens, 1995. 9(10): p. 791-6.

[62] Fisher, N.D. and N.K. Hollenberg, Renin inhibition: what are the therapeutic opportunities? J Am Soc Nephrol, 2005. 16(3): p. 592-9.

[63] Brown, N.J., Aldosterone and vascular inflammation. Hypertension, 2008. 51(2): p. 161-7.

[64] Farquharson, C.A. and A.D. Struthers, Spironolactone increases nitric oxide bioactivity, improves endothelial vasodilator dysfunction, and suppresses vascular angiotensin

I/angiotensin II conversion in patients with chronic heart failure. Circulation, 2000. 101(6): p. 594-7.
[65] Parving, H.H., et al., Aliskiren combined with losartan in type 2 diabetes and nephropathy. N Engl J Med, 2008. 358(23): p. 2433-46.
[66] Cleland, J.G., et al., Clinical trials update from the European Society of Cardiology Congress 2007: 3CPO, ALOFT, PROSPECT and statins for heart failure. Eur J Heart Fail, 2007. 9(10): p. 1070-3.
[67] Wang, X., et al., Assessment of arterial stiffness, a translational medicine biomarker system for evaluation of vascular risk. Cardiovasc Ther, 2008. 26(3): p. 214-23.
[68] Williams, B. and P.S. Lacy, Central aortic pressure and clinical outcomes. J Hypertens, 2009. 27(6): p. 1123-5.
[69] Nelson, M.R., et al., Noninvasive measurement of central vascular pressures with arterial tonometry: clinical revival of the pulse pressure waveform? Mayo Clin Proc, 2010. 85(5): p. 460-72.
[70] Paoletti, R., A.M. Gotto, Jr., and D.P. Hajjar, Inflammation in atherosclerosis and implications for therapy. Circulation, 2004. 109(23 Suppl 1): p. III20-6.
[71] Black, S., I. Kushner, and D. Samols, C-reactive Protein. J Biol Chem, 2004. 279(47): p. 48487-90.
[72] Bautista, L.E., et al., Association between C-reactive protein and hypertension in healthy middle-aged men and women. Coron Artery Dis, 2004. 15(6): p. 331-6.
[73] Dauphinot, V., et al., C-reactive protein implications in new-onset hypertension in a healthy population initially aged 65 years: the Proof study. J Hypertens, 2009. 27(4): p. 736-43.
[74] Abramson, J.L., W.S. Weintraub, and V. Vaccarino, Association between pulse pressure and C-reactive protein among apparently healthy US adults. Hypertension, 2002. 39(2): p. 197-202.
[75] Genest, J., Preventive cardiology: move over low density lipoprotein cholesterol, hello C-reactive protein? Can J Cardiol, 2004. 20 Suppl B: p. 89B-92B.
[76] Savoia, C. and E.L. Schiffrin, Reduction of C-reactive protein and the use of anti-hypertensives. Vasc Health Risk Manag, 2007. 3(6): p. 975-83.
[77] Montecucco, F. and F. Mach, Update on therapeutic strategies to increase adiponectin function and secretion in metabolic syndrome. Diabetes Obes Metab, 2009. 11(5): p. 445-54.
[78] Karthikeyan, V.J. and G.Y. Lip, Antihypertensive treatment, adiponectin and cardiovascular risk. J Hum Hypertens, 2007. 21(1): p. 8-11.
[79] Shargorodsky, M., et al., Adiponectin and vascular properties in obese patients: is it a novel biomarker of early atherosclerosis? Int J Obes (Lond), 2009. 33(5): p. 553-8.
[80] Makita, S., et al., Potential effects of angiotensin II receptor blockers on glucose tolerance and adiponectin levels in hypertensive patients. Cardiovasc Drugs Ther, 2007. 21(4): p. 317-8.
[81] Ylinen, E.A., et al., Cystatin C as a marker for glomerular filtration rate in pediatric patients. Pediatr Nephrol, 1999. 13(6): p. 506-9.

[82] Laterza, O.F., C.P. Price, and M.G. Scott, Cystatin C: an improved estimator of glomerular filtration rate? Clin Chem, 2002. 48(5): p. 699-707.

[83] Massey, D., Commentary: clinical diagnostic use of cystatin C. J Clin Lab Anal, 2004. 18(1): p. 55-60.

[84] Kniepeiss, D., et al., Serum cystatin C is an easy to obtain biomarker for the onset of renal impairment in heart transplant recipients. J Thorac Cardiovasc Surg, 2010.

[85] Mena, C., et al., Cystatin c and blood pressure: results of 24 h ambulatory blood pressure monitoring. Eur J Intern Med, 2010. 21(3): p. 185-90.

[86] Prats, M., et al., Cystatin C and cardiac hypertrophy in primary hypertension. Blood Press, 2010. 19(1): p. 20-5.

[87] Matthews, D.R., et al., Homeostasis model assessment: insulin resistance and beta-cell function from fasting plasma glucose and insulin concentrations in man. Diabetologia, 1985. 28(7): p. 412-9.

[88] Cooper-DeHoff, R.M., M.A. Pacanowski, and C.J. Pepine, Cardiovascular therapies and associated glucose homeostasis: implications across the dysglycemia continuum. J Am Coll Cardiol, 2009. 53(5 Suppl): p. S28-34.

[89] Szmigielski, C., et al., Metabolism of collagen is altered in hypertensives with increased intima media thickness. Blood Press, 2006. 15(3): p. 157-63.

[90] Ishikawa, J., et al., Collagen metabolism in extracellular matrix may be involved in arterial stiffness in older hypertensive patients with left ventricular hypertrophy. Hypertens Res, 2005. 28(12): p. 995-1001.

[91] Lopez, B., et al., The use of collagen-derived serum peptides for the clinical assessment of hypertensive heart disease. J Hypertens, 2005. 23(8): p. 1445-51.

[92] Cesari, M., et al., Inflammatory markers and cardiovascular disease (The Health, Aging and Body Composition [Health ABC] Study). Am J Cardiol, 2003. 92(5): p. 522-8.

[93] Williams, B., et al., Differential impact of blood pressure-lowering drugs on central aortic pressure and clinical outcomes: principal results of the Conduit Artery Function Evaluation (CAFE) study. Circulation, 2006. 113(9): p. 1213-25.

[94] Neal, D.A., et al., Hemodynamic effects of amlodipine, bisoprolol, and lisinopril in hypertensive patients after liver transplantation. Transplantation, 2004. 77(5): p. 748-50.

[95] Takami, T. and Y. Saito, Effects of Azelnidipine plus OlmesaRTAn versus amlodipine plus olmesartan on central blood pressure and left ventricular mass index: the AORTA study. Vasc Health Risk Manag, 2011. 7: p. 383-90.

[96] Morgan, T., et al., Effect of different antihypertensive drug classes on central aortic pressure. Am J Hypertens, 2004. 17(2): p. 118-23.

[97] Kagota, S., et al., Peroxynitrite is Involved in the dysfunction of vasorelaxation in SHR/NDmcr-cp rats, spontaneously hypertensive obese rats. J Cardiovasc Pharmacol, 2007. 50(6): p. 677-85.

[98] Ferguson, J.M., et al., Effects of a fixed-dose ACE inhibitor-diuretic combination on ambulatory blood pressure and arterial properties in isolated systolic hypertension. J Cardiovasc Pharmacol, 2008. 51(6): p. 590-5.

[99] Ishii, H., T. Tsukada, and M. Yoshida, Angiotensin II type-I receptor blocker, candesartan, improves brachial-ankle pulse wave velocity independent of its blood pressure lowering effects in type 2 diabetes patients. Intern Med, 2008. 47(23): p. 2013-8.

[100] Nakamura, M., et al., Brachial-ankle pulse wave velocity as a risk stratification index for the short-term prognosis of type 2 diabetic patients with coronary artery disease. Hypertens Res, 2010. 33(10): p. 1018-24.

[101] Kinouchi, K., et al., Differential Effects in Cardiovascular Markers between High-Dose Angiotensin II Receptor Blocker Monotherapy and Combination Therapy of ARB with Calcium Channel Blocker in Hypertension (DEAR Trial). Int J Hypertens, 2011. 2011: p. 284823.

[102] Miyoshi, T., et al., Olmesartan reduces arterial stiffness and serum adipocyte fatty acid-binding protein in hypertensive patients. Heart Vessels, 2011. 26(4): p. 408-13.

[103] Takiguchi, S., et al., Olmesartan improves endothelial function in hypertensive patients: link with extracellular superoxide dismutase. Hypertens Res, 2011. 34(6): p. 686-92.

[104] Koh, K.K., et al., Additive beneficial effects of atorvastatin combined with amlodipine in patients with mild-to-moderate hypertension. Int J Cardiol, 2011. 146(3): p. 319-25.

[105] Li, M., et al., Impact of combination therapy with amlodipine and atorvastatin on plasma adiponectin levels in hypertensive patients with coronary artery disease: combination therapy and adiponectin. Postgrad Med, 2011. 123(6): p. 66-71.

[106] Yilmaz, R., et al., Impact of amlodipine or ramipril treatment on left ventricular mass and carotid intima-media thickness in nondiabetic hemodialysis patients. Ren Fail, 2010. 32(8): p. 903-12.

[107] de Vinuesa, S.G., et al., Insulin resistance, inflammatory biomarkers, and adipokines in patients with chronic kidney disease: effects of angiotensin II blockade. J Am Soc Nephrol, 2006. 17(12 Suppl 3): p. S206-12.

[108] Martinez-Martin, F.J., et al., Olmesartan/amlodipine vs olmesartan/hydrochlorothiazide in hypertensive patients with metabolic syndrome: the OLAS study. J Hum Hypertens, 2011. 25(6): p. 346-53.

[109] Derosa, G., et al., Differential effects of candesartan and olmesartan on adipose tissue activity biomarkers in type II diabetic hypertensive patients. Hypertens Res, 2010. 33(8): p. 790-5.

[110] Doi, M., et al., Combination therapy of calcium channel blocker and angiotensin II receptor blocker reduces augmentation index in hypertensive patients. Am J Med Sci, 2010. 339(5): p. 433-9.

[111] Ishimitsu, T., et al., Angiotensin-II receptor antagonist combined with calcium channel blocker or diuretic for essential hypertension. Hypertens Res, 2009. 32(11): p. 962-8.

[112] Fukao, K., et al., Effects of calcium channel blockers on glucose tolerance, inflammatory state, and circulating progenitor cells in non-diabetic patients with essential hypertension: a comparative study between Azelnidipine and amlodipine on glucose tolerance and endothelial function - a crossover trial (AGENT). Cardiovasc Diabetol, 2011. 10: p. 79.

[113] Martinez-Martin, F.J., et al., Effects of manidipine and its combination with an ACE inhibitor on insulin sensitivity and metabolic, inflammatory and prothrombotic markers in hypertensive patients with metabolic syndrome: the MARCADOR study. Clin Drug Investig, 2011. 31(3): p. 201-12.

[114] Igarashi, M., et al., Dual blockade of angiotensin II with enalapril and losartan reduces proteinuria in hypertensive patients with type 2 diabetes. Endocr J, 2006. 53(4): p. 493-501.

[115] Matsui, Y., et al., Urinary albumin excretion during angiotensin II receptor blockade: comparison of combination treatment with a diuretic or a calcium-channel blocker. Am J Hypertens, 2011. 24(4): p. 466-73.

[116] Sugihara, M., et al., Safety and efficacy of antihypertensive therapy with add-on angiotensin II type 1 receptor blocker after successful coronary stent implantation. Hypertens Res, 2009. 32(7): p. 625-30.

[117] Sardo, M.A., et al., Effects of the angiotensin II receptor blocker losartan on the monocyte expression of biglycan in hypertensive patients. Clin Exp Pharmacol Physiol, 2010. 37(9): p. 933-8.

[118] Aksnes, T.A., et al., Improved insulin sensitivity by the angiotensin II-receptor blocker losartan is not explained by adipokines, inflammatory markers, or whole blood viscosity. Metabolism, 2007. 56(11): p. 1470-7.

[119] Ruilope, L.M., et al., Efficacy and tolerability of combination therapy with valsartan plus hydrochlorothiazide compared with amlodipine monotherapy in hypertensive patients with other cardiovascular risk factors: the VAST study. Clin Ther, 2005. 27(5): p. 578-87.

[120] Tomiyama, H., et al., Discrepancy between improvement of insulin sensitivity and that of arterial endothelial function in patients receiving antihypertensive medication. J Hypertens, 2007. 25(4): p. 883-9.

[121] Navalkar, S., et al., Irbesartan, an angiotensin type 1 receptor inhibitor, regulates markers of inflammation in patients with premature atherosclerosis. J Am Coll Cardiol, 2001. 37(2): p. 440-4.

[122] Martinez Martin, F.J., Manidipine in hypertensive patients with metabolic syndrome: the MARIMBA study. Expert Rev Cardiovasc Ther, 2009. 7(7): p. 863-9.

[123] Masajtis-Zagajewska, A., J. Majer, and M. Nowicki, Effect of moxonidine and amlodipine on serum YKL-40, plasma lipids and insulin sensitivity in insulin-resistant hypertensive patients-a randomized, crossover trial. Hypertens Res, 2010. 33(4): p. 348-53.

[124] Ge, C.J., et al., Synergistic effect of amlodipine and atorvastatin on blood pressure, left ventricular remodeling, and C-reactive protein in hypertensive patients with primary hypercholesterolemia. Heart Vessels, 2008. 23(2): p. 91-5.

[125] Rizos, C.V., et al., Combining rosuvastatin with sartans of different peroxisome proliferator-activated receptor-gamma activating capacity is not associated with different changes in low-density lipoprotein subfractions and plasma lipoprotein-associated phospholipase A(2). Metab Syndr Relat Disord, 2011. 9(3): p. 217-23.

[126] Negro, R., G. Formoso, and H. Hassan, The effects of irbesartan and telmisartan on metabolic parameters and blood pressure in obese, insulin resistant, hypertensive patients. J Endocrinol Invest, 2006. 29(11): p. 957-61.

[127] Kintscher, U., et al., Irbesartan for the treatment of hypertension in patients with the metabolic syndrome: a sub analysis of the Treat to Target post authorization survey. Prospective observational, two armed study in 14,200 patients. Cardiovasc Diabetol, 2007. 6: p. 12.

[128] Krikken, J.A., et al., Antiproteinuric therapy decreases LDL-cholesterol as well as HDL-cholesterol in non-diabetic proteinuric patients: relationships with cholesteryl ester transfer protein mass and adiponectin. Expert Opin Ther Targets, 2009. 13(5): p. 497-504.

[129] Negro, R. and H. Hassan, The effects of telmisartan and amlodipine on metabolic parameters and blood pressure in type 2 diabetic, hypertensive patients. J Renin Angiotensin Aldosterone Syst, 2006. 7(4): p. 243-6.

[130] Nishimura, H., et al., Losartan elevates the serum high-molecular weight-adiponectin isoform and concurrently improves insulin sensitivity in patients with impaired glucose metabolism. Hypertens Res, 2008. 31(8): p. 1611-8.

[131] Derosa, G., et al., Different actions of losartan and ramipril on adipose tissue activity and vascular remodeling biomarkers in hypertensive patients. Hypertens Res, 2011. 34(1): p. 145-51.

[132] Huang, Y.Y., et al., [Effect of losartan on renal expression of monocyte chemoattractant protein-1 and transforming growth factor-beta(1) in rats after unilateral ureteral obstruction]. Nan Fang Yi Ke Da Xue Xue Bao, 2011. 31(8): p. 1405-10.

[133] Matsumoto, S., K. Takebayashi, and Y. Aso, The effect of spironolactone on circulating adipocytokines in patients with type 2 diabetes mellitus complicated by diabetic nephropathy. Metabolism, 2006. 55(12): p. 1645-52.

[134] Piecha, G., et al., Indapamide decreases plasma adiponectin concentration in patients with essential hypertension. Kidney Blood Press Res, 2007. 30(3): p. 187-94.

[135] Yilmaz, M.I., et al., Effect of antihypertensive agents on plasma adiponectin levels in hypertensive patients with metabolic syndrome. Nephrology (Carlton), 2007. 12(2): p. 147-53.

[136] Koh, K.K., et al., Distinct vascular and metabolic effects of different classes of anti-hypertensive drugs. Int J Cardiol, 2010. 140(1): p. 73-81.

[137] Guo, L.L., Y. Pan, and H.M. Jin, Adiponectin is positively associated with insulin resistance in subjects with type 2 diabetic nephropathy and effects of angiotensin II type 1 receptor blocker losartan. Nephrol Dial Transplant, 2009. 24(6): p. 1876-83.

[138] Albayrak, S., et al., Effect of olmesartan medoxomil on cystatin C level, left ventricular hypertrophy and diastolic function. Blood Press, 2009. 18(4): p. 187-91.

[139] Koc, Y., et al., Effect of Olmesartan on serum cystatin C levels in the patients with essential hypertension. Eur Rev Med Pharmacol Sci, 2011. 15(12): p. 1389-94.

[140] Ogino, K., et al., Addition of losartan to angiotensin-converting enzyme inhibitors improves insulin resistance in patients with chronic heart failure treated without beta-blockers. Circ J, 2010. 74(11): p. 2346-52.

[141] Bahadir, O., et al., Effects of telmisartan and losartan on insulin resistance in hypertensive patients with metabolic syndrome. Hypertens Res, 2007. 30(1): p. 49-53.

[142] Lan, J., et al., The relationship between visfatin and HOMA-IR in hypertensive patients, and the effect of antihypertensive drugs on visfatin and HOMA-IR in hypertensive patients with insulin resistance. Diabetes Res Clin Pract, 2011. 94(1): p. 71-6.

[143] De Luis, D.A., et al., Effects of olmesartan vs irbesartan on metabolic parameters and visfatin in hypertensive obese women. Eur Rev Med Pharmacol Sci, 2010. 14(9): p. 759-63.

[144] Dohi, T., et al., Effects of olmesartan on blood pressure and insulin resistance in hypertensive patients with sleep-disordered breathing. Heart Vessels, 2011. 26(6): p. 603-8.

[145] Enjoji, M., et al., Therapeutic effect of ARBs on insulin resistance and liver injury in patients with NAFLD and chronic hepatitis C: a pilot study. Int J Mol Med, 2008. 22(4): p. 521-7.

[146] Jin, H.M. and Y. Pan, Angiotensin type-1 receptor blockade with losartan increases insulin sensitivity and improves glucose homeostasis in subjects with type 2 diabetes and nephropathy. Nephrol Dial Transplant, 2007. 22(7): p. 1943-9.

[147] Watanabe, S., et al., The effect of losartan and amlodipine on serum adiponectin in Japanese adults with essential hypertension. Clin Ther, 2006. 28(10): p. 1677-85.

[148] Fogari, R., et al., Effect of valsartan and ramipril on atrial fibrillation recurrence and P-wave dispersion in hypertensive patients with recurrent symptomatic lone atrial fibrillation. Am J Hypertens, 2008. 21(9): p. 1034-9.

[149] Ishimitsu, T., et al., Protective effects of an angiotensin II receptor blocker and a long-acting calcium channel blocker against cardiovascular organ injuries in hypertensive patients. Hypertens Res, 2005. 28(4): p. 351-9.

[150] Diez, J., et al., Losartan-dependent regression of myocardial fibrosis is associated with reduction of left ventricular chamber stiffness in hypertensive patients. Circulation, 2002. 105(21): p. 2512-7.

[151] Dziadzio, M., et al., Losartan therapy for Raynaud's phenomenon and scleroderma: clinical and biochemical findings in a fifteen-week, randomized, parallel-group, controlled trial. Arthritis Rheum, 1999. 42(12): p. 2646-55.

[152] Lorenzen, J.M., et al., Angiotensin II receptor blocker and statins lower elevated levels of osteopontin in essential hypertension--results from the EUTOPIA trial. Atherosclerosis, 2010. 209(1): p. 184-8.

[153] Fogari, R., et al., Hydrochlorothiazide added to valsartan is more effective than when added to olmesartan in reducing blood pressure in moderately hypertensive patients inadequately controlled by monotherapy. Adv Ther, 2006. 23(5): p. 680-95.

[154] Park, H., et al., Relationship between insulin resistance and inflammatory markers and anti-inflammatory effect of losartan in patients with type 2 diabetes and hypertension. Clin Chim Acta, 2006. 374(1-2): p. 129-34.

[155] Navarro-Gonzalez, J., et al., Serum and gene expression profile of tumor necrosis factor-alpha and interleukin-6 in hypertensive diabetic patients: effect of amlodipine administration. Int J Immunopathol Pharmacol, 2010. 23(1): p. 51-9.
[156] Ruilope, L.M., et al., 24-hour ambulatory blood-pressure effects of valsartan and hydrochlorothiazide combinations compared with amlodipine in hypertensive patients at increased cardiovascular risk: a VAST sub-study. Blood Press Monit, 2005. 10(2): p. 85-91.